T0226510

Management of Heart Failure in the Emergent Situation

Guest Editors

JAMES F. NEUENSCHWANDER II, MD, FACEP

W. FRANK PEACOCK, MD, FACEP

HEART FAILURE CLINICS

www.heartfailure.theclinics.com

Consulting Editors
RAGAVENDRA R. BALIGA, MD, MBA
JAMES B. YOUNG, MD

Founding Editor
JAGAT NARULA, MD, PhD

January 2009 • Volume 5 • Number 1

SAUNDERS an imprint of ELSEVIER, Inc.

W.B. SAUNDERS COMPANY
A Division of Elsevier Inc.

1600 John F. Kennedy Boulevard • Suite 1800 • Philadelphia, Pennsylvania 19103-2899

http://www.theclinics.com

HEART FAILURE CLINICS Volume 5, Number 1
January 2009 ISSN 1551-7136, ISBN-13: 978-1-4377-0484-6, ISBN-10: 1-4377-0484-0

Editor: Barbara Cohen-Kligerman

Heart Failure Clinics (ISSN 1551-7136) is published quarterly by Elsevier Inc., 360 Park Avenue South, New York, NY 10010-1710. Months of publication are January, April, July, and October. Business and editorial offices: 1600 John F. Kennedy Boulevard, Suite 1800, Phliadelphia, PA 19103-2899. Customer service office: 11830 Westline Industrial Drive, St. Louis, MO 63146. Application to mail at periodicals postage rates is pending at New York, NY and additional mailing offices. Subscription prices are USD 193.00 per year for US individuals, USD 320.00 per year for US institutions, USD 67.00 per year for US students and residents, USD 232.00 per year for Canadian individuals, USD 367.00 per year for Canadian institutions, USD 247.00 per year for international individuals, USD 367.00 per year for international institutions, and USD 85.00 per year for Canadian and foreign students/ residents. To receive student and resident rate, orders must be accompanied by name of affiliated institution, date of term, and the *signature* of program/residency coordinator on institution letterhead. Orders will be billed at individual rate until proof of status is received. Foreign air speed delivery is included in all *Clinics* subscription prices. All prices are subject to change without notice. **POSTMASTER:** Send address changes to *Heart Failure Clinics*, Elsevier Journals Customer Service, 11830 Westline Industrial Drive, St. Louis, MO 63146. **Customer Service: 1-800-654-2452 (US and Canada). From outside of the US and Canada, call 314-453-7041. Fax: 314-453-5170. For print support, e–mail: JournalCustomerService-usa@elsevier.com. For online support, e-mail: JournalsOnlineSupport-usa@elsevier.com.**

Reprints. For copies of 100 or more of articles in this publication, please contact the Commercial Reprints Department, Elsevier Inc., 360 Park Avenue South, New York, NY 10010-1710. Tel.: 212-633-3812; Fax: 212-462-1935; E-mail: reprints@elsevier.com.

Heart Failure Clinics is covered in *MEDLINE/PubMed (Index Medicus).*

Printed and bound in the United Kingdom
Transferred to Digital Print 2011

Cover artwork courtesy of Umberto M. Jezek.

Contributors

CONSULTING EDITORS

RAGAVENDRA R. BALIGA, MD, MBA
Director, Section of Cardiovascular Medicine, University Hospital East; and Clinical Professor of Internal Medicine, The Ohio State University, Columbus, Ohio

JAMES B. YOUNG, MD
Chairman and Professor, Department of Medicine, Lerner College of Medicine; and George and Linda Kaufman Chair, Cleveland Clinic Foundation, Case Western Reserve University; Cleveland, Ohio

GUEST EDITORS

JAMES F. NEUENSCHWANDER II, MD, FACEP
Assistant Professor, Department of Emergency Medicine, The Ohio State University, Columbus, Ohio

W. FRANK PEACOCK, MD, FACEP
Department of Emergency Medicine, The Cleveland Clinic, Cleveland, Ohio

AUTHORS

EZRA AMSTERDAM, MD
Professor of Internal Medicine and Associate Chief for Academic Affairs, Division of Cardiovascular Medicine, Department of Internal Medicine, University of California Davis School of Medicine and Medical Center, Sacramento, California

PAUL CHACKO, MD
Division of Hospital Medicine, Department of Internal Medicine, The Ohio State University College of Medicine, Columbus, Ohio

ANNA MARIE CHANG, MD
Department of Emergency Medicine, University of Pennsylvania, Philadelphia, Pennsylvania

SEAN P. COLLINS, MD, MSc
Assistant Professor, Department of Emergency Medicine, University of Cincinnati School of Medicine, Cincinnati, Ohio

DEBORAH DIERCKS, MD, MSc
Associate Professor, Department of Emergency Medicine, University of California Davis Medical Center, Sacramento, California

CHARLES L. EMERMAN, MD
Professor and Chairperson, Department of Emergency Medicine, MetroHealth Medical Center, Case Western Reserve University School of Medicine, Cleveland, Ohio

GERASIMOS FILIPPATOS, MD
Heart Failure Clinic and Second Department of Cardiology, Attikon University Hospital, Athens, Greece

MIHAI GHEORGHIADE, MD
Professor of Medicine and Surgery and Associate Chief, Division of Cardiology; and Chief, Clinical Cardiology and Telemetry Service, Feinberg School of Medicine, Northwestern University, Northwestern Memorial Hospital, Chicago, Illinois

GARY B. GREEN, MD, MPH, MBA
Associate Professor and Vice-Chairman, Department of Emergency Medicine, New York University School of Medicine, New York, New York

BRIAN C. HIESTAND, MD, MPH, FACEP
Assistant Professor, Department of Emergency Medicine, The Ohio State University, Columbus, Ohio

JUDD E. HOLLANDER, MD
Professor of Emergency Medicine, Department of Emergency Medicine, University of Pennsylvania, Philadelphia, Pennsylvania

PREETI JOIS-BILOWICH, MD
Clinical Assistant Professor, University of Florida, Department of Emergency Medicine, Gainesville, Florida

J. DOUGLAS KIRK, MD
Professor and Vice-Chair of Clinical Operations, Department of Emergency Medicine, University of California Davis, School of Medicine, Sacramento, California

BENJAMIN LAWNER, DO, EMT-P
Clinical Instructor, Department of Emergency Medicine, University of Maryland School of Medicine, Baltimore, Maryland

ALAN S. MAISEL, MD, FACC
Professor of Medicine, Department of Medicine (Cardiology), San Diego Veterans Affairs Medical Center, University of California, San Diego, California

AMAL MATTU, MD, FACEP, FAAEM
Associate Professor and Residency Program Director, Department of Emergency Medicine, University of Maryland School of Medicine, Baltimore, Maryland

MARK G. MOSELEY, MD, MHA
Assistant Professor, Department of Emergency Medicine, The Ohio State University; and Medical Director, Emergency Department and Clinical Decision Unit, The Ohio State University Medical Center, Columbus, Ohio

JAMES F. NEUENSCHWANDER II, MD, FACEP
Assistant Professor, Department of Emergency Medicine, The Ohio State University, Columbus, Ohio

PETER S. PANG, MD
Assistant Professor of Emergency Medicine and Associate Medical Director, Feinberg School of Medicine, Northwestern University, Northwestern Memorial Hospital, Chicago, Illinois

SHIBU PHILIP, MD
Hospitalist, Department of Cardiothoracic Surgery, Jeanes Hospital, Temple University Health System, Philadelphia, Pennsylvania

JOHN T. PARISSIS, MD
Heart Failure Clinic and Second Department of Cardiology, Attikon University Hospital, Athens, Greece

JON W. SCHROCK, MD
Assistant Professor, Department of Emergency Medicine; and Director, Clinical Decision Unit, MetroHealth Medical Center, Case Western Reserve University School of Medicine, Cleveland, Ohio

ELSIE M. SELBY, MSN, ARNP, CCRN, CCNS
Director, Cardiopulmonary and Laboratory Services; and Director, Sleep Disorders Center and Diabetes and Endocrinology Center, Ephraim McDowell Regional Medical Center, Danville, Kentucky

SANDRA G. SIECK, RN, MBA
President and Chief Executive Officer, Sieck HealthCare Consulting, Mobile, Alabama

ALAN B. STORROW, MD
Associate Professor and Director of Research, Department of Emergency Medicine, Vanderbilt University School of Medicine, Nashville, Tennessee

RICHARD L. SUMMERS, MD
Professor of Emergency Medicine, Department of Emergency Medicine, University of Mississippi Medical Center, Jackson, Mississippi

ROBIN J. TRUPP, PhD(c), MSN, ARNP, CCRN
President, Comprehensive CV Consulting LLC; and The Ohio State University, College of Nursing, Columbus, Ohio

Contents

> It is widely recognized that the impact of heart failure on society is enormous. The research community has responded, resulting in an ongoing period of rapid advancement across a wide range of fields. The pace of progress is perhaps most apparent in the barrage of new and revised terminology appearing in the heart failure literature. Although sometimes confusing, the complexity of nomenclature directly reflects a growing appreciation that the symptom complex previously labeled "heart failure" is actually a spectrum of complex multisystem pathologies. Accordingly, clinicians must adopt a more sophisticated and more effective approach to evaluation and treatment that is increasingly based on objective measurement of outcome-linked physiologic parameters rather than the subjectively described symptom constellations relied on previously.

> This article provides a comprehensive review of acute decompensated heart failure (ADHF). It begins with a historical review, defines ADHF, and describes the many factors that may precipitate it.

> The evolution of prehospital treatment of decompensated congestive heart failure has in some ways come full circle: rather than emphasizing a battery of new pharmacotherapies, out-of-hospital providers have a renewed focus on aggressive use of nitrates, optimization of airway support, and rapid transport. The use of furosemide and morphine has become de-emphasized, and a flurry of research activity and excitement revolves around the use of noninvasive positive-pressure ventilation. Further research will clarify the role of bronchodilators and angiotensin-converting enzyme inhibitors in the prehospital setting.

This article presents a basic understanding of the reasons for implantation, how the devices function, and what to do to help improve patient care if a problem occurs.

The emergency department evaluation and management of patients who have potential acute heart failure syndromes (AHFS) has remained a significant challenge for decades. The emergency physician's diagnostic tools for heart failure have remained limited, and the complexity of the syndrome itself has led to risk-averse practice styles with extremely high admission rates. Recently, new diagnostic markers and technology have become promising and even commonplace to assist emergency physicians in risk prediction for patients who have AHFS. Familiarity with these approaches is essential for improved care for patients who have heart failure and for resource use. This article reviews the available literature and describes patient features that need to be accounted for in disposition decision-making.

Acute decompensated heart failure (ADHF) is a common illness presenting to the emergency department (ED) that is amenable to observation unit (OU) treatment. As the number of baby boomers continues to grow and the incidence of heart failure increases, the financial implications of ADHF treatment will become more prominent. Obtaining institutional support and developing a good working relationship with cardiology colleagues is vital to creating workable ADHF protocols for whichever type of OU an institution decides to use.

With an aging population, the United States health care delivery system is struggling to handle an onslaught of chronic disease burden. The current process of regulatory oversight and pay-for-performance reimbursement is a reality in today's health care delivery system. To maintain profitability, facilities must be willing to implement new strategies that marry operational redesign, quality care, and cost-effective treatment. As payers increasingly favor outpatient strategies for patient management, inpatient facilities must develop effective strategies to shift inpatient care into ambulatory settings. This article presents a model, based on acute heart failure, that offers a solution that is fixed on process improvement techniques that levy positive economic impact.

Hospitalization for acute heart failure syndromes (AHFS) results in substantial in-hospital and postdischarge morbidity and mortality. Management of AHFS presents significant challenges, given the heterogeneity of the patient population and the differing etiologies underlying why patients present with acute decompensation. Arrhythmias in the setting of AHFS, such as atrial fibrillation and wide complex tachycardia, present additional challenges. Compounding this challenge is the paucity of evidence on which to base early management. General principles for the

Heart Failure Clinics

THE CLINICS ARE NOW AVAILABLE ONLINE!

Access your subscription at:
www.theclinics.com

Editorial

The Race to Tissue Oxygenation: Special Teams *GoGoGo*

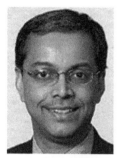 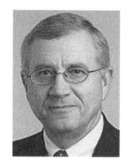

Ragavendra R. Baliga, MD, MBA   James B. Young, MD
Consulting Editors

More than 50,000 patients die every year from acute decompensated heart failure. It is the most common reason for hospital admissions of patients 65 years of age and older, and half these patients who are older than 70 years of age are readmitted within 90 days. One million patients are hospitalized every year with this condition and 20% of them are rehospitalized for this condition within 30 days of the initial admission.[1] One year from index hospitalization, mortality is about 30%, whereas the mortality rate at 1 year for ambulatory New York Heart Association (NYHA) class III heart failure is substantially less than 10%. The event rate for patients hospitalized for heart failure resembles the postmyocardial infarction curve—with a very high event rate in the first 60 days, followed by a relatively flat curve.[2]

Acute decompensated heart failure may present as pulmonary edema, features of decreased cardiac output, or hypoperfusion. In these patients, the need to restore tissue oxygenation is urgent. The approach to restoration of tissue oxygenation includes restoring euvolemia by relieving congestion, addressing etiologic and precipitating factors (**Box 1**), and strategies to prevent recurrence of heart failure.[3] Typically, in the absence of guidelines and paucity of evidence-based therapy recommendations for management of acute decompensated heart failure, the care provided has been disparate.

With a view toward reducing the length of stay and preventing rehospitalization, hospitals are increasingly forming 24-hour on-call special teams, known as Heart Failure Response Teams, to manage these patients. A typical in-patient Heart Failure Response Team comprises one of the hospitalists on-call and two heart failure nurses during business hours. This special team is typically activated within 30 minutes after the patient is admitted to the emergency department (ED) and works, initially, with the ED physicians to stabilize the patient; this strategy is based on an alogrithm previously prepared by a team of cardiologists, ED physicians, and hospitalists (**Fig. 1**). The nurses ensure that all patients receive a discharge summary explaining in detail dietary restrictions, including sodium restriction, medications and dosages, and instructions on whom to contact in case of weight gain or other symptoms; both patients and physicians must sign the forms. The nurses also ensure that a follow-up appointment with the primary care physician is scheduled for 72 hours postdischarge. In the case of a scheduling conflict within this 72-hour window, the patient is scheduled for follow up at a hospital-based clinic. In one hospital, the length of stay decreased by one half of a day and the readmission rate (readmitted for any reason) fell from 22% in 2006 to 18.7% in 2007. Heart failure readmissions falling

Heart Failure Clin 5 (2009) xi–xiv
doi:10.1016/j.hfc.2008.10.001

Box 1
Causes and precipitating factors of acute heart failure

Ischemic heart disease
- Acute coronary syndromes
- Mechanical complications of acute MI
- Right ventricular infarction

Valvular
- Valve stenosis
- Valvular regurgitation
- Endocarditis
- Aortic dissection

Myopathies
- Postpartum cardiomyopathy
- Acute myocarditis

Hypertension/arrhythmia
- Hypertension
- Acute arrhythmia

Circulatory failure
- Septicemia
- Thyrotoxicosis
- Anemia
- Shunts
- Tamponade
- Pulmonary embolism

Decompensation of pre-existing chronic HF
- Lack of adherence
- Volume overload
- Infections, especially pneumonia
- Cerebrovascular insult
- Surgery
- Renal dysfunction
- Asthma, COPD
- Drug abuse
- Alcohol abuse

From Dickstein K, Cohen-Solal A, Filippatos G, et al. Task Guidelines for the diagnosis and treatment of acute and chronic heart failure 2005: the Force for Diagnosis and Treatment of Acute and Chronic Heart Failure 2008 of the European Society of Cardiology. Developed in collaboration with the Heart Failure Association of the ESC (HFA) and endorsed by the European Society of Intensive Care Medicine (ESICM). Eur Heart J 2008;29(19):2388–42; with permission.

review utilization of angiotensin-converting enzyme inhibitor or angiotensin receptor blocker (or to ensure accurate and timely documentation of omission rationale); to screen for risk of deep vein thrombosis and apply prophylaxis; to provide dietary counseling; to promote immunization against pneumococcus or influenza; and to apply strategies to prevent hospitalization.[6] All of these patients were discharged to a dedicated heart failure clinic to help patients self-manage euvolemia. After continuous process improvement, this consortium of hospitals was able to standardize delivery of all these process measures and to reduce readmission rates from 25% in 2004 to 10% in 2007.

One of the main goals of the Heart Failure Response Team is to rapidly restore tissue oxygenation by achieving euvolemia when there is vascular congestion or improve hemodynamics when there is hypoperfusion. In this issue, James F. Neunschwander II and W. Frank Peacock have assembled a team of experts who have very succinctly discussed these challenges in managing acute decompensated heart failure. Increasingly, it is becoming clear that the management of acute decompensated heart failure requires offense, defense, and special teams to restore tissue oxygenation including achieving euvolemia and to reduce length of stay and re-hospitalizations. Emergency department physicians are akin to the offensive line; hospitalists are the defensive line; cardiologists, heart failure nurses, and heart failure disease management programs are the coaches; and the Heart Failure Response Teams are the special teams. Successful management of these patients requires skillful deployment of all teams, and the role of each team has to be tailored to each patient's needs. In our opinion, Heart Failure Response Teams add value in the management of acute decompensated heart failure to promote rapid utilization of diuretics, restore tissue perfusion, and reduce length of stay, re-admissions, and early mortality. *GoGoGo* to these special teams.

Ragavendra R. Baliga, MD, MBA
The Ohio State University
Columbus, OH, USA

James B. Young, MD
Division of Medicine and Lerner College of Medicine
Cleveland Clinic
Cleveland, OH, USA

E-mail addresses:
Ragavendra.Baliga@osumc.edu (R.R. Baliga)
YOUNGJ@ccf.org (J.B. Young)

under diagnosis-related group 127 fell from 10.5% in 2006 to 6.4% in 2007.[4]

The Institute of Medicine, in a bid to reduce medical errors and improve quality, has been championing special response teams to manage critical patients.[5] The establishment of a typical Heart Failure Response Team involves developing reliable processes, systems, or interventions to determine left ventricular function; to provide patients with smoking cessation counseling; to

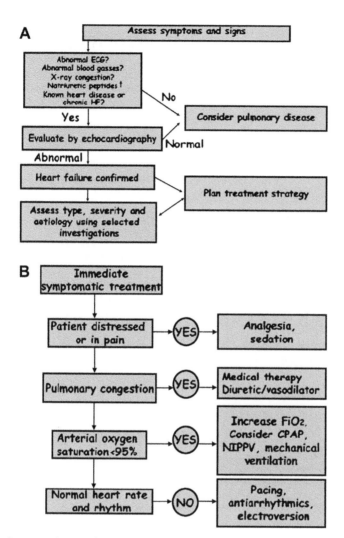

Fig 1. (*A*) Evaluation of suspected acute decompensated heart failure. (*B*) Initial treatment algorithm for management of acute decompensated heart failure. (*From* Dickstein K, Cohen-Solal A, Filippatos G, et al. Guidelines for the diagnosis and treatment of acute and chronic heart failure 2005: the Force for Diagnosis and Treatment of Acute and Chronic Heart Failure 2008 of the European Society of Cardiology. Developed in collaboration with the Heart Failure Association of the ESC (HFA) and endorsed by the European Society of Intensive Care Medicine (ESICM). Eur Heart J 2008;29(19):2388–42; with permission.)

REFERENCES

1. Rosamond W, Flegal K, Furie K, et al. Heart disease and stroke statistics—2008 update: a report from the American Heart Association Statistics Committee and Stroke Statistics Subcommittee. Circulation 2008;117(4):e25–e146.
2. Friedewald VE, Gheorghiade M, Yancy CW, et al. The editor's roundtable: acute decompensated heart failure. Am J Cardiol 2007;99(11):1560–7.
3. Dickstein K, Cohen-Solal A, Filippatos G, et al. Task Guidelines for the diagnosis and treatment of acute and chronic heart failure 2005: the Force for Diagnosis and Treatment of Acute and Chronic Heart Failure 2008 of the European Society of Cardiology. Developed in collaboration with the Heart Failure Association of the ESC (HFA) and endorsed by the European Society of Intensive Care Medicine (ESICM). Eur Heart J 2008;29(19):2388–442.
4. Agency for Healthcare Research and Quality. 24-hour Heart Failure Response Team decreases length of stay and readmission rates. Available at: http://www. innovations.ahrq.gov/content.aspx?id=1820. Accessed November 4, 2008.

5. Institute for Healthcare Improvement. Deliver reliable, evidence-based care for congestive heart failure. Available at http://www.ihi.org/IHI/Programs/Campaign/CHF.htm. Accessed November 4, 2008.

6. Institute for Healthcare Improvement. Mentor hospital registry: congestive heart failure. Available at: http://www.ihi.org/IHI/Programs/Campaign/mentor_registry_chf.htm. Accessed November 4, 2008.

Preface

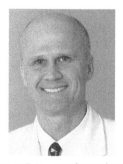

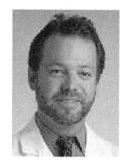

James F. Neuenschwander II,
MD, FACEP

W. Frank Peacock, MD, FACEP

Guest Editors

Acute heart failure has only recently been recognized as a presentation that is unique within the continuum of heart failure. It is characterized by markedly acute symptom exacerbation, the result of a mismatch between circulatory resistance and inadequate myocardial function to meet the metabolic needs of the corpus. With this new perspective, the literature is only recently catching up to its clinical need. Much of the diagnostic and therapeutic science applied to the acute presentation of heart failure is taken from well-done randomized clinical trials of patients who have chronic heart failure. Emergency Physician Arjun Chanmugan once said, "If we don't own acute heart failure, we sure borrow it a lot," which seems to be an accurate characterization. This important distinction emphasizes that, in the acute situation, patients present to the emergency department (ED) when they cannot breathe, and their pathophysiology is not the same as that of the group of patients sitting in an office lobby.

With improvements in the chronic management of heart failure, greater numbers of patients are surviving only to suffer from acute decompensation. This results in a greater need for emergent ambulance transport. The importance of a well-trained emergency medical service system is covered and presented as an outline for other systems to emulate. Once the patient is in the ED, sorting of the undifferentiated dyspneic patient is challenging. The potentially difficult task of accurately diagnosing heart failure is detailed, covering both new strategies and their current controversies. And, as all patients diagnosed with acute heart failure do not require ICU admission or even hospitalization, accurate risk stratification guiding both disposition and therapy selection is detailed.

In this issue of *Heart Failure Clinics*, we also present a historical perspective and overview of the complexities of heart failure pathophysiology. It is pointed out in the issue that heart failure is not a singular entity with a unique cause, and thus its treatment regimens vary greatly. Because the entire developing world is currently confronting a heart failure epidemic, the costs of this entity represent one of the greatest burdens to the entire medical system. We therefore detail the economics of this disease process and engage in a comprehensive discussion regarding the appropriate use of the heart failure observation unit. As the goals of the observation unit are limited, specific acute heart failure treatments are covered. The pharmacology and impact of comorbidities, such as atrial fibrillation, in the total management strategy are addressed.

Additionally, advanced treatments regarding left ventricular assist devices, balloon pumps, pacemakers, internal cardioverter defibrillators, and ultrafiltration are included. This then leads to a separate article covering the difficulties of managing cardiac transplant patients presenting with acute heart failure.

Finally, to a great extent, nursing care drives both in-hospital and postdischarge quality of life in acute heart failure, even more than the pathophysiology of the disease itself. Because of this, we have included an article highlighting the importance of the health team collaboration from the initiation of the patient's care in the prehospital environment, all the way through to discharge planning.

Overall, this issue of *Heart Failure Clinics* has something for almost everyone involved in the spectrum of treating heart failure patients. We hope you enjoy it and we welcome your feedback.

Heart Failure Clin 5 (2009) xv–xvi
doi:10.1016/j.hfc.2008.08.014
1551-7136/08/$ – see front matter

I want to dedicate this book to my beautiful wife Colleen and our three wonderful children Elias, Arel, and Gabriel (J.F.N.).

And thanks to my family, without whom I would get nowhere (W.F.P.).

James F. Neuenschwander II, MD, FACEP
The Ohio State University Medical Center
Emergency Department
376 West 10th Avenue
Columbus, Ohio 43210-1252, USA

W. Frank Peacock, MD, FACEP
The Cleveland Clinic
Department of Emergency Medicine
9500 Euclid Avenue, Desk E-19
Cleveland, OH 44195, USA

E-mail addresses:
James.Neuenschwander@osumc.edu
(J.F. Neuenschwander)
PEACOCW@ccf.org (W.F. Peacock)

Heart Failure and the Emergency Department: Epidemiology, Characteristics, and Outcomes

Gary B. Green, MD, MPH, MBA*

KEYWORDS

- Acute heart failure syndromes • Emergency department
- Epidemiology

TERMINOLOGY AND DEFINITIONS

A common language always greatly facilitates communication, whereas ambiguous or ill-defined terms are often a significant barrier to meaningful idea exchange. This observation is especially apparent at the forefront of any rapidly evolving field of inquiry and is certainly the case for heart failure (HF). Accordingly, considerable effort has been made in recent years among HF researchers, professional societies, and policy makers to establish consensus concerning the most appropriate diagnostic terms and their definitions. Although progress has certainly been made, as the science of HF has progressed it has also become increasingly clear that this is not a monolithic disease with a single common pathway but rather a diverse and complex spectrum of pathologies historically bound by a limited number of shared clinical characteristics. The nomenclature used continues to rapidly expand and evolve as clinical syndromes are increasingly differentiated based on measurable physiologic parameters and outcomes rather than the more subjective characteristics relied on in the past.

HF itself has been most recently redefined by the American College of Cardiology/American Heart Association (ACC/AHA) task force on practice guidelines as "a complex clinical syndrome that can result from any structural or functional cardiac disorder that impairs the ability of the ventricle to fill with or eject blood." Because volume overload is not uniformly present in all patients or at all presentations, use of the older term "congestive heart failure" is to be discouraged.[1] Various authors have used overlapping diagnostic terms to stratify HF presentations by onset or temporal pattern, sometimes contributing more confusion than clarity. For example, The European Society of Cardiology defines the term acute heart failure as "the rapid onset of symptoms and signs secondary to abnormal cardiac function," reserving the more specific term acute decompensated heart failure for "those patients with known HF who experience acute or subacute worsening of their HF state."[2] Many United States authors have used the same terms somewhat differently, describing acute heart failure as "new onset of decompensated HF or decompensation of chronic, established HF with symptoms sufficient to warrant hospitalization."[3] To resolve this diagnostic ambiguity, a 2005 international working group recommended adoption of the inclusive term acute heart failure syndromes, defined as "gradual or rapid deterioration in HF signs and symptoms resulting in a need for urgent therapy."[4] Most recently, the 2007 American College of Emergency Physicians Clinical Policies Committee has also endorsed the term "acute heart

New York University Langone Medical Center, New York, NY, USA
* Department of Emergency Medicine, New York University Langone Medical Center, Bellevue Hospital Administration Building A345, New York, NY 10016.
E-mail address: gary.green@med.nyu.edu

Heart Failure Clin 5 (2009) 1–7
doi:10.1016/j.hfc.2008.08.001
1551-7136/08/$ – see front matter © 2008 Elsevier Inc. All rights reserved.

failure syndromes" as defined by the international working group, and this term is used here.[5]

Although the clinical syndrome of HF is most often caused by myocardial disease, it may also be due to pericardial, endocardial, or great vessel pathology. Further, although most HF patients do have some degree of left ventricular impairment, the causes and characteristics of ventricular functional abnormality are diverse. It is important that the term HF be differentiated from the more specific physiologic descriptor, left ventricular dysfunction, and also not be confused with cardiomyopathy, defined by the AHA as any "disease of the myocardium associated with mechanical and/or electrical dysfunction."[1,6]

In the past, it had been believed that HF was uniformly related to a decreased left ventricular ejection fraction (LVEF). Through further study and more routine use of echocardiography, it has now become apparent that a large proportion of patients who have HF actually have a normal or near-normal LVEF. Until recently, these patients were given the diagnosis of diastolic dysfunction, described as "prolonged, slowed, or incomplete ability [of the myocardium to] generate force, shorten and return to an unstressed length."[7] Recognition that diastole is an active and complex physiologic process rather than simply the passive absence of contraction was and remains a critical concept in the understanding of HF. However, more rigorous study has demonstrated that diastolic functional abnormalities also frequently occur among patients who have reduced LVEF. Diastolic and systolic dysfunctions are thus not mutually exclusive and therefore diastolic dysfunction should no longer be used as a differentiating term. Accordingly, it is now recommended that all patients who have HF undergo echocardiography soon after diagnosis and be classified as having either left ventricular systolic dysfunction (LVSD) or preserved systolic function (PSF). This more physiologically accurate nomenclature will likely have increasingly significant clinical implications, including implications for emergency department (ED) treatment, as ongoing trials focused on each of these groups are completed.[8] Predictably, some diagnostic controversy does remain, particularly concerning the most appropriate threshold EF below which a HF patient should be classified as having LVSD. Although some investigations have used a cutoff of EF less than 50%, the largest United States HF data registries, OPTIMIZE-HF and Acute Decompensated Heart Failure National Registry (ADHERE), currently define LVSD based on an EF less than 40%.[9–11]

EPIDEMIOLOGY AND IMPACT

HF has emerged as a significant public health problem whose impact on quality of life, the health care system, and the economy is already staggering and continues to grow each year as the population ages. The current prevalence of HF within the United States is 5.3 million, or 2.5% of the entire adult population, and it is estimated that 660,000 new cases will be diagnosed this year.[12] Among those older than 65, nearly 1 in 10 are newly diagnosed annually, and in this age group HF is the leading cause of hospitalization.[13,14] In 1979, HF accounted for just 400,000 United States hospital discharges. This number has increased to 1.1 million hospitalizations a year for a primary diagnosis of HF and a total of 3.6 million annual hospitalizations with HF as either a primary or secondary cause, corresponding to an annual direct cost of $23 billion.[1,12] Beyond this, there are greater than 3.4 million ambulatory care visits annually for HF, including approximately 1.1 million ED visits.[12,14] The total cost (direct and indirect) for HF in the United States continues to steadily increase and is currently estimated to be $35 billion to $60 billion.[1,12]

Beyond hospital days and dollars, the human cost of HF is devastating and frequently underappreciated. The natural course of the disease is characterized by inevitable deterioration, with progressive decline in functional capacity exacerbated by frequent episodes of acute, sometimes life-threatening, decompensation requiring repeated ED visits and prolonged hospitalizations. Although somewhat variable based on cause and comorbidity, once diagnosed with HF the prognosis remains grim, with overall mortality rates similar to and sometimes surpassing those of many other disease states routinely labeled as terminal, such as HIV/AIDS and many types of cancer.[12] In the Framingham Heart Study, 80% of men and 70% of women diagnosed with HF died within 8 years, whereas the 1-year mortality approached 20%.[15] Nationally, HF is recorded as the primary cause in 2.2% of all deaths, and one in eight death certificates (284,365 deaths in 2004) list heart failure as either a primary or contributory cause.[12]

Within this context of high overall morbidity and mortality among patients who have chronic HF, an ED visit caused by an acute heart failure syndrome (AHFS) indicates a period of greatly increased short-term mortality risk. Fully 80% of patients who have AHFS require admission and various studies have reported in-hospital mortality rates of 2% to 20%.[16,17] Among those requiring intensive care unit admission from the ED, in-hospital mortality is greater than 10%,[17] whereas an ED presentation of acute pulmonary edema signals a particularly poor prognosis. Twelve percent of these patients do not leave the hospital alive and the 1-year mortality among this subgroup is greater than 40%.[18] Of those surviving to hospital discharge after any AHFS presentation, 11% die within 30 days, 44% require rehospitalization within 6 months, and 33% do not survive 1 year after discharge.[16]

Although the overall burden of disease on society because of HF clearly continues to increase over time, a review of outcomes investigations suggest recent treatment advances may be having a positive effect. Despite a significant increase in disease prevalence, total United States HF-related deaths in 2004 (284,365) were nearly identical to those of 1994 (284,087).[12] Further, although a previous study of nearly 4 million Medicare patients did not show improvement in 30-day mortality between 1992 and 1999,[19] overall survival did improve over a 2-decade period among a community-based longitudinal cohort.[20] The most encouraging data to date concern in-hospital outcomes and are from the ADHERE, which analyzed trends from January, 2002 to December, 2004 among 159,168 HF patients admitted from 285 hospitals. During the 3-year study period the multivariate risk-adjusted mortality rate declined from 4.5% to 3.2%, the need for mechanical ventilation was reduced from 5.3% to 3.4%, and hospital length of stay was reduced from a mean of 6.3 to 5.5 days. Although causation for these improvements cannot be demonstrated, inotrope use decreased during the study period and significant advances were also made in compliance with recently adopted HF quality metrics, including routine assessment of left ventricular function and beta-blocker use.[21]

DEMOGRAPHICS

Although HF can occur at any age because of several structural and functional cardiac abnormalities, statistically speaking it is primarily a disease of the aged. The estimated prevalence of HF among those aged 20 to 39 years old is less than 0.3%, approaches 2% among those 40 to 59, reaches 6% from 60 to 79, and exceeds 12% in those more than 80 years old.[12] The mean age reported for ED patients who had AHFS in the ADHERE database was 72.4 years,[17] similar to the 74.3 years mean age reported among ED HF visits in the National Hospital Ambulatory Care Survey (NHAMCS).[14]

Women and men have an equal lifetime risk for developing HF (one in five), and the proportion of ED visits and hospitalizations for AHFS among women roughly mirrors the gender distribution of the population at a similar age.[12,22] Gender differences do exist, however, in HF pathophysiology and clinical characteristics. Women who have HF are generally older at disease onset compared with men and they have lower rates of coronary artery disease and renal insufficiency. In contrast, women who have HF are more likely to have hypertension and, consistent with this risk profile, a higher proportion of women who have HF have PSF compared with men. Women also have a higher mean LVEF.[22] Studies evaluating gender disparities in outcomes have reported conflicting results.[22,23] Several clinical trials of patients who have chronic HF have suggested that women who have HF have a lower mortality risk.[23–25] Women were uniformly underrepresented in these studies, however, and selection bias may have influenced the results. Gender analysis of the ADHERE database, adjusted for other predictive variables, found similar in-hospital mortality and equivalent rates of dialysis and mechanical ventilation among women and men.[22,26] Further, a prospective investigation of dyspneic ED patients identified as having AHFS by a B-type natriuretic peptide (BNP) measurement greater than 500 found that women actually had a significantly higher 24-month mortality compared with men.[26]

Nearly 1 million African Americans have HF, corresponding to a 50% higher incidence of disease compared with the general population.[12] Overall, black patients develop HF symptoms at an earlier age and their disease progresses more rapidly compared with whites, yet they are generally diagnosed at a more advanced stage of disease.[27–29] There have been many investigations reporting on comparative mortality rates for blacks who have HF but they have provided conflicting results and adequate comparative data is not available concerning HF among Hispanic, Asian, or other ethnic groups. There remains no clear consensus concerning the influence of race/ethnicity on overall HF outcomes.[1,30]

Two recent studies have focused on the complex role of race in the ED evaluation and treatment of AHFS. Hugli and colleagues[14] analyzed data from all ED visits for AHFS in the NHAMCS database from 1992 to 2001. They found a 53% higher ED visit rate for AHFS among blacks compared with whites but a 13% lower hospitalization rate despite a similar proportion of black patients receiving an urgent triage classification. After adjusting for other predictive variables, whites were still 1.7 times more likely to be admitted compared with blacks. Further, only 68% of blacks who had AHFS received a chest radiograph in the ED compared with 80% of whites.[14] Although various explanations for this apparent bias can be postulated, the data suggest a disturbing disparity in the ED physicians' perception of AHFS disease severity between black and white patients that is not supported by existing physiologic or clinical data. Further insight into this issue is provided by a recent subgroup analysis of data from a trial of serum BNP measurement in the evaluation of patients who had HF, the Rapid Emergency Department Heart Failure Outpatient Trial (REDHOT). BNP measurement is a robust predictor of HF severity and it is equally predictive of outcome among black and white patients. In the REDHOT study, BNP levels of black patients were not significantly different from those of white patients. However, whites were significantly more likely to be rated by ED physicians as having more severe HF by New York Heart Association classification (class III or IV), whereas blacks were more likely to be perceived as having milder heart failure (class I or II). Further, although as expected admitted white patients had higher BNP levels than those discharged, black patients who were discharged home actually had higher BNP levels compared with admitted blacks.[30] This "perceptual bias," in which disease severity is systematically underestimated among blacks compared with whites, has also been reported in the evaluation of ED patients presenting with chest pain.[31]

COMORBIDITIES

Coronary artery disease (CAD) is the single greatest contributor to HF morbidity and mortality at all stages of disease. Among those who have LVSD, CAD is identified as the primary etiologic trigger in approximately two thirds of patients. Although other pathology, such as hypertension, valve disease, and atrial fibrillation, is more often cited as the underlying cause in those who have PSF, 30% of these patients also have a preceding diagnosis of myocardial infarction (MI) or angina and at autopsy a majority of patients who have HF have CAD.[1,9–11,17,32] In HF registries and other studies enrolling patients hospitalized for an AHFS, a past history of MI is reported in 31% to 48% and a previous diagnosis of CAD is documented in 57% to 65%.[10,11] Beyond this role in HF initiation, CAD also accelerates disease progression subsequent to HF onset through new infarction, acute or chronic ischemic dysfunction (ie, myocardial stunning or hibernation), and continued endothelial activation of adverse neurohormonal response cascades. Not surprisingly, the effect of CAD on outcome among patients who have HF is devastating. Longitudinal studies have consistently demonstrated that the presence of CAD increases overall mortality by 50% or more. CAD is also a powerful independent predictor of mortality among patients presenting to the ED with AHFS. In one European ED study, after adjusting for all other known prognostic risk factors, the presence of a CAD history increased the risk for death during the study period by 224%.[33]

Like CAD, hypertension (HTN) is both a causative agent and comorbidity in HF. In cohort studies, the presence of either systolic or diastolic HTN significantly increases the risk for a subsequent HF diagnosis, whereas long-term treatment of HTN dramatically reduces the likelihood of HF development.[34–36] The major pathophysiologic link between HTN and HF is HTN-induced left ventricular hypertrophy (LVH), which is itself an independent risk factor for MI and HF.[37] Overall, the contribution of HTN to the burden of HF disease is dramatic, with untreated or inadequately treated HTN estimated to account for approximately 40% of cases in men and approximately 60% in women.[1] Consistent with this, ED-based investigations have found that 53% to 73% of all patients presenting with AHFS have a history of HTN,[16,21] with this risk being somewhat more predominant among those who have PSF than among those who have LVSD (76% versus 66%, $P < .0001$).[11]

Although eliciting a previous history of HTN may provide insight into the likely cause of HF in a given patient, presenting blood pressure in the ED is a more meaningful guide to risk stratification and treatment in those presenting with AHFS. Low systolic blood pressure in the ED is a strong negative prognostic indicator. The high morbidity and mortality in this group is a result of a heightened state of neurohormonal activation and the consequent cascade of increased fluid retention, hyponatremia, renal insufficiency, and treatment resistance.[38] Conversely, patients who have AHFS and an elevated blood pressure on ED presentation are generally characterized by shorter duration of symptoms before arrival and are more likely to be female and older, consistent with a greater likelihood of having PSF rather than LVSD. The implication is that fluid maldistribution rather than fluid overload may be the predominant problem in this group and therefore a treatment focus on vasodilators rather than diuretics may be more effective. Such a directed approach to ED treatment based on presenting blood pressure and other physiologic parameters has been suggested but not yet operationally defined and has not been prospectively studied.[8]

Cardiovascular and renal disease often occur concomitantly and each disease state has a negative effect on the other. Renal impairment is a risk factor for all-cause mortality in a wide variety of cardiovascular diseases and, conversely, cardiovascular disease is the most common cause of death among patients who have chronic kidney disease (CKD) and end-stage renal disease (ESRD), accounting for 50% of their mortality.[39,40] A similar relationship is seen between renal disease and HF. Approximately 50% of all patients who have HF have an impaired glomerular filtration rate, and concomitant HF is reported in up to 40% of those who have ESRD.[40] In the ADHERE registry of ED patients who had AHFS, a history of CKD was recorded in 30%, 21% had a creatinine greater than 2.0 mg/dL in the ED, and 5% were undergoing dialysis.[17] Impaired renal function is also strongly associated with poorer outcome among patients who have HF, even after adjusting for all known covariates. This negative effect on prognosis is independent of LVEF and is of equivalent magnitude among patients who have LVSD and those who have PSF.[39]

The coexistence of HF and renal impairment is usually the result of one or more underlying vascular insults, such as HTN, diabetes, or atherosclerosis. A mutually reinforcing effect on disease progression is observable across the entire spectrum of disease severity but is most apparent and most harmful in those approaching end-stage disease states as manifested by the cardiorenal syndrome. Although a consensus definition does not yet exist, the syndrome has been described as a state of advanced cardiorenal dysregulation occurring in patients who have HF and concomitant renal disease characterized by worsening renal function and diuretic resistance during the treatment of AHFS.[41] Although elucidation of the complex physiology of the cardiorenal syndrome has become an increasingly active area of investigation, the implications of syndrome recognition on ED treatment decisions remains unclear at this time.[40,41]

Other conditions have also been found to have a significant impact on development, progression, or prognosis of HF. A history of atrial fibrillation was present in 31% of patients who had HF enrolled in the ADHERE registry and longitudinal studies report an increasing prevalence of atrial fibrillation with increasing severity of LVSD.[42] Anemia is reported in up to 45% of patients who have HF and occurs as frequently among those who have reduced and preserved LVSF. Anemia and atrial fibrillation are also each associated with significantly increased mortality among patients who have HF.[42,43] Various other investigations have reported a worse prognosis among patients who have HF with diabetes, liver disease, chronic obstructive pulmonary disease, cerebrovascular disease, cancer, and dementia.[14,16,17]

Obesity is highly associated with increased risk for a wide variety of cardiovascular events, including the onset of HF. Surprisingly, among patients already diagnosed with HF, a higher body mass index (BMI) actually seems to have a protective effect. Among nearly 110,000 patients who had AHFS included in the ADHERE registry, in-hospital mortality was inversely related to BMI across all BMI quartiles. This effect persists after adjustment for all other known prognostic factors and occurs among those who have both LVSD and PSF. The physiologic basis of this observation, labeled the obesity paradox, remains unclear at this time but is the subject of much speculation among HF investigators.[44]

SUMMARY AND CLINICAL IMPLICATIONS

Whether measured in deaths or dollars, it is now widely recognized that the impact of heart failure on society is enormous. Through government funding and market forces the research community has responded, resulting in an ongoing period of rapid advancement across a wide range of fields from myocardial cell biology and neurohormonal physiology to HF epidemiology and behavioral interactions. The pace of progress is perhaps most apparent in the barrage of new and revised terminology appearing in the HF literature as researchers and professional societies struggle to quickly translate emerging knowledge into clinical practice. Although sometimes confusing, the complexity of nomenclature directly reflects a growing appreciation that the symptom complex previously labeled "heart failure" does not in fact represent a single disease state but is actually a spectrum of complex multisystem pathologies. Accordingly, clinicians must adopt a more sophisticated and more effective approach to evaluation and treatment that is increasingly based on objective measurement of outcome-linked physiologic parameters rather than the subjectively described symptom constellations relied on previously.

Because HF prevalence continues to increase with the aging population and its natural course is marked by frequent and often life-threatening acute decompensation, ED visits for AHFS will likely continue to increase in the future, further challenging our resources and skills. Each ED presentation of AHFS also represents an opportunity to intervene at a critical stage of illness and the potential to make a dramatic positive impact on duration and quality of life. Emergency physicians must therefore remain on the cutting edge of this rapidly evolving field as real-time stratification of patients who have AHFS into physiologic- and risk-based subgroups becomes a routine part of ED evaluation and increasingly directs the application of emerging therapeutic approaches.

REFERENCES

1. Hunt SA, American College of Cardiology, American Heart Association Task Force on Practice Guidelines. ACC/AHA 2005 guideline update for the diagnosis and management of chronic heart failure in the adult: a report of the American College of Cardiology/American Heart Association Task Force on Practice Guidelines. J Am Coll Cardiol 2005;46:e1–82.
2. Nieminen MS. The task force on acute heart failure of the European Society of Cardiology. Executive summary of the guidelines on the diagnosis and treatment of acute heart failure. Eur Heart J 2005;26: 384–416.
3. Fonarow GC, Adams KF Jr, Abraham WT, et al. Risk stratification for in-hospital mortality in acutely decompensated heart failure: classification and regression tree analysis. JAMA 2005;293:572–80.
4. Gheorghiade M, Zannad F, Sopko G, et al. International working group on acute heart failure syndromes. Acute heart failure syndromes: current state and framework for future research. Circulation 2005;112:3958–68.
5. Silvers SM, ACEP. Clinical Policies Subcommittee on Acute Heart Failure Syndromes. Clinical policy: critical issues in the evaluation and management of adult patients presenting to the emergency department with acute heart failure syndromes. Ann Emerg Med 2007;49:627–69.
6. Maron BJ, Towbin JA, Thiene G, et al. Contemporary definitions and classification of the cardiomyopathies: an AHA scientific statement from the Council on Clinical Cardiology, Heart Failure and Transplantation Committee; Quality of Care and Outcomes Research and Functional Genomics and Translational Biology Interdisciplinary Working Groups; and Council on Epidemiology and Prevention. Circulation 2006;113:1807–16.
7. Zile MR, Brutsaert DL. New concepts in diastolic dysfunction and diastolic heart failure: Part I: diagnosis, prognosis and measurements of diastolic function. Circulation 2002;105:1387–93.
8. Collins S, Storrow AB, Kirk JD, et al. Beyond pulmonary edema: diagnostic, risk stratification, and treatment challenges of acute heart failure management in the emergency department. Ann Emerg Med 2008;51:45–57.
9. Redfield MM, Jocobson SJ, Burnett JC Jr, et al. Burden of systolic and diastolic ventricular dysfunction in the community: appreciating the scope of the heart failure epidemic. JAMA 2003;289:194–202.
10. Yancy CW, Lopatin M, Stevenson LW, et al. Clinical presentation, management and in-hospital outcomes of patients admitted with acute decompensated heart failure with preserved systolic function; a report from the ADHERE database. J Am Coll Cardiol 2006;47: 76–84.
11. Fonarow GC, Stough WG, Abraham WT, et al. Characteristics, treatments and outcomes of patients with preserved systolic function hospitalized for heart failure: report from the OPTIMIZE-HF registry. J Am Coll Cardiol 2007;50:768–77.
12. Rosamond W, Flegal K, Furie K, et al. Heart disease and stroke statistics 2008 update: a report from the American Heart Association Statistics Committee and Stroke Statistics Committee. Circulation 2008; 117:e25–146.
13. O'Connell JB. The economic burden of heart failure. Clin Cardiol 2000;23(Suppl. 3):6–10, III.
14. Hugli O, Braun JE, Kim S, et al. US emergency department visits for decompensated HF, 1992–2001. Am J Cardiol 2005;96:1537–42.
15. Lloyd-Jones DM, Larson MG, Leip EP, et al. Framingham Heart Study. Lifetime risk for developing congestive heart failure: The Framingham Heart Study. Circulation 2002;106:3068–72.
16. Fonarow GC. Epidemiology and risk stratification in acute heart failure. Am Heart J 2008;155:200–7.
17. Adams KF, Fonarow GC, Emerman CL, et al. Characteristics and outcomes of patients hospitalized for heart failure in the US: rationale, design and preliminary observations from the first 100,000 cases in the Acute Decompensated Heart Failure National Registry [ADHERE]. Am Heart J 2005;149: 209–16.
18. Roguiin A, Behar D, Ben Ami H, et al. Long-term prognosis of acute pulmonary edema—an ominous outcome. Eur J Heart Fail 2000;2:137–44.
19. Kaiborod M, Lichtman JH, Heidenreich PA, et al. National trends in outcomes among elderly patients with heart failure. Am J Med 2006;119:e1–7.
20. Forger VL, Weston SA, Redfield MM, et al. Trends in HF incidence and survival in a community-based population. JAMA 2004;292:344–50.
21. Fonarow GC, Heywood T, Heidenreich PA, et al. Temporal trends in clinical characteristics, treatments, and outcomes for heart failure hospitalizations, 2002 to 2004: findings from the Acute Decompensated Heart Failure National Registry (ADHERE). Am Hear J 2007;153:1021–8.
22. Diercks DB, Fonarow GC, Kirk D, et al. Risk stratification in women enrolled in the acute decompensated heart failure national registry emergency module (ADHERE – EM). Acad Emerg Med 2008; 15:151–8.
23. Galvao M, Kalman J, DeMarco T, et al. Gender differences in in-hospital management and outcomes in patients with decompensated heart failure: analysis from the Acute Decompensated Heart Failure National Registry (ADHERE). J Card Fail 2006;12: 100–7.

24. Gustafsson F, Torp-Pederson C, Burchardt H, et al. Female sex is associated with a better long-term survival in patients hospitalized with congestive heart failure. Eur Heart J 2004;25:129–35.

25. Ghali JK, Krause-Steinfauf HJ, Adams KF, et al. Gender differences in advanced heart failure: Insights from the BEST study. J Am Coll Cardiol 2003;42:2128–34.

26. Christ M, Laule-Kilian K, Hochholzer W, et al. Gender specific risk stratification with BNP levels in patients with acute dyspnea. J AM Coll Cardiol 2006;48:1808–12.

27. Alexander M, Grumbach K, Remy L, et al. Congestive heart failure hospitalizations and survival in California: patterns according to race/ethnicity. Am Heart J 1999;137:919–27.

28. Yancy CW. Heart failure in African Americans: a cardiovascular enigma. J Card Fail 2000;6:183–6.

29. Alexander M, Grumbach K, Selby J, et al. Hospitalization for congestive heart failure. Explaining racial differences. JAMA 1995;274:1037–42.

30. Daniels LB, Bhalla V, Clopton P, et al. B-type natriuretic peptide levels and ethnic disparities in perceived severity of heart failure: results from the Rapid Emergency Department Heart Failure Outpatient Trial (RED-HOT) multicenter study of BNP levels and emergency department decision making in patients presenting with shortness of breath. J Card Fail 2006;12:281–5.

31. Keyle PM, Pezzin LE, Green GB. Disparities in the emergency department evaluation of chest pain patients. Acad Emerg Med 2007;14(2):149–56.

32. Gheorghiade M, Bonow RO. Chronic heart failure in the United States: a manifestation of coronary artery disease. Circulation 1998;97:282–9.

33. Purek L, Laule-Kilian K, Christ A, et al. Coronary artery disease and outcome in acute congestive heart failure. Heart 2006;92:598–602.

34. Levy D, Larson MG, Vasan RS, et al. The progression from hypertension to congestive heart failure. JAMA 1996;275:1557–62.

35. Wilhelmsin L, Rosengren A, Eriksson H, et al. Heart failure in the general population of men: morbidity, risk factors and prognosis. J Intern Med 2001;249:253–61.

36. Kostis JB, Davis BR, Cutler J, et al. Prevention of heart failure by antihypertensive treatment in older persons with isolated systolic hypertension. JAMA 1997;278:212–6.

37. Vakili BA, Okin PM, Devereux RB. Prognostic implications of left ventricular hypertrophy. Am Heart J 2001;141:334–41.

38. Gheorghiade M, Abramson WT, Albert NM, et al. Systolic blood pressure at admission, clinical characteristics and outcome in patients hospitalized with acute heart failure. JAMA 2006;296:2217–26.

39. Hillege HL, Nitsch D, Pfeffer MA, et al. Renal function as a predictor of outcome in a broad spectrum of patients with heart failure. Circulation 2006;113:671–8.

40. Obialo CI. Cardiorenal consideration as a risk factor for heart failure. Am J Cardiol 2007;99(Suppl):21D–4D.

41. Liang KV, Williams AW, Greene EL, et al. Acute decompensated heart failure and the cardiorenal syndrome. Crit Care Med 2008;36(Suppl):S75–88.

42. Parkish R, Maisel WH, Toca FM, et al. Atrial fibrillation in heart failure: high mortality risk even if ventricular function is preserved. Am Heart J 2005;150:701–6.

43. Berry C, Norrie J, Hogg K, et al. The prevalence, nature and importance of hematologic abnormalities in heart failure. Am Heart J 2006;151:1313–21.

44. Fonarow GC, Srikanthan P, Cosantzo MR, et al. An obesity paradox in acute heart failure: analysis of body mass index and inhospital mortality for 108,927 patients in the Acute Decompensated Heart Failure National Registry. Am Heart J 2007;153:74–81.

Pathophysiology of Acute Decompensated Heart Failure

Richard L. Summers, MD[a],*, Ezra Amsterdam, MD[b]

KEYWORDS

- Acute heart failure • Pathophysiology
- Emergency medicine

A disease condition synonymous with heart failure was recognized as early as the ancient Egyptian and Byzantine Empires.[1] Early descriptions of the condition focused on the outward signs of edema, and the resulting diagnosis was often referred to as the dropsy from the Greek word hydrops meaning water.[2] An understanding of the etiology and pathophysiologic mechanisms involved were unknown at that time, however.

It was not until the early 17th century after William Harvey's work in defining the functioning of the circulation, that the heart was implicated in this disease process. In light of these emerging concepts, another English physician, William Withering, first documented a successful treatment for this condition, in which the circulation was targeted with the use of foxglove (digitalis purpura).[3]

By the 20th century, fewer people were dying of infectious diseases, and heart failure became a more commonplace source of morbidity and mortality. Most early descriptions were very cardiocentric, and the dropsy diagnosis was replaced with the more descriptive term congestive heart failure, emphasizing what was considered at that time a central role of the heart in the pathophysiology.

Since that time, the definition of heart failure has evolved as knowledge and understanding of the pathophysiology of the condition have changed. By the latter half of the 20th century, Arthur C. Guyton provided a description of the quantitative physiologic relationships between cardiac output, extracellular fluid volume, and blood pressure control, with a central role for the kidneys in long-term regulation.[4–6] This work was centered on the premise that the primary goal of the circulation was to provide fluids and nutrients to the tissues of the body. A description of heart failure that emerged from these concepts viewed this disease process as a more generalized failure of the circulation from a system's perspective.[4,6] Continuing basic science research and clinical investigations have resulted in the cardiorenal model of heart failure, in which inappropriately elevated neurohormonal (NH) activity is pivotal in both the etiology and progression of the disorder.[7,8] Also evident from this conceptual construct is an understanding that the pathophysiology of acute decompensated heart failure (ADHF) is somewhat different from the chronic form of the disease. The physiologic systems involved overlap, however, and a modern-day approach to managing ADHF requires an understanding of this interplay of disease states.[9]

DEFINITION OF ACUTE DECOMPENSATED HEART FAILURE AND PATHOPHYSIOLOGIC OVERVIEW

From an analysis of the various clinical circumstances that potentially can lead to a condition of heart failure, it is obvious that this pathology is really a spectrum of disease states. Therefore, a more generalized pathophysiologic definition of heart failure should be based upon a broad-based consideration of the function of the circulation as a whole. Using the Guytonian framework of

[a] University of Mississippi Medical Center, Jackson, MS, USA
[b] University of California School of Medicine (Davis) and Medical Center, Sacramento, CA, USA
* Corresponding author. Department of Emergency Medicine, University of Mississippi Medical Center, 2500 North State Street, Jackson, MS 39216.
E-mail address: rsummers@pol.net (R.L. Summers).

Heart Failure Clin 5 (2009) 9–17
doi:10.1016/j.hfc.2008.08.005

circulatory control, a comprehensive modern-day definition of acute heart failure might be considered as follows:

"Acute decompensated heart failure is a hemodynamic state in which the systemic circulation is unable to meet the immediate needs of the body tissues secondary to a destabilization of the complex physiologic interactions between the heart, peripheral vasculature, and their supporting neurohormonal systems."[10–12]

Acute heart failure is characterized by a rapid downward trending of cardiac output values paralleled by an ongoing retention of fluid in an attempt to compensate and maintain blood flow to the tissues. As fluid is retained and pulmonary edema and hypoxia ensue, there is a continuing downward spiral in cardiac and circulatory functioning that is driven by positive feedback. This hemodynamic profile differs from chronic heart failure, in which steady-state circulatory conditions are maintained by an interplay of compensatory physiologic mechanisms that result in a stable (although often tenuous) hemodynamic status. In this state, the cardiac output and arterial pressure are normalized at the cost of accumulation of excess body fluid volume. In practice, the differentiation between the two states (acute versus chronic) is not demarcated clearly. In actuality, acute heart failure usually occurs in the context of an ongoing chronic heart failure condition. Time constants of the action of the physiologic mechanisms controlling cardiac output account for the apparent clinical differences. The moment-to-moment hemodynamic state is controlled by short-term physiologic control mechanisms that determine the flows, resistances, and pressures of the circulation.[13] These factors are the evident determinants of the acute condition. Not so obvious are the NH and renal mechanisms that control the long-term circulatory state and determine the background conditions in which the short-term controllers function.[14]

HEMODYNAMICS OF ACUTE DECOMPENSATED HEART FAILURE

General hemodynamic and cardiac output control can be illustrated in **Fig. 1** using the classic Guyton diagrams equating the flow out of the heart (as depicted by the Starling contractility curve) with flow into the heart from the peripheral circulation (venous return).[5,13] The mean circulatory filling pressure is the driving force for venous return and filling of the atria and ventricles. The filling pressures in turn establish the stroke volume and

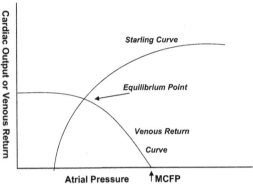

Fig. 1. Graphical analysis of cardiac output as determined by the intersection between the Starling and the venous return curves. This equilibrium point defines the steady-state cardiac output at a specific atrial pressure. The venous return (and cardiac output) becomes zero when the atrial pressure equals the mean circulatory filling pressure (MCFP).

cardiac output by the Starling mechanism. The balance between these functional relationships determines the cardiac output and venous return at a specific atrial pressure (the equilibrium point). The structure and form of the relationships determining cardiac output are shaped by both acute and chronic physiologic regulatory mechanisms. The factors adjusting moment-to-moment changes in contractility and venous compliance acutely determine the flows, pressures, and resistances in the circuit. Intermediate and long-term regulatory mechanisms establish the baseline reactivity of the kidneys and vasculature and the total amount of fluid within the system.

The sequence of pathophysiologic events typical of acute heart failure is depicted in **Fig. 2**. The normal equilibrium between the Starling and venous return curves (A) is shifted by a depression in cardiac contractility[1] to form a new balance (B) at a lower cardiac output and a higher atrial pressure. The lower cardiac output and the resultant lower perfusion pressures initiate a cascade of compensatory physiologic mechanisms of an NH nature (catecholamines, aldosterone, and renin/angiotensin). These regulatory factors produce a retention of fluid to increase the venous return (curve shift 2) and bring cardiac output back to normal levels (C). The cost of this compensation is an even higher atrial pressure. Diastolic dysfunction is characterized by normal cardiac contractility and a diminished ventricular compliance.[15,16] This often is seen in conditions of obesity and longstanding hypertension.[16–18] The reduced compliance limits filling of the atria and ventricles.[19] An accumulation of fluid in the venous system therefore is required to increase the driving

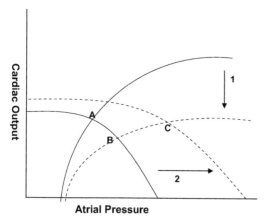

Fig. 2. As ventricular contractility is depressed (1) cardiac output is reduced, and atrial pressures are elevated as the equilibrium moves from point A to point B. The reduced cardiac output results in less perfusion of the kidneys and retention of fluid. This fluid retention shifts the venous return curve (2) to restore the cardiac output to a normal state. The cost of the shift is a higher atrial pressure at the equilibrium point C. If the higher atrial pressure produces pulmonary edema, hypoxia, and further reductions in cardiac function, a vicious cycle can occur.

pressure for venous return and cardiac filling (**Fig. 3**). When this fluid accumulation occurs in the peripheral circulation, there is potential for the development of edema in the extremities. Likewise, left ventricular diastolic dysfunction can produce pulmonary congestion.

Atrial pressures and pressures within the venous vasculature are the major determinants of pressure at the level of the pulmonary capillary.[20] This pressure is the driving force for the formation of pulmonary edema during acute

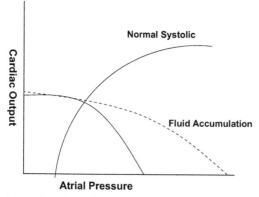

Fig. 3. Diastolic dysfunction is characterized by normal cardiac contractility and diminished ventricular compliance. An accumulation of fluid in the venous system is required to increase the driving pressure for venous return and cardiac filling.

decompensation. By the Starling equation:
$$J_v = K_f\,([P_c - P_i] - \sigma\,[\pi_c - \pi_i])$$
where:

J_v is the net fluid movement between compartments.

K_f is the filtration coefficient.

P_c is the pulmonary capillary hydrostatic pressure.

P_c is the interstitial hydrostatic pressure.

π_c is the pulmonary capillary osmotic pressure.

π_i is the interstitial osmotic pressure.

σ is the reflection coefficient.

If the atrial or venous pressures become high enough to cause pulmonary edema and hypoxia, there is further suppression of cardiac contractility and the Starling curve, with an ensuing vicious cycle of progressive decompensation.[13] A comprehension of the integration of both acute and chronic dynamics is important for understanding modern strategies for managing these patients.

THE ROLE OF NEUROHORMONAL AND CYTOKINE ACTIVATION IN ACUTE DECOMPENSATED HEART FAILURE

As noted in the previous section, the homeostatic regulation of mammalian salt and water metabolism, circulatory function, and blood pressure depends on the integration of multiple physiologic mechanisms. NH controls play an essential role in these processes through the activity of the sympathetic nervous system (SNS), renin angiotensin aldosterone system (RAAS), arginine vasopressin (AV), and natriuretic peptides (NP). Endothelium-derived vasoactive factors and other mediators also contribute to this physiologic organization. Several of these systems augment cardiac contractility, blood volume, sodium retention, and blood pressure, and others provide a counterbalance by promoting opposite cardiocirculatory effects. Under normal physiologic conditions, these mechanisms act in concert to modulate cardiac, renal, and vascular function for maintaining appropriate blood volume, perfusion pressure, cardiac output, and its distribution. When an impairment of myocardial function results in reduced blood supply to end organs, however, NH activity is augmented as a compensatory response to support circulatory function by maintaining cardiac output and perfusion pressure. Whereas this activation may be helpful for limited periods, the deleterious effects of excessive and prolonged NH activation now are considered to be central to the pathophysiology of heart failure.[9]

Conceptual models of heart failure have evolved over the last 50 years to explain the deranged physiology of this syndrome. According to the early form of the cardiorenal model, heart failure was viewed as a state of excessive fluid retention related to inadequate cardiac pump function. This was followed by the hemodynamic model, in which abnormal cardiac function resulted in altered loading conditions, which were responsible for the accompanying signs and symptoms. Subsequent basic and clinical investigations, including therapeutic trials, have resulted in the NH model of heart failure, in which inappropriately elevated NH activity is pivotal in the etiology and progression of the disorder (**Fig. 4**).[8]

NEUROHORMONAL ACTIVATION IN CARDIAC DYSFUNCTION
Sympathetic Nervous System

The initial stimulus for activation of the NH systems is impairment of left ventricular function, which may be related to injury from ischemia, infarction, inflammation, valvular disease or cardiomyopathy. Elevated plasma norepinephrine was one of the earliest findings in studies of NH activation in heart failure. Not only are high levels of plasma norepinephrine characteristic of chronic heart failure, but the degree of elevation correlates closely with the severity of cardiac dysfunction and also is related to impaired prognosis.[21,22] Indeed, 1-year survival of patients who had plasma norepinephrine greater than 800 pg/mL was less than 40%.[21] Further, multivariate analysis of five univariate predictors of survival (heart rate, plasma rennin activity, serum sodium, stroke work index, and plasma norepinephrine) demonstrated that norepinephrine was the sole significant factor.[21]

Norepinephrine is directly toxic to cardiac myocytes, the mechanism of which has been attributed to calcium overload or apoptosis. It also induces several alterations in signal transduction, including down-regulation of β1 adrenergic receptors, uncoupling of β2 adrenergic receptors, and increased activity of inhibitory G-protein.[23] The changes in β1 receptors promote myocardial hypertrophy, which, when chronic, progresses to ventricular remodeling, dilation, and progressive functional impairment.[24] Further and interrelated deleterious effects of SNS activation include tachycardia and vasoconstriction, causing increased myocardial oxygen demand; ischemia, infarction, and arrhythmias; and myocyte apoptosis, all of which contribute to further activation of the SNS in the pattern of a vicious cycle (see **Fig. 4**). Additionally, norepinephrine directly and indirectly (through its adverse circulatory effects) activates the RAAS.

Renin Angiotensin Aldosterone System

Heart failure is associated with marked elevations of each of the components of the RAAS.[25] Renin is released from the juxtaglomerular apparatus in response to sympathetic stimulation and reduced renal blood flow.[14] Renin cleaves angiotensinogen to form the decapeptide angiotensin I, from which the angiotensin-converting enzyme induces formation of the octapeptide angiotensin II, a potent vasoconstrictor with multiple additional actions. These include augmentation of sympathetic tone, release of arginine vasopressin, synthesis and secretion of aldosterone by the zona glomerulosa of the adrenal cortex, and renal sodium and water retention. In addition to circulating angiotensin II, cardiac and vascular tissue renin angiotensin systems have been identified that induce

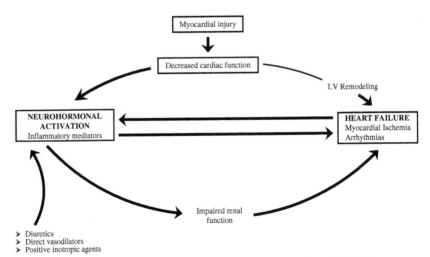

Fig. 4. Cardiac dysfunction and neurohormonal activation promote a cycle of deleterious consequences that contribute to the pathophysiology of heart failure. See text for details.

remodeling of these organs.[26] Angiotensin II has direct myocardial toxic effects that include hypertrophy and apoptosis, and its plasma levels correlate with the severity of cardiac dysfunction and prognosis.[27,28] Aldosterone is synthesized in numerous tissues, including the heart and blood vessels, and the adrenal cortex, suggesting a paracrine effect of the hormone. It has potent renal sodium retaining actions and promotes cardiac and vascular fibrosis, endothelial dysfunction, myocardial infarction, cardiac hypertrophy, and mortality.[29,30]

Arginine Vasopressin

Vasopressin, a potent vasoconstrictor and important regulator of plasma osmolality and free water clearance, is secreted by the pituitary gland and is elevated in patients who have heart failure. Its release is influenced by osmotic and nonosmotic stimuli and is promoted by angiotensin II and activation of osmotic receptors. Vasopressin is inhibited by baroreceptor stimulation and natriuretic peptides. It induces vasoconstriction by activating vasopressin 1 receptors, and promotes renal water reabsorption and secretion of renin by stimulating vasopressin 2 receptors. Vasopressin levels more than twice those in control subjects have been reported in patients who have heart failure.[28] In a study of the relative contributions of specific NH systems to the augmented systemic vascular resistance in patients who had heart failure, it was found that the SNS contribution was highest; the RAAS was also important, and vasopressin's effect was least, suggesting that this hormone likely contributes significantly to vasoconstriction in heart failure only when its levels are elevated markedly.[31]

Natriuretic Peptides

The major peptides of this family of compounds are atrial natriuretic peptide (ANP) and brain (B-type) natriuretic peptide (BNP). They are activated by atrial and ventricular volume and pressure receptors and are elevated in heart failure. These peptides promote natriuresis, reduce SNS and RAAS activity, inhibit vasopressin and endothelin, decrease systemic vascular resistance, and induce venodilation. The effects of BNP are particularly prominent in this regard. The natriuretic peptides, however, probably play little physiologic role in the control of the circulation or in the amelioration of ADHF.[32] The clinical importance of these peptides is with regard to their use as a diagnostic tool and therapeutic potentials when used in pharmacologic doses.[32] BNP initially was identified in porcine brain but later found to be produced in much greater concentrations in human ventricular myocardium. It is initially synthesized as a 134 amino acid peptide (preproBNP) from which is cleaved proBNP, which is cleaved further to form active BNP and the inactive N-terminal (NT)-proBNP. The significance of this degradation is the diagnostic implications of the differential half-lives of these compounds: BNP, 22 minutes; NT-proBNP, 120 minutes. Levels of the natriuretic peptides increase in proportion to the severity of the underlying cardiac disease. Further, in one study, multivariate analysis of patients who had heart failure revealed that a high level of BNP was the only independent NH factor predictive of mortality.[33] BNP has assumed important diagnostic, therapeutic, and prognostic roles for managing patients who have heart failure.[34,35]

Inflammatory Mediators

Recent studies have implicated these agents in the pathophysiology of heart failure. The following is a brief presentation of several of the major inflammatory mediators that have been demonstrated to influence the course of patients who have heart failure.

Endothelin

The endothelins, produced by endothelial cells, are potent vasoconstrictors and are involved in maintaining vascular tone and blood pressure. The major agent of this group is ET-1. This peptide causes several important cardiovascular effects, including vasoconstriction, renal sodium retention, and production of tumor necrosis factor (TNF)-α. It also has growth factor properties. ET-1 is elevated in heart failure in which its major source is the pulmonary vasculature. High levels of ET-1 are associated with increased mortality in this setting.[36]

Tumor necrosis factor

TNF-α plays an important role in the systemic inflammatory response. This mediator produces cardiac structural and functional alterations, including fibrosis, remodeling, and apoptosis.[37] It is elevated in heart failure, in which its levels correlate with the severity of cardiac impairment and mortality.[38]

Interleukins

Interleukins (IL), which are produced by various cells, are prominent mediators in the pathogenesis of heart failure. Both IL-1 and IL-6 are increased in heart failure. IL-1 depresses myocardial contractility, inhibits myocyte responsiveness to β-adrenergic stimulation, and promotes myocyte apoptosis.[39]

Elevated levels of IL-6 are associated with unfavorable clinical findings in patients who have heart failure.[40]

ROLE OF NEUROHORMONAL ACTIVITY AND INFLAMMATION IN ACUTE DECOMPENSATED HEART FAILURE

NH mechanisms generally are considered long-term controllers of the circulation, and their role is well known in patients who have chronic heart failure. Most of the facts in the preceding section were derived from studies of patients who had chronic heart failure. There is less information regarding the contribution of these maladaptive mechanisms in ADHF; however, it appears that they are also prominent in this setting. Although ADHF typically occurs as an exacerbation of compensated chronic cardiac failure, the clinical presentation may be de novo cardiac decompensation. Precipitating factors of ADHF are numerous and include noncompliance with diet and medication; uncontrolled hypertension; cardiac ischemia and arrhythmias; pulmonary embolism; infection; and other systemic illnesses.

In patients who have ADHF, there is evidence of increased NH activation,[41–43] as reflected by elevated levels of norepinephrine, renin activity, aldosterone, ET-1 and other cytokines. These mediators are associated with vasoconstriction, fluid retention, and cardiac arrhythmias.[42] In addition, increased levels of cytokines have been documented in patients who have ADHF and correlate with prognosis.[44–46] These recent findings support the role of NH activation and augmented cytokine activity in the pathogenesis of ADHF and have important implications for diagnosis, prognosis, and treatment.

Cardiorenal Syndrome

As is clear from the foregoing, activation of the SNS, RAAS, vasopressin, and inflammatory markers in patients with heart failure has a profound and adverse effect on cardiac and renal function. Whether worsening renal function specifically contributes to the progression of heart failure or is a marker of advanced cardiac and kidney impairment is unclear.[47] The combination of this dual organ malfunction, however, has been termed the cardiorenal syndrome.[7] It is associated with diuretic resistance and is common in ADHF. The pathophysiology of this syndrome appears to be related to a complex interplay of NH and hemodynamic mechanisms. It has important therapeutic and prognostic implications, because conventional therapy is limited. Additionally, clinical outcomes are poor.

Clinical Pathophysiology of Acute Heart Failure

In a typical clinical scenario, a patient who has chronic heart failure will preserve a stable condition unless there is some perturbation (such as an increased fluid intake, worsening cardiac function, or noncompliance with medications) that requires the systemic physiology to activate an adjustment.[48] A crescendoing activation of the long-term cardiac output control mechanisms seeking to maintain stability in response to a perturbation ultimately can overwhelm the short-term controllers and result in the development of ADHF. When a patient arrives in the emergency department in the acute throes of a decompensated heart failure event, the critical efforts in the resuscitative process are directed toward a rapid relief of the pulmonary edema and an improvement in central oxygenation for vital organ support. This goal requires that the physician create an immediate change in the hemodynamic state in a way that promptly reduces the atrial pressures and alleviates the pulmonary congestion. From a pathophysiologic perspective, the time-urgent nature of the condition obviates a role for the long-term controllers of the circulation in the primary phase of ADHF management. A treatment scheme targeting the plumbing of the intravascular pressures and flows should be the first consideration in the emergent stabilization of the ADHF patient.[48] This objective often can be achieved by measures that reduce afterload or preload conditions in an attempt to reduce the atrial pressure and forces driving fluid extravasations at the level of the capillary. Although it is common to observe a rapid resolution of the patient's congestion and hypoxia with these treatments, the physiologic adjustments in hemodynamics initiated by most conventional acute therapies do not provide for long-term circulatory stability.[48,49] The derangements in the neurohormonal axis and other chronic control mechanisms that led to the decompensated state are usually still present after the primary resuscitation and drive a continued fluid retention by the kidneys even in the face of the initial acute management. Therefore, it is important to immediately begin to address the physiologic mechanisms responsible for the chronic regulation of the circulation in a secondary phase of resuscitation of these patients.

Therapeutic implications of neurohormonal activation in heart failure

Based on an understanding of the NH model of heart failure and the pharmacologic actions of current therapeutic modalities, the limitations and potentially deleterious role of these approaches can be understood. Thus, although diuretics, vasodilators, and positive inotropic agents may afford symptomatic relief, they tend to exacerbate underlying detrimental NH overactivity on the myocardium, vasculature, kidney, and fluid and electrolyte balance. Diuretics stimulate further activation of the RAAS, SNS, vasopressin, and endothelin, as do direct vasodilators (see **Fig. 4**).[50] The unfavorable myocardial effects of positive inotropic agents are similar to those of the endogenous catecholamines described previously. These considerations have stimulated concern for judicious and physiologically rational application of these therapeutic approaches based on underlying pathophysiology to mitigate their undesirable effects.[51]

Special Pathophysiologic Conditions of Heart Failure

The diverse physiologic factors affecting an overlapping and time-varying control of cardiac output and general circulatory functioning can result in an incongruence between a patient's ventricular function, body fluid volume status, and state of heart failure. There are several common clinical scenarios in which such paradoxes can arise.

Pathophysiology of fluid volume overload heart failure

Even when there is normal cardiac function, it is still possible to overwhelm the circulation with fluid to a point where the heart is ineffective as a pump. When this happens, the circulation becomes congested, and edema can develop. If the volume overload is prolonged, the heart function can begin to deteriorate under the strain, and a vicious cycle begins.[52] Chronic renal failure is the most common clinical condition in which patients present with fluid volume overload. In these cases, a manipulation of the hemodynamics may be all that is possible until the excess fluid is removed by dialysis or some other method. If the renal failure is in the end stages, the NH systems have little or no role in the pathophysiology of the heart failure.

Pathophysiology of acute heart failure in the dehydrated patient

Heart failure is typically thought of as a condition of fluid volume excess.[53] Elderly bed-ridden patients who have marginal ventricular function and an ongoing treatment with diuretics, however, can present with a paradoxical condition, in which they have evidence of pulmonary congestion and yet are volume contracted.[10] Just as pulmonary edema can lead to myocardial hypoxia and worsening contractility, a progressing dehydration can result in a decrease in coronary perfusion and

precipitate an acute heart failure event. Although it is counterintuitive, it may be necessary to begin a fluid bolus as a part of the initial resuscitation of these patients. This rehydration process, however, should be done judiciously and with a concurrent manipulation of the hemodynamics to optimize flow around the circuit.

Pathophysiology of diuretic-resistant heart failure

Most forms of acute heart failure are very responsive to diuretic treatment in the primary phase of resuscitation. As noted previously, however, continued aggressive treatment with diuretics can stimulate an already activated NH response further. Increasing levels of angiotensin and catecholamines can restrict renal blood flow severely, while an elevated serum aldosterone enhances fluid reabsorption in the distal tubule. This pathophysiologic condition attenuates the effectiveness of subsequent doses of diuretics and results in limited urine output.[48] If the patient is not volume contracted, therapies targeting the NH systems might be used to enhance the effectiveness of the diuretic.

REFERENCES

1. Saba MM, Ventura HO, Saleh M, et al. Ancient Egyptian medicine and the concept of heart failure. J Card Fail 2006;12:416–21.
2. Lutz JE. A XII century description of congestive heart failure. Am J Cardiol 1988;61(6):494–5.
3. Breckenridge A. William Withering's legacy—for the good of the patient. Clin Med 2006;6(4):393–7.
4. Guyton AC, Coleman TG, Granger HJ. Circulation: overall regulation. Annu Rev Physiol 1972;34:13–46.
5. Guyton AC. The systemic venous system in cardiac failure. J Chronic Dis 1959;9:465–75.
6. Montani JP, Adair TH, Summers RL, et al. A simulation support system for solving large physiological models on microcomputers. Int J Biomed Comput 1989;24:41–54.
7. Bongartz LG, Cramer MJ, Doevendans PA, et al. The severe cardiorenal syndrome: Guyton revisited. Eur Heart J 2005;26:11–7.
8. Mann DL, Bristow MR. Mechanisms and models in heart failure: the biomechanical model and beyond. Circulation 2005;111(21):2837–49.
9. Braunwald E, Bristow MR. Congestive heart failure: fifty years of progress. Circulation 2000;102(4):IV14–23.
10. Summers RL. Rapid clinical assessment of hemodynamic profiles and targeted treatment of patients with acutely decompensated heart failure: wet and cold profile. Clin Cardiol 2004;27(Suppl V):V10–1.

11. Summers RL. Cardiovascular emergencies: chapter 32: future diagnostics: impedance cardiography in the assessment and management of acute heart failure. New York: McGraw-Hill Companies; 2006. 357–63.

12. Summers RL. Emerging diagnostics: impedance cardiography in the assessment and management of acute heart failure. Critical Pathways in Cardiology 2005;4:134–9.

13. Guyton AC, Jones CE, Coleman TG. Circulatory physiology: cardiac output and its regulation. (2nd edition). Philadelphia: W.B. Saunders; 1973.

14. Hall JE, Guyton AC, Mizelle HL. Role of the renin–angiotensin system in control of sodium excretion and arterial pressure. Acta Physiol Scand Suppl 1990;591:48–62.

15. Andrew P. Diastolic heart failure demystified. Chest 2003;124:744–53.

16. Summers RL, Kolb JC, Woodward LH, et al. Differentiating systolic from diastolic heart failure using impedance cardiography. Acad Emerg Med 1999; 6(7):693–9.

17. Carroll JF, Summers RL, Dzielak DJ, et al. Diastolic compliance is reduced in obese rabbits. Hypertension 1999;33:811–5.

18. Summers RL, Kolb JC. Left ventricular hypertrophy as a marker of diastolic dysfunction in patients with acute congestive heart failure. Eur J Emerg Med 2002;9(4):351.

19. Summers RL, Montani JP. Computer model of cardiac diastolic dynamics. Comput Cardiol 1992;19: 697–700.

20. Gaar KA Jr, Taylor AE, Owens LJ. Effect of capillary pressure and plasma protein on development of pulmonary edema. Am J Phys 1967;213(1):79–82.

21. Cohn JN, Levine TB, Olivari MT, et al. Plasma norepinephrine as a guide to prognosis in patients with chronic congestive heart failure. N Engl J Med 1984;311(13):819–23.

22. Francis GS, Benedict C, Johnstone DE, et al. Comparison of neuroendocrine activation in patients with left ventricular dysfunction with and without congestive heart failure. A substudy of the studies of left ventricular dysfunction (SOLVD). Circulation 1990; 82(5):1724–9.

23. Mann DL, Kent RL, Parsons B, et al. Adrenergic effects on the biology of the adult mammalian cardiocyte. Circulation 1992;85(2):790–804.

24. Adams JW, Sakata Y, Davis MG, et al. Enhanced Galpha q signaling: a common pathway mediates cardiac hypertrophy and apoptotic heart failure. Proc Natl Acad Sci U S A 1998;95(17):10140–5.

25. Anand IS, Ferrari R, Kalra GS, et al. Edema of cardiac origin. Studies of body water and sodium, renal function, hemodynamic indexes, and plasma hormones in untreated congestive cardiac failure. Circulation 1989;80(2):299–305.

26. Bader M, Jörg P, Ovidiu B, et al. Tissue renin–angiotensin systems: new insights from experimental animal models in hypertension research. J Mol Med 2001;9(2):76–102.

27. Tan LB, Jalil JE, Pick R, et al. Cardiac myocyte necrosis induced by angiotensin II. Circ Res 1991; 69(5):1185–95.

28. Francis GS, Cohn JN, Johnson G. Plasma norepinephrine, plasma renin activity, and congestive heart failure. Relations to survival and the effects of therapy in V-HeFT II. The V-HeFT VA Cooperative Studies Group. Circulation 1993;87(Suppl. 6):V140–8.

29. Loskutoff D, Quigley J. PAI-1, fibrosis, and the elusive provisional fibrin matrix. J Clin Invest 2000; 106(12):1441–3.

30. Swedberg K, Eneroth P, Kjekshus J, et al. Hormones regulating cardiovascular function in patients with severe congestive heart failure and their relation to mortality. CONSENSUS Trial Study Group. Circulation 1990;82(5):1730–6.

31. Creager M, Faxon D, Cutler S. Contribution of vasopressin to vasoconstriction in patients with congestive heart failure: comparison with the renin–angiotensin system and the sympathetic nervous system. J Am Coll Cardiol 1986;7(4):758–65.

32. Summers RL, Montani JP. Computer model of ANP-hemodynamic interactions. Comput Cardiol 1991; 18:697–700.

33. Tsutamoto T, Wada A, Maeda K, et al. Attenuation of compensation of endogenous cardiac natriuretic peptide system in chronic heart failure: prognostic role of plasma brain natriuretic peptide concentration in patients with chronic symptomatic left ventricular dysfunction. Circulation 1997;96(2):509–16.

34. Colucci WS, Elkayam U, Horton DP, et al. Intravenous nesiritide, a natriuretic peptide, in the treatment of decompensated congestive heart failure. N Engl J Med 2000;343(4):246–53.

35. Maisel AS, McCord J, Nowak RM, et al. Bedside B-type natriuretic peptide in the emergency diagnosis of heart failure with reduced or preserved ejection fraction: results from the breathing not properly multinational study. J Am Coll Cardiol 2003;1(11):2010–7.

36. Wei CM, Lerman A, Rodeheffer RJ, et al. Endothelin in human congestive heart failure. Circulation 1994; 89(4):1580–6.

37. Bradham WS, Bozkurt B, Gunasinghe H, et al. Tumor necrosis factor-alpha and myocardial remodeling in progression of heart failure: a current perspective. Cardiovasc Res 2002;53(4):822–30.

38. Torre-Amione G, Kapadia S, Benedict C, et al. Proinflammatory cytokine levels in patients with depressed left ventricular ejection fraction: a report from the studies of left ventricular dysfunction (SOLVD). J Am Coll Cardiol 1996;27(5):1201–6.

39. Francis SE, Holden H, Holt CM, et al. Interleukin-1 in myocardium and coronary arteries of patients with

dilated cardiomyopathy. J Mol Cell Cardiol 1998; 30(2):215–23.

40. Aukrust P, Ueland T, Lien E, et al. Cytokine network in congestive heart failure secondary to ischemic or idiopathic dilated cardiomyopathy. Am J Cardiol 1999;83(3):376–82.

41. Aronson D, Burger AJ. Neurohormonal prediction of mortality following admission for decompensated heart failure. Am J Cardiol 2003;91(2):245–8.

42. Aronson D, Burger AJ. Neurohumoral activation and ventricular arrhythmias in patients with decompensated congestive heart failure: role of endothelin. Pacing Clin Electrophysiol 2003;26(3):703–10.

43. Milo O, Cotter G, Kaluski E, et al. Comparison of inflammatory and neurohormonal activation in cardiogenic pulmonary edema secondary to ischemic versus nonischemic causes. Am J Cardiol 2003; 92(2):222–6.

44. Chin. Interleukin-6, tissue factor and von Willebrand factor in acute decompensated heart failure: relationship to treatment and prognosis. Blood 2003;14(6):515.

45. Mueller C, Laule-Kilian K, Christ A, et al. Inflammation and long-term mortality in acute congestive heart failure. Am Heart J 2006;151(4):845–50.

46. Peschel T, Schonauer M, Thiele H, et al. Invasive assessment of bacterial endotoxin and inflammatory cytokines in patients with acute heart failure. Eur J Heart Fail 2003;5(5):609–14.

47. Liang K, Williams A, Greene E. Acute decompensated heart failure and the cardiorenal syndrome. Crit Care Med 2008;36(1 Suppl):S75–88.

48. Peacock WF, Allegra J, Ander D, et al. Management of acute decompensated heart failure in the emergency department. Congest Heart Fail 2003; 9(Suppl 1):3–18.

49. Rame JE, Sheffield MA, Dries DL, et al. Outcomes after emergency department discharge with a primary diagnosis of heart failure. Am Heart J 2001; 142:714–9.

50. Shah M, Ali V, Lamba S, et al. Pathophysiology and clinical spectrum of acute congestive heart failure. Rev Cardiovasc Med 2001;(Suppl):9–18.

51. Burger AJ. A review of the renal and neurohormonal effects of B-type natriuretic peptide. Congest Heart Fail 2005;11(1):30–8.

52. Cotter G, Felker GM, Adams KF, et al. The pathophysiology of acute heart failure—is it all about fluid accumulation? Am Heart J. 2008;155:9–18.

53. Cotter G, Metra M, Milo-Cotter O, et al. Fluid overload in acute heart failure—redistribution and other mechanisms beyond fluid accumulation. Eur J Heart Fail 2008;10(2):165–9.

Prehospital Management of Congestive Heart Failure

Amal Mattu, MD, FACEP, FAAEM*, Benjamin Lawner, DO, EMT-P

KEYWORDS

- Congestive heart failure • Pulmonary edema
- Prehospital • Noninvasive ventilation

The prehospital evaluation and treatment of decompensated congestive heart failure (CHF) is as varied as there are emergency medical services (EMS) providers. The nation's EMSs encompass a diverse group of volunteers, career professionals, paraprofessionals, and physicians. The scope of practice for management of decompensated CHF changes varies across jurisdictions and is subject to change according to a medical director's level of comfort and preference. A major reason for the disparities between practices is the limited availability of data from the prehospital setting. Most treatment protocols are based on research on in-hospital patients that has been extrapolated to the prehospital setting. The few prehospital studies that do exist are relatively small and usually retrospective in nature. This article highlights some of those prehospital studies on which many treatment protocols are based. A detailed discussion of the pathophysiology of decompensated CHF and the mechanisms underlying common treatments is found in other articles in this issue.

PREHOSPITAL PERSONNEL AND TRAINING

Physicians who interact with prehospital personnel should have an understanding of the different levels of prehospital care providers, their training, and their capabilities. Basic life support treatment is generally provided at the emergency medical technician (EMT)–basic level. The National Highway Traffic and Safety Administration (NHTSA) recommends a 110-hour curriculum, but this standard is not uniformly followed.[1] State EMS offices often modify the national curriculum to suit their particular needs. For the purposes of this article, basic life support (BLS) treatment refers to prehospital care that is noninvasive. First responders, basic-level EMTs, and ambulance attendants deliver BLS care.

The paramedic provider is the product of a prehospital training system that is still in evolution. In an effort to promote a more advanced prehospital level of care, the Los Angeles County Fire Department began training individuals in the 1970s to go beyond simple BLS by administering intravenous fluids and medications in the out-of-hospital setting. Later, the city of Miami instituted the first organized prehospital advanced life support (ALS) system. Paramedics and intermediate-level EMTs in this system functioned at the ALS level and performed intravenous medication therapy, defibrillation, endotracheal intubation, and external cardiac pacing. This system was gradually adopted around the country, and the NHTSA has endorsed a national standard curriculum for paramedic training that requires 1000 to 1200 hours of classroom instruction.[2]

Despite advanced training and an expanded scope of practice, paramedics still encounter significant challenges in diagnosis and management of decompensated CHF. The diagnosis of a heart failure syndrome is complicated by the often austere out-of-hospital environment. Patients in extremis are often unable to provide an adequate history, and paramedics must rely on clinical presentation to formulate an initial diagnostic impression. The lack of adequate lighting and

University of Maryland School of Medicine, Baltimore, MD, USA
* Corresponding author. Department of Emergency Medicine, University of Maryland School of Medicine, 110 South Paca Street, 6th Floor, Suite 200, Baltimore, MD 21201.
E-mail address: amattu@smail.umaryland.edu (A. Mattu).

Heart Failure Clin 5 (2009) 19–24
doi:10.1016/j.hfc.2008.08.004

even basic diagnostic testing (eg, thermometer, chest radiology, B-type natriuretic peptide test) further obfuscates the identification of an acute heart failure syndrome from noncardiac causes of dyspnea. Because of these challenges, paramedics may adopt a "shotgun-type" approach to the management of the patient in respiratory distress with the use of multiple, rather than targeted, therapies. Unfortunately, there is a relatively high misdiagnosis rate for prehospital patients who have presumed decompensated CHF; when patients are treated in this shotgun type of manner, misdiagnosed patients suffer adverse consequences. Paramedic training is beginning to address some of these issues through improved education, and an increasing number of state protocols are more frequently requiring discussion with or preauthorization by a physician for certain medications that were once considered basic (eg, furosemide). Many ALS systems still function under the doctrine of off-line medical control, however, which permits paramedics and EMT-intermediates to treat patients according to preapproved algorithms.

BASIC LIFE SUPPORT INTERVENTION

Unfortunately the first responder and EMT-basic have a limited arsenal of tools at their disposal. BLS treatment is generally noninvasive and therefore focuses on rapid transport to a hospital. EMTs and first responders are educated in signs and symptoms suggestive of heart failure and severe respiratory distress. Recognition of abnormal vital signs may prompt a BLS crew to expedite transport to an emergency department or request assistance from an ALS provider. In more rural areas of the country, this practice of ALS intercept functions to deliver paramedic-level care to patients who are farther away from definitive therapy.

Oxygen remains the mainstay of BLS-level therapy. First responders are trained to administer high-flow oxygen by way of non-rebreather mask to patients in severe respiratory distress. Should a patient's respiratory status further deteriorate, the BLS provider is capable of assisting respirations by way of a bag-valve mask device. Adjuncts, such as nasopharyngeal and oropharyngeal airways, are available to BLS crews who encounter a patient in cardiorespiratory arrest. Cardiopulmonary resuscitation and automated external defibrillation would also be within the basic provider's scope of practice should the patient who has acute heart failure decompensate further.

ADVANCED LIFE SUPPORT INTERVENTION—AIRWAY SUPPORT

Paramedics clearly have greater resources at their disposal when caring for the patient who has decompensated heart failure. Although the administration of high-flow oxygen by way of a non-rebreather mask is still routine, the use of noninvasive positive pressure ventilation (NIPPV) is gaining attention and popularity in prehospital systems. The two main modalities of delivering NIPPV are by continuous positive pressure ventilation (CPAP) and bi-level positive pressure ventilation (BiPAP). Three recent meta-analyses of studies evaluating NIPPV have demonstrated that the use of either CPAP or BiPAP for patients who have decompensated CHF is associated with decreased need for intubation, reduced ICU and hospital length of stay, reduced costs, and decreased mortality.[3–5] The studies on which these meta-analyses are based primarily evaluated emergency department and in-hospital patients. Based on these ED and in-hospital studies, many EMS systems enthusiastically adopted NIPPV for prehospital use also. Most of these systems have chosen to use CPAP over BiPAP because of its ease of use, and recent studies evaluating prehospital use of CPAP have demonstrated encouraging results.

In 2001 Kosowsky and colleagues[6] published a case series of 19 patients demonstrating the usefulness of prehospital CPAP. Cincinnati Fire Department paramedics were authorized to implement CPAP "at their discretion" for patients believed to be suffering from acute cardiogenic pulmonary edema. CPAP was administered by face mask and maintained at a fixed pressure of 10 cm H_2O. CPAP was discontinued if the patient could not tolerate the face mask or experienced further deterioration. Emergency department physicians corroborated the field diagnosis of pulmonary edema in 13 of 19 patients receiving CPAP. Patients undergoing CPAP therapy were less likely to require intubation on hospital arrival and experienced a reduced length of stay.

In 2006 Hubble and colleagues[7] conducted a nonrandomized trial that included 120 patients and examined endotracheal intubation as the primary endpoint. Other surrogate markers of treatment efficacy that were included were respiratory rate, subjective dyspnea score, hospital length of stay, and mortality. Similar to Kosowsky's series, paramedics administered CPAP by way of face mask at a fixed pressure. The authors found that patients treated with CPAP experienced decreased need for intubation, hospital length of stay, and mortality.

A more recent study by Plaisance and colleagues[8] evaluated early prehospital use of CPAP (within 15 minutes of ambulance arrival) versus delayed use of CPAP (30–45 minutes after arrival). Medical therapies, including use of nitrates and diuretics, were also evaluated in various combinations with early and delayed CPAP. Early administration of CPAP with or without medications demonstrated superior outcomes when compared with medical therapy alone or delayed CPAP with medications. Early use of CPAP was associated with greater improvements in oxygenation, dyspnea, and tracheal intubation rates. Investigators also discovered a trend toward decreased mortality. The study emphasized the importance of early application of CPAP, because even a 15-minute delay in application of CPAP was associated with worse outcomes. CPAP continues to gain widespread support for the prehospital setting, and studies that seek to affirm its effectiveness are ongoing. Although CPAP protocols exist in many ALS jurisdictions, NIPPV is still not considered the standard of prehospital care.

Prehospital care providers should be aware of not only the indications of NIPPV but also the contraindications and shortcomings. NIPPV therapy should be avoided in patients who have vomiting or altered mental status. Some patients may also be unable to tolerate the face mask because of claustrophobia, and thick beards may make a tight seal impossible. Finally, if a patient is in extremis and is rapidly decompensating, definitive airway control with endotracheal intubation should not be delayed with a trial of NIPPV as long as the prehospital care providers have expertise in endotracheal or nasotracheal intubation. A more detailed discussion of NIPPV is provided in other articles in this issue.

ADVANCED LIFE SUPPORT INTERVENTION—MEDICAL THERAPIES

For hypertensive patients who have acute heart failure, EMS systems have traditionally embraced the use of a triple cocktail of nitroglycerine, morphine, and furosemide. This treatment has recently fallen under increased scrutiny, however. A paucity of data supports the routine administration of opiates and diuretics to prehospital patients who have decompensated CHF.[9] On the contrary, studies have demonstrated that these medications may actually be harmful, especially when the prehospital diagnosis is incorrect. Hoffman and colleagues[10] compared nitroglycerin (NTG), furosemide, and morphine in 57 patients who had presumed decompensated CHF. The best outcomes in dyspnea and hospital morbidity (respiratory

depression, dehydration, prolonged in-hospital course) were associated with NTG. The use of furosemide was associated with significant electrolyte abnormalities in some patients, and more than 25% of patients later required fluid repletion because of dehydration and hypotension. Of note, 23% of patients were misdiagnosed and did not have pulmonary edema. In these patients who were inappropriately treated, the use of furosemide and morphine was associated with increased dyspnea and morbidity. Even in these misdiagnosed patients, however, the use of NTG alone was not associated with any adverse effects.

Wuerz and colleagues[11] conducted the largest prehospital study evaluating the use of medications in the management of 599 patients who had presumed decompensated CHF. Once again, a significant number of patients (18%) were misdiagnosed and inappropriately treated for CHF. Most of these misdiagnosed patients were eventually found to have acute asthma, chronic obstructive pulmonary disease (COPD), pneumonia, or bronchitis. In these misdiagnosed patients, if NTG was the sole prehospital treatment, the patients had a 2.2% mortality. In contrast, if these patients were treated with morphine or furosemide (with or without NTG), the mortality was found to be 21.7%.

A recent prehospital study of presumed decompensated CHF was conducted by Jaronik and colleagues.[12] They evaluated 144 prehospital patients who were treated with furosemide. They found that 42% of the patients were misdiagnosed and did not actually have CHF. In fact 17% of the patients were diagnosed as having sepsis, dehydration, or pneumonia (without CHF) and in these patients the administration of furosemide was considered "potentially harmful." Nine study patients died, 7 of whom were in the group of misdiagnosed patients who had received furosemide "inappropriately."

Although the total number of patients in these studies is relatively small, several important conclusions can be made nevertheless. First, prehospital health care providers often misdiagnose patients as having decompensated CHF, with misdiagnosis rates as high as 42%. Second, administration of furosemide or morphine to these misdiagnosed patients is associated with adverse consequences. This finding should be no surprise; patients who have acute asthma or COPD exacerbations or pneumonia are often dehydrated because of poor oral intake and the insensible fluid losses associated with tachypnea and fever. Diuretics exacerbate fluid and electrolyte imbalance; furthermore, morphine, especially in patients who have COPD exacerbations, promotes respiratory depression. Even in patients who are correctly diagnosed, more than half of patients who have severely decompensated heart failure are not actually fluid overloaded, but rather have pulmonary edema because of fluid maldistribution.[13-15] The focus of therapy for these patients should be vascular redistribution rather than diuresis, and in fact, they may actually suffer adverse neurohumoral and renal effects from aggressive diuresis. Third, it seems that the use of NTG is without significant adverse consequences even when the prehospital diagnosis is incorrect. If the diagnosis of decompensated CHF is correct, then NTG is clearly beneficial by providing rapid preload reduction and needed vascular redistribution.

In addition to the evidence demonstrating adverse consequences of diuretics and morphine when the diagnosis is incorrect, there is also a lack of evidence suggesting that these medications are quickly beneficial when the diagnosis is correct. Patients who have decompensated CHF and especially cardiogenic pulmonary edema have decreased renal blood flow because of markedly increased afterload.[13] As a result, the diuretic and preload-reducing effect of furosemide may be delayed 90 to 120 minutes.[16-18] Unless transport times are extremely long, furosemide is unlikely to exert a beneficial effect before hospital arrival and may actually be harmful. Obstacles to accurate diagnosis, coupled with the lack of immediate benefit, urge prehospital medical directors to reconsider the priority of diuresis.

Morphine also has limited benefit even in correctly diagnosed patients who have decompensated CHF. The traditional teaching that morphine produces rapid preload reduction is not supported by studies that used invasive hemodynamic monitoring, and in fact those studies indicate that morphine is associated with transient increases in right heart filling pressure and reductions in cardiac index.[19,20] An ED-based retrospective study by Sacchetti and colleagues[21] suggested that the routine use of morphine in the early management of patients who had cardiogenic pulmonary edema was associated with a fivefold increase in ICU use and intubation rates. Although morphine is also promoted because of its anxiolytic effect, this can actually be accomplished quickly and more safely with small dosages of benzodiazepines when anxiolysis is truly necessary. In all but rare cases, however, rapid treatment of hypoxia results in resolution of anxiety, and additional pharmacologic agents targeted at anxiety are usually not needed.

The use of bronchodilators is also common among prehospital providers when caring for patients who have undifferentiated dyspnea. Because patients who have decompensated CHF may present with wheezing, bronchodilators are also commonly used in these patients. The prehospital study by Wuerz and colleagues[11] suggested that bronchodilators were safe in all types of patients who had dyspnea. There was no increase in mortality when patients were treated with bronchodilators, regardless of the final diagnosis.[22] A recent study by Singer and colleagues,[22] however, has suggested otherwise. They evaluated more than 10,000 patients from the Acute Decompensated Heart Failure National Registry Emergency Module who were provided bronchodilators during acute treatment, in the prehospital setting or in the ED. They found that the use of bronchodilators in patients who did not have a history of COPD was associated with a slightly greater need for "aggressive interventions," including mechanical ventilation. Whether the bronchodilator use was causing adverse outcomes or was simply a marker of sicker patients is unclear from this nonrandomized, retrospective study. Nevertheless, the study does raise concerns regarding the liberal use of bronchodilators in the management of prehospital patients who have undifferentiated dyspnea, especially if the presumptive diagnosis is decompensated CHF. Further studies will need to clarify this question.

The use of angiotensin-converting enzyme (ACE) inhibitors in patients who have decompensated CHF in the ED has gained support in recent years.[13,15,23-30] A series of small studies has demonstrated that early use of ACE inhibitors in the sublingual (captopril) or intravenous (captopril, enalapril) formulation are associated with rapid improvements in preload, afterload, cardiac output, and dyspnea,[23-30] and perhaps also a significant decrease in need for ICU use and intubation.[21] Prehospital studies of ACE inhibitors are lacking; however, some prehospital systems are now using ACE inhibitors for hypertensive patients when the diagnosis of decompensated CHF is strongly suspected.[9] In the state of Maryland, for example, the administration of 25 mg sublingual captopril is incorporated into the standing protocol for patients who have decompensated CHF after the aggressive use of nitrates (see **Box 1**). Prehospital providers should be cautious to only use these medications in patients in whom the diagnosis is nearly certain, and only in patients who remain normotensive or hypertensive after nitrate therapy. ACE inhibitors must also be avoided in patients who have had prior adverse reactions (eg, angioedema). Further research is needed before the prehospital use of ACE inhibitors is widely recommended.

Patients who have concurrent hypotension and decompensated CHF pose a unique challenge for

The following protocol is for adult patients.

- Continuous positive airway pressure (CPAP) should be considered for moderate dyspnea and must be implemented in severe dyspnea. Use early; administer 3 doses of NTG while setting up, acclimatizing the patient and applying CPAP.
- Perform 12 lead ECG (if available) and in the face of inferior wall with posterior wall extension MI, consider lowering the second dosing of NTG
- If patient has a prescription or previous history of nitroglycerin use, administer nitroglycerin per dosing below. May be repeated if symptoms persist, and BP is greater than 90 mm HG, and pulse is greater than 60 bpm, to a maximum dose of 4 mg. If BP drops below 90 mm Hg, treat with medical fluid bolus(es) [initial bolus 250–500 cc; may repeat x 1].
- If patient does not have a prescription or previous history of nitroglycerin use, an IV must be established prior to administration; then administer nitroglycerin as below.
- Initiate lactated ringer's keep vein open
- If IV cannot be established, nitroglycerin may be administered with medical consultation
- Nitrogylcerin

  1) Asymptomatic (dyspnea on exertion, not at rest) – apply oxygen per GPC to maintain O$_2$ saturation greater than 93%.
  2) Mild symptoms (mild dyspnea at rest, despite O$_2$ treatment; able to speak full sentences) – administer low dose NTG 0.4 mg SL at 3-5 minute intervals
  3) Moderate symptoms (moderate dyspnea; O$_2$ saturation less than 93% on O$_2$; unable to speak full sentences; normal mental status; SBP will generally be greater than 150 mm Hg)-High Dose NTG (assess BP before each administration)-with CPAP: administer initial dose of 0.4 mg SL followed in 3 minutes by high dose NTG 0.8 mg SL repeat 0.8 mg once in 3-5 minutes (complete dose = 2.0 mg)-without CPAP: administer initial dose of 0.4 mg NTG SL; then every 3-5 minutes give 0.8 mg NTG SL to a maximum dose of 4.4 mg without medical consult.
  4) Severe symptoms (O$_2$ saturation less than 90% [hypoxia]; one word sentences, altered sensorium, diaphoresis; SBP will generally be greater than 180 mm Hg)-Treat with High Dose NTG as…above
  5) Consider additional nitroglycerin
  6) Consider albuterol for wheezing
  7) Administer captopril 25 mg SL for moderate or severe symptoms so long as SBP $\geq$ 110 mm Hg after NTG administration

- (Medical Control Option) Consider furosemide 0.5–1.0 mg/kg slow IV push
- If blood pressure low: consider fluid boluses followed by dopamine

field providers. Treatment is directed toward expeditious transport and blood pressure support. Some ALS providers are authorized to administer a judicious bolus of intravenous fluids and dopamine infusion. The use of inotropes in the prehospital setting should ideally involve on-line medical control. The administration of any other vasoactive medications besides NTG and dopamine often lies outside the ordinary scope of practice of prehospital provider and is, therefore, not an option.

SUMMARY

The evolution of prehospital treatment of decompensated CHF has in some ways come full circle: rather than emphasizing a battery of new pharmacotherapies, out-of-hospital providers have a renewed focus on aggressive use of nitrates, optimization of airway support, and rapid transport. The use of furosemide and morphine has become de-emphasized, and a flurry of research activity and excitement revolves around the use of NIPPV. Further research will clarify the role of bronchodilators and ACE inhibitors in the prehospital setting.

The out-of-hospital environment is often chaotic and unpredictable. Paramedics operate without the support of ancillary personnel and cannot rely on laboratory or radiographic data to solidify an initial diagnostic impression. As technology evolves and disseminates into the out-of-hospital arena, it will therefore be important to adopt strategies grounded in not only solid physiologic principles but also safety and simplicity.

REFERENCES

1. Emergency medical technician—basic: national standard curriculum. Available at: http://www.nhtsa.gov/. Accessed January 31, 2008.
2. Emergency medical technician—paramedic: national standard curriculum. Available at: http://www.nhtsa.gov. Accessed January 31, 2008.

3. Masip J, Roque M, Sanchez B, et al. Noninvasive ventilation in acute cardiogenic pulmonary edema: a systematic review and meta-analysis. JAMA 2005;294:3124–30.

4. Peter JV, Moran JL, Phillips-Hughes J, et al. Effect of non-invasive positive pressure ventilation (NIPPV) on mortality in patients with acute cardiogenic pulmonary oedema: a meta-analysis. Lancet 2006;367:1155–63.

5. Collins SP, Mielniczuk LM, Whittingham HA, et al. The use of noninvasive ventilation in emergency department patients with acute cardiogenic pulmonary edema: a systematic review. Ann Emerg Med 2006;48:260–9.

6. Kosowsky J, Stephanides S, Branson R, et al. Prehospital use of continuous positive airway pressure for presumed pulmonary edema: a preliminary case series. Prehosp Emerg Care 2001;5:190–6.

7. Hubble M, Richards M, Jarivs R, et al. Effectiveness of prehospital continuous positive airway pressure in the management of acute pulmonary edema. Prehospital Emergency Care 2006;10:430–9.

8. Plaisance P, Pirracchio R, Berton C, et al. A randomized study of out-of-hospital continuous positive airway pressure for acute cardiogenic pulmonary oedema: physiological and clinical effects. Eur Heart J 2007;28:2895–901.

9. Mosesso V, Dunford J, Blackwell T, et al. Prehospital therapy for acute congestive heart failure: state of the art. Prehospital Emergency Care 2003;7:13–23.

10. Hoffman JR, Reynolds S. Comparison of nitroglycerin, morphine and furosemide in treatment of presumed pre-hospital pulmonary edema. Chest 1988;92:586–93.

11. Wuerz RC, Meador SA. Effects of prehospital medications on mortality and length of stay in congestive heart failure. Ann Emerg Med 1992;21:669–74.

12. Jaronik J, Mikkelson P, Fales W, et al. Evaluation of prehospital use of furosemide in patients with respiratory distress. Prehospital Emergency Care 2006;10(2):194–7.

13. Mattu A, Martinez JP, Kelly BS. Modern management of cardiogenic pulmonary edema. Emerg Med Clin North Am 2005;23:1105–25.

14. Cotter G, Felker GM, Adams KF, et al. The pathophysiology of acute heart failure—Is it all about fluid accumulation? Am Heart J 2008;155:9–18.

15. Collins S, Storrow AB, Kirk JD, et al. Beyond pulmonary edema: diagnostic, risk stratification, and treatment challenges of acute heart failure management in the emergency department. Ann Emerg Med 2008;51:45–57.

16. Francis GS, Siegel RM, Goldsmith SR, et al. Acute vasoconstrictor response to intravenous furosemide in patients with chronic congestive heart failure. Ann Intern Med 1985;103:1–6.

17. Ikram H, Chan W, Espiner EA, et al. Haemodynamic and hormone responses to acute and chronic frusemide therapy in congestive heart failure. Clin Sci 1980;59:443–9.

18. Nelson GI, Silke B, Ahuja RC, et al. Haemodynamic advantages of isosorbide dinitrate over frusemide in acute heart-failure following myocardial infarction. Lancet 1983;1(8327):730–3.

19. Lappas DG, Geha D, Fischer JE, et al. Filling pressures of the heart and pulmonary circulation of the patient with coronary artery disease after large intravenous doses of morphine. Anesthesiology 1975;42:153–9.

20. Timmis AD, Rothman MT, Henderson MA, et al. Haemodynamic effect of intravenous morphine in patients with acute myocardial infarction complicated by severe left ventricular failure. Br Med J 1980;280:980–2.

21. Sacchetti A, Ramoska E, Moakes ME, et al. Effect of ED management on ICU use in acute pulmonary edema. Am J Emerg Med 1999;17:571–4.

22. Singer AJ, Emergman C, Char DM, et al. Bronchodilator therapy in acute decompensated heart failure patients without a history of chronic obstructive pulmonary disease. Ann Emerg Med 2008;51:25–34.

23. Annane D, Bellissat E, Pussare E, et al. Placebo-controlled, randomized, double-blind study of intravenous enalaprilat efficacy and safety in acute cardiogenic pulmonary edema. Circulation 1996;94:1316–24.

24. Barnett JC, Zink KM, Touchon RC. Sublingual captopril in the treatment of acute heart failure. Curr Ther Res 1991;49:274–81.

25. Brivet F, Delfraissy JF, Giudicelli JF, et al. Immediate effects of captopril in acute left ventricular heart failure secondary to myocardial infarction. Eur J Clin Invest 1981;11:369–73.

26. Haude M, Steffen W, Erbel R, et al. Sublingual administration of captopril versus nitroglycerin in patients with severe congestive heart failure. Int J Cardiol 1990;27:351–9.

27. Hamilton RJ, Carter WA, Gallagher EJ. Rapid improvement of acute pulmonary edema with sublingual captopril. Acad Emerg Med 1996;3:205–12.

28. Langes K, Siebels J, Kuck KH. Efficacy and safety of intravenous captopril in congestive heart failure. Curr Ther Res 1993;53:167–76.

29. Tohmo H, Karanko M, Korpilahti K. Haemodynamic effects of enalaprilat and preload in acute severe heart failure complicating myocardial infarction. Eur Heart J 1994;15:523–7.

30. Varriale P, David W, Chryssos BE. Hemodynamic response to intravenous enalaprilat in patients with severe congestive heart failure and mitral regurgitation. Clin Cardiol 1993;16:235–8.

Diagnosis of Heart Failure

Anna Marie Chang, MD[a],*, Alan S. Maisel, MD, FACC[b],
Judd E. Hollander, MD[a]

KEYWORDS

- Heart failure • BNP • Nt-pro BNP
- Diagnosis of heart failure

Heart failure is a major public health concern, with 1.5 million new cases diagnosed and more than 1 million hospital admissions yearly as a result of heart failure.[1–5] Most cases are admitted through the emergency department. Patients may complain of dyspnea, which is the subjective feeling of difficulty breathing, or an awareness of respiratory distress. The differential diagnosis of dyspnea is vast, however, and includes not only congestive heart failure (CHF) but also chronic obstructive pulmonary disease (COPD), pneumonia, asthma, acute coronary syndrome, and neuromuscular disorders (**Table 1**). It is often difficult to distinguish heart failure from other causes of acute dyspnea. Failure to diagnose heart failure increases mortality, prolongs hospital stay, and increases treatment costs.[1–5] Clinicians rely on the history and physical examination and laboratory and radiographic tests.

HISTORY AND PHYSICAL EXAMINATION

Several studies have examined the accuracy and reliability of history and physical examination findings for the diagnosis of CHF. Wang and colleagues[4,5] conducted a MEDLINE search of articles published between 1966 and 2005 and performed a meta-analysis of 18 studies that evaluated the usefulness of clinical history, physical examination, and basic tests and reported likelihood ratios for proper diagnosis of heart failure (**Table 2**). They found that a past medical history of heart failure was the most useful historical parameter. Risk factors for heart failure that also may be helpful include hypertension, diabetes,

valvular heart disease, old age, male sex, and obesity.[6–9] The symptom with the highest sensitivity for a diagnosis of heart failure was dyspnea on exertion, but orthopnea and edema are also useful symptoms to assess.[4,5] The most specific symptoms were paroxysmal nocturnal dyspnea, orthopnea, and edema,[4,5] which increased the likelihood of heart failure. In the meta-analysis by Wang et al, the overall clinical gestalt of the emergency physician was also associated with high sensitivity and specificity (LR +, 4.4);[4] however, others have found that it was accurate approximately half the time.[10]

On physical examination, the presence of a third heart sound had the highest likelihood ratio positive (11) but was not useful as a negative predictor (LR−, 0.88).[4] Jugular venous distension, rales, and lower extremity edema are other useful findings that should be ascertained.[4,5] Jugular venous distension correlates with an elevated right-sided atrial pressure, which may occur secondary to elevated left-sided filling pressure.[11–14] Butman and colleagues[15] found that the presence of jugular venous distension was specific and sensitive for an elevated pulmonary capillary wedge pressure. A third heart sound is related to rapid filling of a poorly compliant ventricle or increased filling pressure.[12] These physical examination findings are indicative of unfavorable prognosis in patients with heart failure. Drazner and colleagues[11] found that even after adjusting for other signs of severe heart failure, elevated jugular venous pressure and a third heart sound were independently associated with an increased risk of hospitalization for heart failure, death or hospitalization for heart

a University of Pennsylvania, Philadelphia, PA, USA
b San Diego VA Medical Center, San Diego, USA
* Corresponding author. Department of Emergency Medicine, Ground Floor, Ravdin Building, University of Pennsylvania, Ground Ravdin, 3400 Spruce Street, Philadelphia, PA 19104-4283.
E-mail address: changam@uphs.upenn.edu (A.M. Chang).

Heart Failure Clin 5 (2009) 25–35
doi:10.1016/j.hfc.2008.08.013
1551-7136/08/$ – see front matter © 2008 Published by Elsevier Inc.

Table 1
Differential diagnosis of dyspnea

Cardiac	Mixed Cardiac or Pulmonary
Congestive heart failure	COPD with pulmonary hypertension and cor pulmonale
Coronary artery disease	Deconditioning
Myocardial infarction	Chronic pulmonary emboli
Cardiomyopathy	Trauma
Valvular dysfunction	**Noncardiac or nonpulmonary**
Left ventricular hypertrophy	Metabolic conditions (eg, acidosis)
Asymmetric septal hypertrophy	Pain
Pericarditis	Neuromuscular disorders
Arrhythmias	Otorhinolaryngeal disorders
Pulmonary	Functional
COPD	Anxiety
Asthma	Panic disorders
Restrictive lung disorders	Hyperventilation
Hereditary lung disorders	
Pneumothorax	

failure, and death from pump failure. The interrater reliability of a third heart sound has been shown in studies to be low to moderate, however.[16–19] It is often difficult to assess a third heart sound in many patients with confounding diseases, such as COPD and obesity, or in the loud chaotic environment of the emergency department.

Studies that have addressed the correlation between physical examination findings and more invasive measures, such as pulmonary capillary wedge pressure, have produced variable results. Stevenson and Perloff[20] prospectively compared physical examination findings with hemodynamic measurements in 50 patients with known chronic heart failure and a low ejection fraction and found that rales, edema, and elevated mean jugular venous pressure were absent in almost half of patients with elevated pulmonary capillary wedge pressures. Chakko and colleagues[21] examined 52 patients with CHF and found that physical and radiographic signs of congestion were more common in patients with elevated pulmonary capillary wedge pressure, but positive findings had poor predictive power. The Evaluation Study of Congestive Heart Failure and Pulmonary Artery Catheterization Effectiveness (ESCAPE) trial demonstrated that the addition of a pulmonary artery catheter to the management of acute decompensated heart failure did not affect overall mortality and hospitalization.[22]

Chest Radiography

Chest radiographs also may be helpful in the diagnosis of heart failure in the emergency department.

Pulmonary venous congestion, cardiomegaly, and interstitial edema were the findings most associated with a final diagnosis of heart failure (**Table 3**).[4] When present, these radiographic signs are highly specific.[3] Collins and colleagues[23,24] found that up to 20% of patients subsequently diagnosed with heart failure had negative chest radiographs at the time of evaluation in the emergency department, however. In patients who have late-stage heart failure, radiographic signs of heart failure can be minimal despite elevated wedge pressures.[3]

Electrocardiograms

The electrocardiogram is more useful for examining the cause or precipitant of heart failure rather than for diagnosing. Electrocardiogam signs of ischemia, acute myocardial infarction, or arrhythmias may point to the precipitating cause of heart failure.[4] The presence of atrial fibrillation had the highest likelihood ratio positive for diagnosis of heart failure; however, new t-wave changes were also associated with the diagnosis of heart failure (**Table 3**).[4] Atrial fibrillation develops in approximately one third of patients with heart failure[25] and often indicates a worse prognosis than sinus rhythm.[26]

Scoring Systems

Multiple scoring systems have been proposed for the diagnosis of heart failure (**Table 4**) using components of the history and physical examination, including the Framingham Criteria, the Boston,

Table 2
Summary of diagnostic accuracy of findings on history and physical examination in emergency department patients presenting with dyspnea

	Pooled		Summary LR (95% CI)	
Finding	Sensitivity	Specificity	Positive	Negative
Initial clinical judgment	0.61	0.86	4.4 (1.8–10.0)	0.45 (0.28–0.73)
History				
Heart failure	0.60	0.90	5.8 (4.1–8.0)	0.45 (0.38–0.53)
Myocardial infarction	0.40	0.87	3.1 (2.0–4.9)	0.69 (0.58–0.82)
Coronary artery disease	0.52	0.70	1.8 (1.1–2.8)	0.68 (0.48–0.96)
Dyslipidemia	0.23	0.87	1.7 (0.43–6.9)	0.89 (0.69–1.1)
Diabetes mellitus	0.28	0.83	1.7 (1.0–2.7)	0.86 (0.73–1.0)
Hypertension	0.60	0.56	1.4 (1.1–1.7)	0.71 (0.55–0.93)
Smoking	0.62	0.27	0.84 (0.58–1.2)	1.4 (0.58–3.8)
COPD	0.34	0.57	0.81 (0.60–1.1)	1.1 (0.95–1.4)
Symptoms				
PND	0.41	0.84	2.6 (1.5–4.5)	0.70 (0.54–0.91)
Orthopnea	0.50	0.77	2.2 (1.2–3.9)	0.65 (0.45–0.92)
Edema	0.51	0.76	2.1 (0.92–5.0)	0.64 (0.39–1.1)
Dyspnea on exertion	0.84	0.34	1.3 (1.2–1.4)	0.48 (0.35–0.67)
Fatigue and weight gain	0.31	0.70	1.0 (0.74–1.4)	0.99 (0.85–1.3)
Cough	0.36	0.61	0.93 (0.70–1.2)	1.0 (0.87–1.3)
Physical examination				
Third heart sound	0.13	0.99	11 (4.9–25.0)	0.88 (0.83–0.94)
Abdominojugular reflux	0.24	0.96	6.4 (0.81–51.0)	0.79 (0.62–1.0)
Jugular venous distension	0.39	0.92	5.1 (3.2–7.9)	0.66 (0.57–0.77)
Rales	0.60	0.78	2.8 (1.9–4.1)	0.51 (0.37–0.70)
Any murmur	0.27	0.90	2.6 (1.7–4.1)	0.81 (0.73–0.90)
Lower extremity edema	0.50	0.78	2.3 (1.5–3.7)	0.64 (0.47–0.87)
Valsalva maneuver	0.73	0.65	2.1 (1.0–4.2)	0.41 (0.17–1.0)
SBP < 100 mm Hg	0.06	0.97	2.0 (0.60–6.6)	0.97 (0.91–1.0)
Fourth heart sound	0.05	0.97	1.6 (0.47–5.5)	0.98 (0.93–1.0)
SBP > 150 mm Hg	0.28	0.73	1.0 (0.69–1.6)	0.99 (0.84–1.2)
Wheezing	0.22	0.58	0.52 (0.38–0.71)	1.3 (1.1–1.7)
Ascites	0.01	0.97	0.33 (0.04–2.9)	1.0 (0.99–1.1)

Abbreviations: LR, likelihood ratio; CI, confidence interval; PND, parosxysmal nocturnal dyspnea; SBP, systolic blood pressure.
Data from Wang CS, Fitzgerald JM, Schulzer M, et al. Does this dyspneic patient in the emergency department have congestive heart failure? JAMA 2005;294:1944–56.

and National Health and Nutrition Examination Survey Criteria. These scoring systems have been prospectively validated, with specificities ranging from 94% to 99% and low sensitivities ranging from 35% to 63%;[3] however, they were mostly designed for the outpatient setting. Hsieh and colleagues[1] recently completed a validation of the acute heart failure index clinical prediction rule. This index identifies a group of patients with heart failure at low risk for inpatient deaths and

serious complications (< 2% risk). In their study, the acute heart failure index had 98% sensitivity and 19% specificity for the specified outcomes, safely identifying a low risk cohort. The computerized algorithm can be accessed at http://www.centerem.com/hfpr/.[1]

B-TYPE NATRIURETIC PEPTIDE

B-type natriuretic peptide (BNP) is released into the bloodstream when there is increased

Table 3
Summary of diagnostic accuracy of findings on chest radiograph and electrocardiogram in emergency department patients presenting with dyspnea

Finding	Pooled		Summary LR (95% CI)	
	Sensitivity	Specificity	Positive	Negative
Chest radiograph				
Pulmonary venous congestion	0.54	0.96	12.0 (6.8–21.0)	0.48 (0.28–0.83)
Interstitial edema	0.34	0.97	12.0 (5.2–27.0)	0.68 (0.54–0.85)
Alveolar edema	0.06	0.99	6.0 (2.2–16.0)	0.95 (0.93–0.97)
Cardiomegaly	0.74	0.78	3.3 (2.4–4.7)	0.33 (0.23–0.48)
Pleural effusion	0.26	0.92	3.2 (2.4–4.3)	0.81 (0.77–0.85)
Any edema	0.70	0.77	3.1 (0.60–16.0)	0.38 (0.11–1.3)
Pneumonia	0.04	0.92	0.50 (0.29–0.87)	1.0 (1.0–1.1)
Hyperinflation	0.03	0.92	0.38 (0.20–0.69)	1.1 (1.0–1.1)
Electrocardiogram				
Atrial fibrillation	0.26	0.93	3.8 (1.7–8.8)	0.79 (0.65–0.96)
New t-wave changes	0.24	0.92	3.0 (1.7–5.3)	0.83 (0.74–0.92)
Any abnormal finding	0.50	0.78	2.2 (1.6–3.1)	0.64 (0.47–0.88)
ST elevation	0.05	0.97	1.8 (0.80–4.0)	0.96 (0.95–1.0)
ST depression	0.11	0.94	1.7 (0.97–2.9)	0.95 (0.90–1.0)

Abbreviations: LR, likelihood ratio; CI, confidence interval.
Data from Wang CS, Fitzgerald JM, Schulzer M, et al. Does this dyspneic patient in the emergency department have congestive heart failure? JAMA 2005;294:1944–56.

myocardial pressure and stretching and physiologically results in vasodilation and natriuresis. It is released as a prohormone and subsequently cleaved into the biologically active BNP and the inactive component, NT-proBNP. The half-lives of BNP and NT-proBNP in the bloodstream are approximately 22 and 120 minutes.[27–30]

The Breathing Not Properly Multinational Study was a large multinational trial that studied more than 1500 patients and demonstrated that BNP was a useful test in patients presenting to the emergency department with undifferentiated shortness of breath.[27] It demonstrated that BNP levels alone were more accurate predictors of the presence or absence of heart failure than any historical factors, physical examination findings, or other laboratory values. BNP was more accurate than emergency physician estimates of the likelihood of heart failure. BNP levels were much higher in patients who were subsequently

Table 4
Comparison of the performance statistics of clinical questionnaires for the diagnosis of chronic heart failure

Questionnaire	Cut-Off	Number of Subjects	Sensitivity	Specificity	PPV	NPV
Boston	≥5(possible)	568	55.1 ± 3.93	96.1 ± 0.59	38.9 ± 4.39	97.9 ± 0.23
	≥8(probable)	296	35.3 ± 4.04	99.1 ± 0.17	63.5 ± 5.80	97.1 ± 0.26
Duke		469	46.1 ± 3.59	84.9 ± 5.57	12.1 ± 4.01	97.2 ± 0.33
Framingham	2 major and minor criteria	982	62.8 ± 3.86	93.7 ± 0.89	30.7 ± 3.53	98.3 ± 0.22
Gheorghiade		718	54.6 ± 4.00	95.1 ± 0.69	33.6 ± 3.88	97.9 ± 0.24
NHANES-I		551	61.7 ± 3.80	94.0 ± 0.68	31.7 ± 3.25	98.2 ± 0.22

Abbreviations: PPV, positive predictive value; NPV, negative predictive value.
Data from Fonseca C, Oliveira AG, Mota T, et al. EPIC investigators. Evaluation of the performance and concordance of clinical questionnaires for the diagnosis of heart failure in primary care. Eur J Heart Failure 2004;6:813–20.

diagnosed with heart failure than in patients diagnosed with noncardiac dyspnea (675 pg/mL versus 110 pg/mL) (**Fig. 1**). A BNP value of more than 500 pg/mL is highly suggestive of heart failure. The negative predictive value of BNP at levels less than 50 pg/mL was very high (96%).[27] Patients with systolic dysfunction also had higher levels of BNP compared with patients with diastolic dysfunction.[28]

McCullough and colleagues[29] did a subset analysis from the Breathing Not Properly Study in which physicians were asked to assess the probability of heart failure as the leading diagnosis for the patients' dyspnea. The addition of BNP levels into the clinical evaluation of HF raised the diagnostic accuracy by 10% in patients for whom the emergency department physician had a high confidence in the diagnosis of heart failure. In the one third of patients for whom the emergency department physician was uncertain of the diagnosis (20%–80% pretest probably of CHF diagnosis), the addition of BNP to clinical judgment correctly classified 74% of the patients and only misclassified 7% of the patients as not having CHF when the final diagnosis was CHF (**Fig. 2**).

The Rapid Emergency Department Heart Failure Outpatient Trial (REDHOT) showed a disconnect between physician assessment of heart failure severity and BNP levels.[31] In the first phase, 464 patients visiting emergency departments with complaints of breathing difficulty had BNP measurements taken on arrival. Physicians were blinded to BNP results; however, inclusion in the trial required a BNP of more than 100 pg/mL. Patients discharged from the emergency department had higher BNP levels than patients admitted to the hospital (976 pg/mL versus 766 pg/mL). With respect to the admitted patients, 11% had BNP levels less than 200 pg/mL, which is indicative of a non–heart failure diagnosis or less severe CHF.

Most of these patients were perceived to have class III or IV heart failure. Mortality rates for these patients were 0% at 30 days and only 2% at 90 days, suggesting that patients with low levels of BNP might have been safe for discharge. With respect to patients who were actually discharged, 78% had BNP levels more than 400 pg/mL. At 90 days, mortality was 9%. There was no mortality of patients discharged with BNP levels less than 400 pg/mL, which suggests that use of BNP in the emergency department might also help determine which well-appearing patients are at high risk for a bad outcome over the short-term (90 days). The finding also suggests that when a clinician thinks a patient is safe for discharge but the BNP is more than 400 pg/mL, the clinician may wish to reconsider the disposition decision. Almost one in ten patients with these characteristics were dead by 90 days. They concluded that BNP levels may be helpful to physicians in making triage decisions about whether to admit or discharge patients.[31]

Elevations of BNP are also useful for assessing risk stratification and prognosis in patients with heart failure. BNP levels are related to changes in limitations of physical activities and functional status. Harrison and colleagues[32] followed 325 patients for 6 months after an index visit to the emergency department for dyspnea. Higher BNP levels were associated with a progressively worse prognosis. In the ESCAPE trial, patients with BNP of more than 1500 pg/mL had greater mortality and longer length of stay than patients with BNP of less than 500 pg/mL.[33]

Mueller and colleagues[34] conducted the B-type Natriuretic Peptide for Acute Shortness of Breath Evaluation (BASEL) study. Patients were randomly assigned to receive a BNP measurement in the emergency department or not. The use of BNP levels reduced the need for hospitalization and

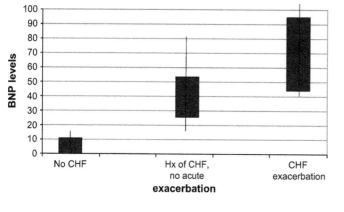

Fig. 1. Results of the Breathing Not Properly Study. Patients with a diagnosis of acute congestive heart failure had mean (± SD) B-type natriuretic peptide levels of 675 pg/mL, whereas patients without congestive heart failure had B-type natriuretic peptide levels of 110 pg/mL. The 72 patients who had baseline ventricular dysfunction without an acute exacerbation had a mean B-type natriuretic peptide level of 346 pg/mL. (*Data from* Maisel AS, Krishnaswamy P, Nowak RM, et al. Rapid measurement of B-type natriuretic peptide in the emergency diagnosis of heart failure. N Engl J Med 2002;347: 161–7.)

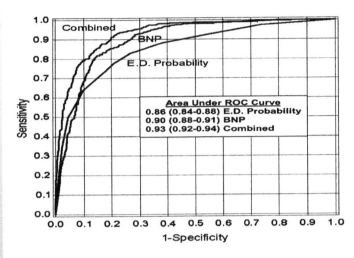

Fig. 2. In the one third of patients for whom the emergency department physician is uncertain of the diagnosis (20%–80% pretest probably of CHF diagnosis), adding BNP to clinical judgment correctly classified 74% of the patients and only misclassified 7% of the patients as not having CHF when the final diagnosis was CHF. Compared through a range of values with the use of ROC curves, the areas under the ROC curve were 0.86, 0.90, and 0.93 for clinical judgment, for BNP, and for both in combination, respectively ($P < .001$ for all). (From McCullough PA, Nowak RM, McCord J, et al. B-type natriuretic peptide and clinical judgment in emergency diagnosis of heart failure: analysis from Breathing Not Properly (BNP) Multinational Study. Circulation 2002;106:416–22; with permission.)

intensive care. The median time to discharge was 3 days shorter in patients who received BNP measurement, and there was a decreased cost of treatment by $1800 with no difference in 30-day mortality rates.[34] Moe and colleagues[35] found that the addition of NT-proBNP reduced the duration of emergency department visit, the number of patients rehospitalized, and direct medical costs over 60 days from enrollment.

This test is also useful in patients with underlying COPD/bronchospastic disorders, because an elevated level may discern between a pulmonary or cardiac cause of the patient's dyspnea. After adjustments for cardiovascular risk factors in patients who have COPD with an elevated BNP, the risk ratio of having heart failure is 4.5 that of controls without COPD, and the rate-adjusted hospital prevalence of heart failure is 3 times greater among patients discharged with a diagnosis of COPD.[36] McCullough and colleagues[37] looked at a subset of patients from the BNP trial who did not have a prior diagnosis of heart failure but did have a prior diagnosis of COPD or asthma. Of these 417 patients, 87 were diagnosed with heart failure. Physician judgment only diagnosed 37% of the patients ultimately diagnosed with heart failure. Mean BNP values were 587 and 109 pg/mL for those with and without heart failure, respectively (**Fig. 3**). At a cutpoint of 100 pg/mL, BNP had a sensitivity of 93.1% and negative predictive value of 97.7%.[37] Caution must be used, however, because BNP is produced by both ventricles and may be elevated in conditions of right ventricular strain, such as pulmonary hypertension, cor pulmonale, or pulmonary embolism.[3] In patients with pulmonary embolism, an elevated BNP above 100 pg/mL or even in the upper normal

range had higher mortality. These low-grade elevations were associated with right ventricular strain and dysfunction.[38]

The Pro-BNP Investigation of Dyspnea in the Emergency Department (PRIDE) study used a similar study design and found that a level of more than 450 pg/mL for patients younger than age 50 and more than 900 pg/mL for patients older than 50 was highly sensitive and specific for the diagnosis of CHF. An NT-proBNP level of less than 300 pg/mL had a high negative predictive value.[30]

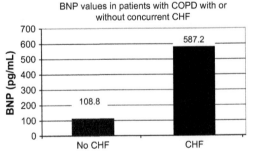

Fig. 3. A subset of patients from the Breathing Not Properly Trial who did not have a prior diagnosis of CHF with a prior diagnosis of COPD or asthma. Mean BNP values were 587 and 109 pg/mL for patients with and without CHF, respectively. At a cutpoint of 100 pg/mL, BNP had a sensitivity 93.1% and negative predictive value 97.7%. (From McCullough PA, Hollander JE, Nowak RM, et al, BNP Multinational Study Investigators. Uncovering heart failure in patients with a history of pulmonary disease: rationale for the early use of B-type natriuretic peptide in the emergency department. Acad Emerg Med 2003;10:198–204; with permission.)

The International Collaborative of NT-proBNP Study took the data from the PRIDE study and combined it with multiple international sites and confirmed that NT-proBNP was useful in the diagnostic evaluation of acute heart failure.[39]

BNP and NT-proBNP must be used in conjunction with physician judgment and other findings.[29,30] Further studies and subset analysis show that NP (natriuretic peptides; either BNP or NTproBNP) are affected by a multitude of factors. NP levels are not affected by the presence of diabetes[40,41] but are lower in overweight and obese individuals, and the test loses sensitivity in this population.[42–44] NPs have ethnic and age differences;[45,46] however, BNP is still effective in decreasing time to discharge and total cost of treatment in women and elderly patients.[46–48] NPs are at least partially renally cleared, which impacts their clinical utility. For BNP, some researchers have suggested using a higher cutoff (200 pg/mL) value for patients with a glomerular filtration rate of less than 60 mL/min.[27] Studies have shown that a reduced baseline glomerular filtration rate is associated with decreased survival in patients with systolic heart failure.[49] It is unclear whether this is caused by poor kidney perfusion secondary to low cardiac output or if it is part of the spectrum of cardiorenal syndrome.[32] BNP is useful in patients with end-stage renal disease on dialysis. It has been shown that levels can drop 20% to 40% after a dialysis session, and BNP could be used as an index of intravascular volume.[49–51]

Limited data directly comparing BNP to NTproBNP are available. Heeschen and colleagues[52] completed a head-to-head comparison of BNP to NT-proBNP for the diagnosis of heart failure. In their study, age, sex, and renal function had no impact on the diagnostic utility of both tests when compared by logistic regression models. BNP and NT-proBNP were found to be equally sensitive and specific[52,53]

PHONOCARDIOGRAPHY

Auscultatory assessment of the S3 heart sound is difficult in the emergency setting. Even when optimal, interobserver concordance is low.[16–19] Phonoelectrocardiographic devices can potentially improve detection of an S3 or S4 heart sound compared with auscultation. The Audicor system is an acoustic cardiogram that replaces the standard V3 and V4 leads with sensors and collects sound and electrical data. Sound data are collected at 10-second intervals and analyzed using a signal-processing algorithm that has been previously validated.[54,55] Peacock and colleagues[55] studied the device and found that in patients with indeterminate BNP levels (100–500 pg/mL), the presence of an S3 increased the positive likelihood ratio to 4.3 for the diagnosis of CHF. Shapiro and colleagues[54] conducted a more invasive study that compared the results of the BNP and computerized phonoelectrocardiographic system to cardiac catheterization and found that it was 88% accurate for diagnosis of left ventricular dysfunction. These studies are small, however, and more data are needed before the usefulness or clinical impact of the Audicor system can be determined.

IMPEDANCE MONITORS

Impedance cardiography is a noninvasive measurement of cardiac output, cardiac index, and thoracic fluid content.[56,57] Electrical impedance

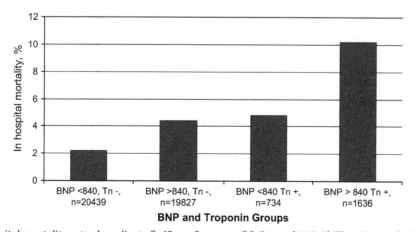

Fig. 4. In-hospital mortality rates (unadjusted). (*From* Fonarow GC, Peacock WF, Phillips CO, et al, ADHERE Scientific Advisory Committee and Investigators. Usefulness of B-type natriuretic peptide and cardiac troponin levels to predict in-hospital mortality from ADHERE. Am J Cardiol 2008;101:231–7; with permission.)

is defined as the resistance to flow of an electrical current. Bone and tissue are poor conductors, whereas blood and fluids are good conductors with lower impedance.[5] The information made available from these devices has been shown to help delineate a diagnosis in the emergency department, identify patients at increased near-term risk of recurrent decompensation, and predict rehospitalization.[56]

Impedance cardiography monitors can be used at the bedside. Impedance is determined by applying four pairs of electrodes to the chest and neck. Because electrical impedance changes proportionally to fluid flow, the machine may then calculate several hemodynamic parameters, including stroke volume, systemic vascular resistance, cardiac output, and an index of thoracic fluid. The increase in thoracic fluid that occurs during a heart failure exacerbation decreases overall average impedance and can suggest a fluid overloaded state.[5,56,57]

Implantable cardioverter/defibrillator devices also can monitor intrathoracic impedance.[58–60] Yu and colleagues[59] conducted a study using the Optivol intrathoracic impedance device (Medtronic, Inc.) in NYHA class III and IV patients and confirmed that there was an inverse correlation between intrathoracic impedance and intracardiac filling pressure. The device recorded measurements starting at 34 days postimplantation and averaged a total of 64 measurements each day between 12PM and 5PM. Impedance measurements decreased (associated with increased thoracic fluid) an average of 2 weeks before symptom onset and hospitalization, suggesting that reporting of these data may make it feasible for physicians to intervene before symptom onset.[60] The default setting for the OptiVol system had a 76.9% sensitivity for predicting hospitalization.[60] Vollman and colleagues[61] found that the device had a sensitivity and positive predictive value of 60% to detect heart failure deterioration but had a 40% false-positive rate. One study showed that the combination of weight gain and a positive BNP had a sensitivity of 55%.[61] This device may not have more diagnostic accuracy but might allow earlier detection. Larger randomized controlled trials are needed to determine their clinical use.

CARDIAC TROPONIN I

Up to 40% of patients admitted for acute decompensated heart failure present with an elevated troponin level.[62–70] Although troponin is useful in the setting of acute coronary syndrome and can help identify acute coronary syndrome as the precipitant of heart failure, it is also useful for risk stratification of patients who have heart failure in the absence of ACS. An elevated cardiac troponin I level is a predictor of 30-day and 1-year mortality, even after adjusting for confounding factors. The ESCAPE and ADHERE trials showed that a multimarker strategy (BNP and troponin) for the assessment of patients hospitalized with heart failure adds incremental prognostic information.[33,67,68] In the ADHERE trial, troponin was increased in 5.6% of 42,636 heart failure episodes. A combination of a BNP above the median (> 840 pg/mL) with increased troponin was associated with twice the in-hospital mortality (**Fig. 4**). After covariate adjustment, mortality was twice as high for patients with elevated BNP and troponin compared with patients with solely elevated BNP.[67]

SUMMARY

The approach to the diagnosis of heart failure is complex, but the diagnostic armamentarium has increased significantly in the past decade. Diagnostic markers such as BNP and NT proBNP have proven value for the diagnosis of heart failure over and above the traditional tools that only included the history, physical examination, and chest radiography. Invasive and noninvasive impedance cardiography can be used to diagnose or even predict development of heart failure, but their role in clinical practice still needs to be better defined.

REFERENCES

1. Hsieh M, Auble TE, Yealy DM. Validation of the acute heart failure index. Ann Emerg Med 2008;51:37–44.
2. Mueller C, Laule-Kilian K, Frana B, et al. Use of B-type natriuretic peptide in the management of acute dyspnea in patients with pulmonary disease. Am Heart J 2006;151:471–7.
3. Collins S, Storrow AB, Kirk JD, et al. Beyond pulmonary edema: diagnostic, risk stratification, and treatment challenges of acute heart failure management in the emergency department. Ann Emerg Med 2008;51:45–57.
4. Wang CS, Fitzgerald JM, Schulzer M, et al. Does this dyspneic patient in the emergency department have congestive heart failure? J Am Med Assoc 2005;294:1944–56.
5. Wong GC, Ayas NT. Clinical approaches to the diagnosis of acute heart failure. Curr Opin Cardiol 2007;22:207–13.
6. Tsuyuki RT, McKelvie RS, Arnold JM, et al. Acute precipitants of congestive heart failure exacerbations. Arch Intern Med 2001;161:2337–42.

7. Levy D, Larson MG, Vasan RS, et al. The progression from hypertension to congestive heart failure. J Am Med Assoc 1996;275:1557–62.

8. Chen YT, Vaccarino V, Williams CS, et al. Risk factors for heart failure in the elderly: a prospective community-based study. Am J Med 1999;106:605–12.

9. Chae CU, Pfeffer MA, Glynn RJ, et al. Increased pulse pressure and risk of heart failure in the elderly. JAMA 1999;28:634–9.

10. Remes J, Miettinen H, Reunanen A, et al. Validity of clinical diagnosis of heart failure in primary health care. Eur Heart J;199(12):315–21.

11. Drazner MH, Rame E, Stevenson LW, et al. Prognostic importance of elevated jugular venous pressure and a third heart sound in patients with heart failure. N Engl J Med 2001;345:574–81.

12. Drazner MH, Hamilton MA, Fonarow G, et al. Relationship between right and left-sided filling pressures in 1000 patients with advanced heart failure. J Heart Lung Transplant 1999;18:1126–32.

13. Collins SP, Lindsell CJ, Peacock WF, et al. The combined utility of an S3 heart sound and B-type natriuretic peptide levels in emergency department patients with dyspnea. J Card Fail 2006;12:286–92.

14. Collins SP, Lindsell CJ, Peacock WF, et al. The effect of treatment on the presence of abnormal heart sounds in emergency department patients with heart failure. Am J Emerg Med 2006;24:25–32.

15. Butman SM, Ewy GA, Standen JR, et al. Bedside cardiovascular examination in patients with severe chronic heart failure: importance of rest or inducible jugular venous distension. J Am Coll Cardiol 1993; 22:968–74.

16. Marcus GM, Vessey J, Jordan MV, et al. Relationship between accurate auscultation of a clinically useful third heart sound and level of experience. Arch Intern Med 2006;166:617–22.

17. Marcus GM, Michaels AD, De Marco TD, et al. Usefulness of the third heart sound in predicting an elevated level of B-type natriuretic peptide. Am J Cardiol 2004;93:1312–3.

18. Ishmail AA, Wing S, Ferguson J, et al. Interobserver agreement by auscultation in the presence of a third heart sound in patients with congestive heart failure. Chest 1987;91:870–3.

19. Mangione S, Neiman LZ. Cardiac auscultatory skills of internal medicine and family practice trainees: a comparison of diagnostic proficiency. JAMA 1997;278:717–22.

20. Stevenson LW, Perloff JK. The limited reliability of physical signs for estimating hemodynamics in chronic heart failure. JAMA 1989;261:884–8.

21. Chakko S, Woska D, Martinez H, et al. Clinical, radiographic, and hemodynamic correlations in chronic congestive heart failure: conflicting results may lead to inappropriate care. Am J Med 1991; 90:353–9.

22. Binanay C, Califf RM, Hasselblad V, et al. ESCAPE Investigators and ESCAPE Study Coordinators. Evaluation study of congestive heart failure and pulmonary artery catheterization effectiveness: the escape trial. J Am Med Assoc 2005;294:1625–33.

23. Collins SP, Lindsell CJ, Abraham WT, et al. The emergency department chest radiograph is unreliable in establishing a diagnosis of heart failure. J Card Fail 2004;10:S30.

24. Collins S, Lindsell CJ, Storrow AB, et al. Prevalence of negative chest radiography in the emergency department patient with decompensated heart failure. Ann Emerg Med 2006;47:13–8.

25. Middlekauff HR, Stevenson WG, Stevenson LW. Prognostic significance of a trial fibrillation in advanced heart failure: a study of 390 patients. Circulation 1991;84:40–8.

26. Mathew J, Hunsberger S, Fleg J, et al. Incidence, predictive factors, and prognostic significance of supraventricular tachyarrhythmias in congestive heart failure. Chest 2000;118:914–22.

27. Maisel AS, Krishnaswamy P, Nowak RM, et al. Breathing Not Properly Multinational Study Investigators. Rapid measurement of b-type natriuretic peptide in the emergency diagnosis of heart failure. N Engl J Med 2002;347:161–7.

28. Maisel AS, McCord J, Nowak RM, et al. Breathing Not Properly Multinational Study Investigators. Bedside b-type natriuretic peptide in the emergency diagnosis of heart failure with reduced or preserved ejection fraction: results from the Breathing Not Properly Multinational Study. J Am Coll Cardiol 2003;41:2010–7.

29. McCullough PA, Nowak RM, McCord J, et al. for the BNP Multinational Study Investigators. B-type natriuretic peptide and clinical judgment in emergency diagnosis of heart failure. Circulation 2002;106:416–22.

30. Januzzi JL Jr, Camargo CA, Anwaruddin S, et al. The N-terminal pro-BNP investigation of dyspnea in the emergency department (PRIDE) study. Am J Cardiol 2005;95:948–54.

31. Maisel AS, Hollander JE, Guss D, et al. Rapid Emergency Department Heart Failure Outpatient Trial Investigators. Primary results of the rapid emergency department heart failure outpatient trial (redhot): a multicenter study of b-type natriuretic peptide levels, emergency department decision making, and outcomes in patients presenting with shortness of breath. J Am Coll Cardiol 2004;44:1328–33.

32. Harrison A, Morrison LK, Krishnaswamy P, et al. B-type natriuretic peptide (BNP) predicts future cardiac events in patients presenting to the emergency department with dyspnea. Ann Emerg Med 2002; 39:131–8.

33. Shah MR, Hasselblad V, Tasissa G, et al. Rapid assay brain natriuretic peptide and troponin I in patients hospitalized with decompensated heart

failure. From the evaluation study of congestive heart failure and pulmonary artery catheterization effectiveness trial. Am J Cardiol 2007;100:1427–33.

34. Mueller C, Scholer A, Laule-Kilian K, et al. Use of B-type natriuretic peptide in the evaluation and management of acute dyspnea. N Engl J Med 2004;350: 647–54.

35. Moe GW, Howlett J, Januzzi JL, et al. Canadian Multicenter Improved Management of Patients with Congestive Heart Failure (improve-chf) Study Investigators. N-terminal pro-b-type natriuretic peptide testing improves the management of patients with suspected acute heart failure: primary results of the Canadian prospective randomized multicenter improve-chf study. Circulation 2007;115: 3103–10.

36. LeJemtel TH, Padeletti M, Jelic S. Diagnostic and therapeutic challenges in patients with coexistent chronic obstructive pulmonary disease and chronic heart failure. J Am Coll Cardiol 2007;49:171–80.

37. McCullough PA, Hollander JE, Nowak RM, et al. BNP Multinational Study Investigators. Uncovering heart failure in patients with a history of pulmonary disease: rationale for the early use of b-type natriuretic peptide in the emergency department. Acad Emerg Med 2003;10:198–204.

38. Wolde M, Tulevski II, Mulder JW, et al. Brain natriuretic peptide as a predictor of adverse outcome in patients with pulmonary embolism. Circulation 2003;107:2082–4.

39. Januzzi JL, Van Kimmenade R, Lainchbury J, et al. NT-proBNP testing for diagnosis and short-term prognosis in acute destabilized heart failure: an international pooled analysis of 1256 patients. The international collaborative of NT-proBNP study. Eur Heart J 2006;27:330–7.

40. Wu AH, Omland T, Duc P, et al. Breathing Not Properly Multinational Study Investigators. The effect of diabetes on B-type natriuretic peptide concentrations in patients with acute dyspnea: an analysis from the Breathing Not Properly Multinational Study. Diabetes Care 2004;27:2398–404.

41. O'Donoghue M, Kenney P, Oestreicher E, et al. Usefulness of aminoterminal pro-brain natriuretic peptide testing for the diagnostic and prognostic evaluation of dyspneic patients with diabetes mellitus seen in the emergency department (from the PRIDE Study). Am J Cardiol 2007;100:1336–40.

42. McCord J, Mundy BJ, Hudson MP, et al, for the BNP Multinational Study Investigators. The relationship between obesity and b-type natriuretic peptide levels. Arch Intern Med 2004;164:2247–52.

43. Mehra MR, Uber PA, Park MH, et al. Obesity and suppressed B-type natriuretic peptide levels in heart failure. J Am Coll Cardiol 2004;43:1590–5.

44. Krauser DG, Lloyd-Jones DM, Chae CU, et al. Effect of body mass index on natriuretic peptide levels in patients with acute congestive heart failure: a proBNP investigation of dyspnea in the emergency department (PRIDE) substudy. Am Heart J 2005;149(4):744–50.

45. Daniels LB, Bhalla V, Clopton P, et al. B-type natriuretic peptide (BNP) levels and ethnic disparities in perceived severity of heart failure: results from the rapid emergency department heart failure outpatient trial (REDHOT) multicenter study of BNP levels and emergency department decision making in patients presenting with shortness of breath. J Card Fail 2006;12:281–5.

46. Mueller C, Laule-Kilian K, Frana B, et al. The use of B-type natriuretic peptide in the management of elderly patients with acute dyspnoea. J Intern Med 2005;258:77–85.

47. Weber M, Hamm C. Role of B-type natriuretic peptide (BNP) and NT-proBNP in clinical routine. Heart 2006;92:843–9.

48. Mueller C, Laule-Kilian K, Scholer A, et al. Use of B-type natriuretic peptide for the management of women with dyspnea. Am J Cardiol 2004;94:1510–4.

49. Dries DL, Exner DV, Domanski MJ, et al. The prognostic implications of renal insufficiency in asymptomatic and symptomatic patients with left ventricular systolic dysfunction. J Am Coll Cardiol 2000;35:681–9.

50. Heywood JT, Fonarow GC, Costanzo MR, et al. ADHERE Scientific Advisory Committee and Investigators. High prevalence of renal dysfunction and its impact on outcome in 118,465 patients hospitalized with acute decompensated heart failure: a report from the adhere database. J Card Fail 2007;13: 422–30.

51. Akiba T, Tachibana K, Togashi K, et al. Plasma human brain natriuretic peptide in chronic renal failure. Clin Nephrol 1995;44(Suppl 1):S61–4.

52. Heeschen C, Hamm CW, Mitrovic V, et al. Platelet Receptor Inhibition in Ischemic Syndrome Management (PRISM) Investigators. Diagnostic accuracy of b type natriuretic peptide and amino terminal proBNP in the emergency diagnosis of heart failure. Heart 2005;91:606–12.

53. National Kidney Foundation. Clinical practice guidelines for chronic kidney disease: evaluation, classification, and stratification. Am J Kidney Dis 2002; 2(Suppl 1):S46–75.

54. Shapiro M, Moyers B, Marcus GM, et al. Diagnostic characteristics of combining phonocardiographic third heart sound and systolic time intervals for the prediction of left ventricular dysfunction. J Card Fail 2007;13:18–24.

55. Peacock WF, Harrison A, Moffa D. Clinical and economic benefits of using audicor s3 detection for diagnosis and treatment of acute decompensated heart failure. Congest Heart Fail 2006;12(Suppl 1): 32–6.

56. Packer M, Abraham WT, Mehra MR, et al. Prospective evaluation and identification of cardiac decompensation by icg test (predict) study investigators and coordinators utility of impedance cardiography for the identification of short-term risk of clinical decompensation in stable patients with chronic heart failure. J Am Coll Cardiol. 2006;47:2245–52.

57. Peacock WF, Summers RL, Vogel J, et al. Impact of impedance cardiography on diagnosis and therapy of emergent dyspnea: the ed-impact trial. Acad Emerg Med 2006;13:365–71.

58. Yamokoski LM, Haas GJ, Gans B, et al. Optivol fluid status monitoring with an implantable cardiac device: a heart failure management system. Expert Rev Med Devices 2007;4:775–80.

59. Yu CM, Wang L, Chau E, et al. Intrathoracic impedance monitoring in patients with heart failure: correlation with fluid status and feasibility of early warning preceding hospitalization. Circulation 2005;112:841–8.

60. Wang L. Fundamentals of intrathoracic impedance monitoring in heart failure. Am J Cardiol 2007;99:3G–10G.

61. Vollmann D, Nägele H, Schauerte P, et al. European IN-SYNC Sentry Observational Study Investigators. Clinical utility of intrathoracic impedance monitoring to alert patients with an implanted device of deteriorating chronic heart failure. Eur Heart J 2007;28:1835–40.

62. Kuwabara Y, Sato Y, Miyamoto T, et al. Persistently increased serum concentrations of cardiac troponin in patients with acutely decompensated heart failure are predictive of adverse outcomes. Circ J 2007;71:1047–51.

63. Heeschen C, Hamm CW, Mitrovic V, et al. Platelet Receptor Inhibition in Ischemic Syndrome Management (PRISM) Investigators. N-terminal pro-B-type natriuretic peptide levels for dynamic risk stratification of patients with acute coronary syndromes. Circulation 2004;110:3206–12.

64. You JJ, Austin PC, Alter DA, et al. Relation between cardiac troponin I and mortality in acute decompensated heart failure. Am Heart J 2007;153:462–70.

65. Sato Y, Kita T, Takatsu Y, et al. Biochemical markers of myocyte injury in heart failure. Heart 2004;90:1110–3.

66. Ishii J, Nomura M, Nakamura Y, et al. Risk stratification using a combination of cardiac troponin T and brain natriuretic peptide in patients hospitalized for worsening chronic heart failure. Am J Cardiol 2002;89:691–5.

67. Fonarow GC, Peacock WF, Phillips CO, et al. ADHERE Scientific Advisory Committee and Investigators. Usefulness of B-type natriuretic peptide and cardiac troponin levels to predict in-hospital mortality from ADHERE. Am J Cardiol 2008;101:231–7.

68. Fonarow GC, Peacock WF, Phillips CO, et al. ADHERE Scientific Advisory Committee and Investigators. Admission B-type natriuretic peptide levels and in-hospital mortality in acute decompensated heart failure. J Am Coll Cardiol 2007;49:1943–50.

69. Horwich TB, Patel J, MacLellan WR, et al. Cardiac troponin I is associated with impaired hemodynamics, progressive left ventricular dysfunction, and increased mortality rates in advanced heart failure. Circulation 2003;108:833–8.

70. Demir M, Kanadasi M, Akpinar O, et al. Cardiac troponin T as a prognostic marker in patients with heart failure: a 3-year outcome study. Angiology 2007;58:603–9.

Emergency Department Stabilization of Heart Failure

Preeti Jois-Bilowich, MD[a],*, Deborah Diercks, MD, MSc[b]

KEYWORDS

- Heart failure • Dyspnea • Nitroglycerin • Diuretics
- Ventilation • Vasodilators • Ultrafiltration • Interventions
- Nesiritide • Morphine • Emergency department
- Stabilization

Patients who have heart failure (HF) make up a clinically diverse population. They are a heterogenous group that has multiple complicating comorbities, various etiologies of HF, and differing pathophysiologic triggers resulting in acute decompensation.[1,2] Increased understanding of the diversity of HF patients has led to new insights in the emergent management of these patients. Physicians and researchers are re-evaluating the properties of intravenous diuretics, vasodilators, and inotropes commonly used to alleviate congestion and restore hemodynamic stability. In particular, the shift has been to re-examine how these therapies should be administered, which HF patients should receive them, and the consequences of these therapeutic decisions.

CLASSIFICATION OF HEART FAILURE

HF patient types have not been well described or tailored with specific treatment strategies in prospective randomized studies. The selection of existing treatments tends to be empiric due to the paucity of randomized clinical trial data. In addition, HF trials have largely focused on enrolling subjects based on prespecified ejection fraction criteria.[3] Some of the HF-specific treatments, when used without caution, may result in myocardial injury,[4] impaired renal function,[5] and increased mortality risk,[6] further complicating therapeutic decisions.

The European Society of Cardiology guidelines were the first to classify patients who have HF into distinct clinical conditions.[7] These guidelines classified patients into clinical conditions based on symptoms and hemodynamic parameters. Despite the publication of these guidelines, there are no inclusive, evidence-, or consensus-based treatment algorithms that address the individual treatment needs of each type of HF patient, particularly in the emergency department (ED) setting. Recommendations should focus on therapeutic management, emphasizing the identification and matching of HF patient types to specific treatment strategies. Management algorithms should supplement these recommendations.

Traditional methods of categorizing HF patient types use classification based on hemodynamic characteristics obtained through invasive monitoring at presentation and a clinical symptom profile that suggests HF: peripheral edema, weight gain, fatigue, dyspnea due to pulmonary congestion, and history of HF.[4,8–12] Although most EDs do not obtain hemodynamic parameters such as pulmonary capillary wedge pressure or cardiac output by way of invasive means, they do rely on an easily obtainable parameter—blood pressure.

Patients can subsequently be classified into normotensive, hypertensive, and hypotensive HF. Although the exact pathophysiology, clinical characteristics, and appropriate treatment options of each of these patient types has yet to be clarified,

[a] University of Florida, Gainesville, FL, USA
[b] University of California–Davis Medical Center, Sacramento, CA, USA
* Corresponding author. University of Florida, Department of Emergency Medicine, 1329 SW 16th Street, Room 4270, Gainesville, FL 32610.
E-mail address: preetijois@yahoo.com (P. Jois-Bilowich).

Heart Failure Clin 5 (2009) 37–42
doi:10.1016/j.hfc.2008.08.006
1551-7136/08/$ – see front matter. Published by Elsevier Inc.

recommendations for the initial treatment, based largely on observational data and expert consensus, can be suggested. Signs, symptoms, and hemodynamic characteristics of the normotensive and hypertensive groups are described in the following paragraphs.

Normotensive Heart Failure

These patients may represent nearly half of the HF population.[2] Blood pressure is normal (systolic blood pressure range of 90–140 mm Hg), and there is usually a history of progressive worsening of chronic HF. In this group, symptoms and signs develop over days, and pulmonary and systemic congestion (seen as jugular venous distension and peripheral edema) are present. Ejection fraction is usually reduced. Management is often difficult because many patients are refractory to therapy and continue to have signs of congestion despite the initial improvement in symptoms. In some patients, the clinical or radiographic signs of pulmonary congestion are not evident despite elevated left ventricular filling pressures.[2,4,7,13] These patients have acute decompensation as a result of their cardiac failure.[14]

Hypertensive Acute Heart Failure

Data from the Acute Decompensated Heart Failure National Registry demonstrates that 50% of HF patients have a systolic blood pressure greater than 140 mm Hg on presentation.[2] These patients are more likely to have diastolic dysfunction with preserved left ventricular ejection fraction, are more often women, and are older.[1,4] Symptom onset is generally acute, with severe dyspnea and signs of end-organ hypoperfusion. Acute pulmonary edema is the hallmark of hypertensive HF and is usually auscultated on examination as rales and identified on chest radiography as pulmonary edema. The clinical target is systemic blood pressure control, with a focus on early, aggressive vasodilation, more so than on diuresis. This holds particularly true when pulmonary congestion is related to fluid maldistribution, rather than an increase in total fluid volume.[4,8] These patients have a syndrome that has been referred to as "acute vascular failure," and the initial treatment in this group reflects that etiology.[14]

The novel concept of identifying and varying treatment based on systemic blood pressure addresses the diversity of the presentation of HF that is often seen in the ED. It is important to note that this classification is not entirely inclusive of all the challenges faced when evaluating patients who have HF but encompasses a large proportion of the patients seen.[12]

MECHANISM OF SYMPTOMS IN HEART FAILURE
Acute Decompensated Cardiac Heart Failure

In the euvolemic state, there is a well-defined balance between the actions of the renin-angiotensin-aldosterone (RAA) system and the natriuretic peptides that maintains fluid status. This perfect homeostasis, however, is lost in disease states such as HF, in which the mechanisms of sodium and water retention far outweigh natriuretic effects. In HF states, excess sodium and fluid retention occurs mainly within the extracellular fluid volume space. This retention results in an equal increase of fluid volume in each of the interstitial and plasma spaces. Despite this rise in total body volume and, therefore, plasma volume (PV), the arterial filling pressure remains low, which in turn continues to stimulate retention of sodium and water.[15]

Patients who have acute decompensated HF have decreased cardiac reserve, and the acute process occurs as progression of this state. Worsening cardiac contractility can be a result of ischemia, arrhythmias, inflammatory activation, or progressive deterioration in myocardial dysfunction due to the underlining mechanism causing the HF process. Subjects who have poor cardiac contractility may also develop decompensation as a result of medication noncompliance and may therefore not have further contractility impairment. The results of this event are worsening forward perfusion, increased left ventricular pressure, and alterations in the neurohormonal states that maintain fluid balance.[14] Increased left ventricular filling pressures influence changes in neurohormonal activation, activation of gene expression programs, and induction of myocte apoptosis in HF patients. Through indirect activation of the RAA, adrenergic, and cytokine systems and by way of a direct effect on myocardial stretch, fluid accumulation fosters left ventricular remodeling. Increased intraventricular pressure can cause coronary hypoperfusion, leading to subendocardial ischemia and, thus, worsening cardiac function.[16]

One study looked at PV in acute HF patients compared with normal subjects. The patients who had acute HF had visible evidence of volume overload, such as peripheral edema, jugular venous distention, and ascites; they also had PV measurements that were 34% higher compared with healthy subjects.[17]

Feigenbaum and colleagues[18] looked at PV in HF patients undergoing treatment and found a 23% PV contraction in patients treated with diuretics. They concluded that standard drug therapy may lead to a contracted PV in chronic HF patients, highlighting an important segment of the HF population in whom PV is contracted even though the overall extracellular fluid volume is elevated. In these patients, therapy other than diuresis alone may be more beneficial.

There are multiple mechanisms responsible for the pathogenesis of HF; however, fluid accumulation is the most common reason for hospitalization of patients who have HF. Dyspnea, rales, and peripheral edema are the most common signs and symptoms found in HF cases. In these patients, there is often an associated gradual increase in body weight and peripheral edema; however, body weight is a fairly insensitive measure of fluid accumulation. Current research focuses on methodologies aimed at earlier outpatient detection of fluid accumulation.[16]

Acute Vascular Failure

Acute vascular failure is usually a result of increased vascular resistance in the setting of reduced cardiac contractility and occurs in the settings of abnormal and normal ejection fraction, although more commonly in the latter. The increased vascular mismatch can result in elevated blood pressure that results in an increase in afterload and diastolic left ventricular failure. In this situation, the rapid change in vascular status results in dyspnea through fluid redistribution into the pulmonary circulation due to increased pulmonary venous pressure. It is important to note that dyspnea in these patients is due to overwhelming the absorptive capacity of the alveolar cells during this redistribution; it is not a result of an overall increase in extracellular fluid volume.[12,14]

EMERGENCY DEPARTMENT MANAGEMENT OF HEART FAILURE: INITIAL INTERVENTIONS
Oxygen Therapy

Most patients who present with HF require some form of oxygen supplementation. Nasal cannula delivery for mild dyspnea and a nonrebreather facemask for moderate dyspnea are usually sufficient modalities of oxygen delivery. In patients who have severe dyspnea, particularly those who have acute pulmonary edema, ventilatory support may be required.

Ventilatory Support

Noninvasive ventilation—continuous positive airway pressure (CPAP) or bilevel positive airway pressure (BiPAP)—has been shown to be effective in reducing the need for intubation, decreasing mortality, and reducing hospital length of stay.[19] Its use should be considered in all patients who

have intact mental status and show early signs of respiratory embarrassment or fatigue. It is imperative to realize that noninvasive ventilation is not an alternative to mechanical ventilation in patients who have respiratory failure. Therefore, it should not be used as a modality to "buy time" in anticipation of endotracheal intubation.

Although both CPAP and BiPAP appear beneficial, there has been no demonstrated superiority of one method. Both act to decrease preload and cardiac filling pressures; however, BiPAP produces a more rapid decrease in blood pressure, whereas CPAP results in a greater initial reduction in mean pulmonary capillary wedge pressure.[20,21] Prior studies have demonstrated more rapid resolution of dyspnea and superior improvement in Po_2 and Pco_2 values with BiPAP.[22,23]

When comparing clinical outcomes, the evidence is confusing and often contradictory. One prospective comparison trial suggested a higher rate of myocardial infarction with the use of BiPAP, but this has not been found in subsequent investigations.[21–23] A recent meta-analysis found a significant mortality reduction for patients treated with CPAP but not with BiPAP, with no overall difference in effect on subsequent intubation rate.[24] In contrast, the 3CPO trial (a randomized controlled trial of continuous positive airway pressure versus noninvasive ventilation versus standard therapy for acute cardiogenic pulmonary edema) demonstrated no significant outcome differences between BiPAP and CPAP and claimed no mortality benefit to noninvasive ventilation in general.[25] This conclusion was supported in another multicenter comparison study conducted in France that showed Boussignac CPAP and BiPAP to be effective in improving respiratory distress even in hypercapnic patients, but with no differences in patient outcomes.[26]

More than one third of acute HF patients who have acute pulmonary edema require mechanical ventilation.[27–29] Tachypnea, diaphoresis, fatigue, and confusion are the ominous signs of impending respiratory failure. In some patients, however, findings may be more subtle, calling on enhanced clinical suspicion from the treating physician. Objective measures can be used to determine the need for mechanical ventilation, including persistent hypoxia ($Sao_2 < 90$) despite supplemental oxygen, hypercarbia ($Paco_2 > 55$ mm Hg), and acidosis (pH < 7.25).[30]

THERAPEUTIC INTERVENTIONS

The initial management of acute HF is focused on improving symptoms and the hemodynamic profile of the patient. Treatment end points vary among clinical trials and often include an assessment of dyspnea in combination with a hemodynamic parameter such as a change in pulmonary artery wedge pressure.[31] Despite clinical trials and clinicians using these parameters as treatment end points, a large number of patients are still symptomatic when discharged from the hospital.[8] Currently, the treatment options in the ED include diuretics and vasodilators.[7,13] Although these agents are commonly used, clinical trial data supporting their use in the ED setting are lacking. Clinical trials largely done in the inpatient setting, however, have shown that these therapies improve hemodynamic function, decrease dyspnea, and diminish signs and symptoms of venous congestion.[32–36] It is important to note that no pharmacologic agent has been shown to reduce mortality when implemented in the ED for treatment of patients who have acute HF. Realizing the limitation of extrapolating the results of clinical trials largely done in the inpatient setting after hours of treatment, guidelines are available that provide some recommendations for pharmacologic treatment in the ED setting.[7,13,37]

Pharmacologic management is discussed elsewhere in this issue; however, a brief discussion of vaptans and ultrafiltration is presented here.

Ultrafiltration

Ultrafiltration allows removal of isotonic fluid and, in contrast to diuretic therapy, does not lead to neurohormonal activation.[38] It has been associated with improved weight loss and decreased incidence of rehospitalization compared with diuretic use.[39] A recent trial of patients who have acute HF with low ejection fraction and signs of congestion randomized to receive ultrafiltration or intravenous diuretics showed no difference in renal hemodynamics between the two groups. In this small trial by Rogers and colleagues[40] in which 19 patients were randomized, the change in glomerular filtration rate was not different between two groups. At 48 hours, however, there was no significant difference in fluid removal. The investigators concluded that ultrafiltration was as effective as standard of care, without an adverse impact on renal hemodynamics.

Vaptans

States of fluid imbalance or retention are often associated with elevation in plasma levels of arginine vasopressin. This neuropeptide is secreted by the hypothalamus and is instrumental in regulation of serum osmolality and circulatory homeostasis. There are three receptors mediating the actions

of arginine vasopressin: V1a, V1b, and V2. V1a receptors are primarily located in vascular smooth muscle cells and respond to vasopressin by vasoconstricting.[41] V1b regulates adrenocorticotropin hormone release. V2 receptor subtypes are found in the renal collecting duct and regulate free water excretion.[42]

Owing to the roles of V1a and V2 receptors in the pathogenesis of HF, recent studies have shown promise using vasopressin antagonism to treat euvolemic hyponatremia. Selective antagonists include relcovaptan (V1a), tolvaptan (V2), and lixivaptan (V2). The nonselective agonist conivaptan (V1a/V2) is the first vaptan approved by the Food and Drug Administration for the treatment of euvolemic hyponatremia.[43,44] Large-scale clinical trials are currently ongoing to evaluate the benefit of vaptan use in patients who have HF.

DIAGNOSIS OF HEART FAILURE: THE IMPORTANCE OF GETTING IT RIGHT

A discussed throughout this article, the signs and symptoms of HF are varied and therefore nonspecific, complicating accurate diagnosis. Several studies have shown the ED misdiagnosis rate of HF to be 10% to 20%.[45,46] ED misdiagnosis amounts to delay in treatment and gaps in appropriate disposition of the patient. In addition, misdiagnosed HF patients accrue roughly $2500 more in-hospital charges than patients who are correctly diagnosed, which is particularly alarming given that the total yearly estimated cost due to HF hospitalization in the United States is $30 billion.[45] For economic and patient outcome reasons, it is clearly important to make an accurate diagnosis of HF and to start early treatment in the ED.

REFERENCES

1. Cleland JG, Swedberg K, Follath F, et al. The Euro-Heart Failure survey programme—a survey on the quality of care among patients with heart failure in Europe. Part 1: patient characteristics and diagnosis. Eur Heart J 2003;24:442–63.
2. Adams KF Jr, Fonarow GC, Emerman CL, et al. Characteristics and outcomes of patients hospitalized for heart failure in the United States: rationale, design, and preliminary observations from the first 100,000 cases in the Acute Decompensated Heart Failure National Registry (ADHERE). Am Heart J 2005;149:209–16.
3. Gheorghiade M, Mebazaa A. The challenge of acute heart failure syndromes. Am J Cardiol 2005; 96(Suppl 6A):86G–9G.
4. Gheorghiade M, De Luca L, Fonarow GC, et al. Pathophysiologic targets in the early phase of acute

heart failure syndromes. Am J Cardiol 2005; 96(Suppl 6A):11G–7G.

5. Sackner-Bernstein JD, Skopicki HA, Aaronson KD. Risk of worsening renal function with nesiritide in patients with acutely decompensated heart failure. Circulation 2005;111:1487–91.

6. Sackner-Bernstein JD, Kowalski M, Fox M, et al. Short-term risk of death after treatment with nesiritide for decompensated heart failure: a pooled analysis of randomized controlled trials. JAMA 2005; 293:1900–5.

7. Nieminen MS, Bohm M, Cowie MR, et al. Executive summary of the guidelines on the diagnosis and treatment of acute heart failure: the Task Force on Acute Heart Failure of the European Society of Cardiology. Eur Heart J 2005;26:384–416.

8. Gheorghiade M, Zannad F, Sopko G, et al. Acute heart failure syndromes: current state and framework for future research. Circulation 2005;112:3958–68.

9. Cotter G, Moshkovitz Y, Milovanov O, et al. Acute heart failure: a novel approach to its pathogenesis and treatment. Eur J Heart Fail 2002;4:227–34.

10. Kirk JD, Costanza MR. Managing patients with acute decompensated heart failure. Clinical Courier 2006; 23(56):1–14.

11. Gheorghiade M, Abraham W, Albert N, et al. for the OPTIMIZE- HF [Organized Program to Initiate Lifesaving Treatment in Hospitalized Patients with Heart Failure] Investigators and Coordinators. Systolic blood pressure at admission, clinical characteristics, and outcomes in patients hospitalized with acute heart failure. JAMA 2006;296:2217–26.

12. Filippatos G, Zannad F. An introduction to acute heart failure syndromes: definition and classification. Heart Fail Rev 2007;12:87–90.

13. Adams KF, Lindenfeld J, Arnold JMO, et al. for the Heart Failure Society of America. HFSA 2006 comprehensive heart failure practice guideline. J Card Fail 2006;12:e1–122.

14. Cotter G, Felker GM, Adams K, et al. The pathophysiology of acute heart failure—is it all about fluid accumulation? Am Heart J 2008;155(1):9–18.

15. Kalra P, Anagnostopoulos C, Bolger A, et al. The regulation and measurement of plasma volume in heart failure. J Am Coll Cardiol 2002;39(12):1901–8.

16. Metra M, Dei Cas L, Bristow M. The pathophysiology of heart failure: it is a lot about fluid accumulation. Am Heart J 2008;155(1):1–5.

17. Anand I, Ferrari R, Kalra G, et al. Edema of cardiac origin. Studies of body water and sodium, renal function, hemodynamic indexes, and plasma hormones in untreated congestive cardiac failure. Circulation 1989;80:299–305.

18. Feigenbaum M, Welsch M, Mitchell M, et al. Contracted plasma and blood volume in chronic heart failure. J Am Coll Cardiol 2000;35:51–5.

19. Collins SP, Mielniczuk LM, Whittingham HA, et al. The use of noninvasive ventilation in emergency department patients with acute cardiogenic pulmonary edema: a systematic review. Ann Emerg Med 2006;48(3):260–9, 9 e1–9 e4.

20. Philip-Joet FF, Paganelli FF, Dutau HL, et al. Hemodynamic effects of bilevel nasal positive airway pressure ventilation in patients with heart failure. Respiration 1999;66(2):136–43.

21. Levitt MA. A prospective, randomized trial of BiPAP in severe acute congestive heart failure. J Emerg Med 2001;21(4):363–9.

22. Mehta S, Jay GD, Woolard RH, et al. Randomized, prospective trial of bilevel versus continuous positive airway pressure in acute pulmonary edema. Crit Care Med 1997;25(4):620–8.

23. Nava S, Carbone G, DiBattista N, et al. Noninvasive ventilation in cardiogenic pulmonary edema: a multicenter randomized trial. Am J Respir Crit Care Med 2003;168(12):1432–7.

24. Masip J, Roque M, Sanchez B, et al. Noninvasive ventilation in acute cardiogenic pulmonary edema: systematic review and meta-analysis. JAMA 2005; 294(24):3124–30.

25. Cleland JG, Abdellah AT, Khaleva O, et al. Clinical trials update from the European Society of Cardiology Congress 2007: 3CPO, ALOFT, PROSPECT and statins for heart failure. Eur J Heart Fail 2007; 9(10):1070–3.

26. Moritz F, Brousse B, Gellee B, et al. Continuous positive airway pressure versus bilevel noninvasive ventilation in acute cardiogenic pulmonary edema: a randomized multicenter trial. Ann Emerg Med 2007;50(6):666–75.

27. Sacchetti A, Ramoska E, Moakes ME, et al. Effect of ED management on ICU use in acute pulmonary edema. Am J Emerg Med 1999;17(6):571–4.

28. Pang D, Keenan SP, Cook DJ, et al. The effect of positive pressure airway support on mortality and the need for intubation in cardiogenic pulmonary edema: a systematic review. Chest 1998;114(4): 1185–92.

29. Yan AT, Bradley TD, Liu PP. The role of continuous positive airway pressure in the treatment of congestive heart failure. Chest 2001;120(5):1675–85.

30. Masip J, Paez J, Merino M, et al. Risk factors for intubation as a guide for noninvasive ventilation in patients with severe acute cardiogenic pulmonary edema. Intensive Care Med 2003;29(11):1921–8.

31. Teerlink JR. Dyspnea as an end point in clinical trials of therapies for acute decompensated heart failure. Am Heart J 2003;145(2):S26–33.

32. Bayram M, De Luca L, Massie MB, et al. Reassessment of dobutamine, dopamine, and milrinone in the management of acute heart failure syndromes. Am J Cardiol 2005;96(Suppl):47G–58G.

33. Brater DC. Diuretic therapy. N Engl J Med 1998;339: 387–95.

34. Stough WG, O'Connor CM, Gheorghiade M. Overview of current noninodilator therapies for acute heart failure syndromes. Am J Cardiol 2005;96(Suppl):41G–6G.

35. Moazemi K, Chana JS, Willard AM, et al. Intravenous vasodilator therapy in congestive heart failure. Drugs Aging 2003;20:485–508.

36. Elkayam U, Bitar F, Akhter MW, et al. Intravenous nitroglycerin in the treatment of decompensated heart failure: potential benefits and limitations. J Cardiovasc Pharmacol Ther 2004;9:227–41.

37. Silvers SM, Howell JM, Kosowsky JM, et al. Clinical policy: critical issues in the evaluation and management of adult patients presenting to the emergency department with acute heart failure syndromes. Ann Emerg Med 2007;49(5):627–69.

38. Marenzi G, Gazi S, Giraldi F, et al. Interrelation of humoral factors, hemodynamics, and fluid and salt metabolism in congestive heart failure: effects of extracorporeal ultrafiltration. Am J Med 1993;94:49–56.

39. Costanzo MR, Guglin ME, Saltzberg MT, et al. Ultrafiltration versus intravenous diuretics for patients hospitalized for acute decompensated heart failure. J Am Coll Cardiol 2007;49:675–83.

40. Rogers H, Marshall J, Bock J, et al. A randomized, controlled trial of the renal effects of ultrafiltration as compared to furosemide in patients with acute decompensated heart failure. J Card Fail 2008; 4(1):1–5.

41. Lee C, Watkins M, Patterson J, et al. Vasopressin: a new target for the treatment of heart failure. Am Heart J 2003;146:9–18.

42. Sanghi P, Uretsky B, Schwarz E. Vasopressin antagonism: a future treatment option in heart failure. Eur Heart J 2005;26:538–43.

43. Lemmens-Gruber R, Kamyar M. Vasopressin antagonists. Cell Mol Life Sci 2006;63(15): 1766–79.

44. Ali F, Raufi M, Washington B, et al. Conivaptan: a dual receptor vasopressin v1a/v2 antagonist. Cardiovasc Drug Rev 2007;25(3):261–79.

45. Dao Q, Krishnaswamy P, Kazanegra R, et al. Utility of B-type natriuretic peptide in the diagnosis of congestive heart failure in an urgent-care setting. J Am Coll Cardiol 2001;37:379–85.

46. Collins S, Lindsell CJ, Storrow AB, et al. Prevalence of negative chest radiography in the emergency department patient with decompensated heart failure. Ann Emerg Med 2006;47:13–8.

Pharmacologic Stabilization and Management of Acute Heart Failure Syndromes in the Emergency Department

J. Douglas Kirk, MD[a],*, John T. Parissis, MD[b],
Gerasimos Filippatos, MD[b]

KEYWORDS
- Heart failure • Emergency department
- Therapeutic options

Acute heart failure (AHF) can be defined as a gradual or rapid change in heart failure signs and symptoms resulting in the need for urgent therapy.[1] Although AHF is a common admission diagnosis associated with high readmission and mortality rates,[2,3] its treatment remains largely empiric and evidence-based clinical practice guidelines that specifically address the management of these patients are lacking.[4,5] The primary short-term therapeutic targets are to stabilize hemodynamics, to alleviate congestion, and to improve symptoms; however, none of the agents used in AHF management have been shown to improve postdischarge clinical outcomes.[6] This finding may be related to the incomplete understanding of the pathophysiology of AHF, which has traditionally been considered a disease of low cardiac output attributable to systolic dysfunction with subsequent fluid overload.[3] Consequently, diuretics and vasodilators became standard of care in the management of acute pulmonary edema, much as inotropes became standard of care in the treatment of hypoperfusion/cardiogenic shock. This pathophysiologic model has been called into question by emerging registry data,[2,3] which suggest that AHF is not represented by a homogeneous group of patients but rather multiple types of patients who have heart failure with various forms of acute decompensation. In addition, the limited AHF treatment success may be associated with the timing and modality of drug administration and patient and endpoint selection.[1] Moreover, some of the drugs may cause myocardial injury,[7] impair renal function,[8] and increase mortality.[9] Despite this lack of evidence-based care and associated poor prognosis, only recently have guidelines[4,5] begun to address management of these patients.

Systolic blood pressure (SBP) at presentation is increasingly shown to be a major prognostic factor in AHF.[10,11] Consequently, it has been recently suggested that patients who have AHF should be classified on the basis of their SBP at presentation into three groups: (1) hypertensive AHF, (2) normotensive AHF, and (3) hypotensive AHF.[7,11–13] This novel classification scheme may facilitate early

[a] University of California Davis, School of Medicine, Sacramento, CA, USA
[b] Attikon University Hospital, Athens, Greece
* Corresponding author. Department of Emergency Medicine, University of California Davis, School of Medicine, Sacramento, CA 95817.
E-mail address: jdkirk@ucdavis.edu (J.D. Kirk).

Heart Failure Clin 5 (2009) 43–54
doi:10.1016/j.hfc.2008.08.003
1551-7136/08/$ – see front matter

risk stratification of patients who have AHF and promote a more targeted treatment strategy.

The suggested use of diuretics, vasodilators, and inotropes provided herein is predicated on this approach.

THERAPEUTIC OPTIONS

The following is an overview of the pharmacologic agents whose use in an emergency department (ED) or observation unit would be appropriate. These recommendations are for the acute and poststabilization care of patients who would be managed in an observation unit or during a prolonged ED stay. They are provided in the context of the aforementioned patient types, with the intent of matching the pathophysiology to the most appropriately tailored therapy. Dosing guidelines, indications, and contraindications for the most commonly used agents are provided in **Table 1**. The recommendations are based largely on observational data and expert consensus, with an emphasis on patient safety and an attempt to minimize the deleterious effects of certain therapies.

Diuretics

Loop diuretics are a central component of AHF management because of their efficacy in inducing diuresis and rapidly reducing systemic volume overload and relieving symptoms. Despite their clinical efficacy, however, these drugs are not devoid of risk. Evidence is emerging to suggest the potential toxicities of these agents, including renal dysfunction, electrolyte abnormalities, orthostatic hypotension, and maladaptive neurohormonal activation, particularly when administered in high doses.[14–17] Unfortunately, there is a paucity of large-scale randomized controlled clinical trials evaluating loop diuretics in the management of AHF. As a result, their use remains largely empiric, without clear recommendations regarding dosing regimens, administration methods, and duration of treatment. Regardless, they remain a central component to AHF management because there are few alternatives and their use is endorsed by current guidelines.[4,5]

A few studies have assessed the potential deleterious effects of high-dose loop diuretics. Cotter and colleagues[18] showed that combined low-dose intravenous dopamine and oral furosemide have similar efficacy in improving symptoms and urine output but cause less renal impairment and hypokalemia than higher doses of intravenous furosemide. Another study by Cotter and coworkers demonstrated that high-dose isosorbide dinitrate plus low-dose furosemide is more effective than high-dose furosemide with low-dose isosorbide nitrate in need for mechanical ventilation and frequency of myocardial infarction in patients who have pulmonary edema.[19] Continuous infusion of furosemide may be superior to intermittent bolus administration in patients who have advanced chronic heart failure.[20,21]

Clinical use of diuretics

Loop diuretic therapy is more beneficial in patients who have volume overload and systemic congestion. These patients usually have normal SBP, gradual worsening of symptoms and signs, and reduced left ventricular ejection fraction. Their management is problematic because many patients continue to have systemic congestion despite the initial symptomatic response.[2,4,5,7] Aggressive diuresis with an aim of improving symptoms and achieving euvolemia seems to be helpful in this clinical setting.

Treatment of these patients is depicted in **Fig. 1**. The lowest intravenous (IV) dose that achieves the desired level of diuretic effect should be administered. Empirically, patients on chronic diuretic therapy may receive a starting dose equivalent to the daily outpatient oral dose. A starting dose of 20 mg of furosemide may be administered intravenously to patients who have never been treated with loop diuretics. High initial doses of loop diuretics should be avoided because they may induce renal dysfunction and decrease a patient's ability to tolerate life-saving therapies, such as angiotensin-converting enzyme inhibitors (ACE-I). The patient's blood pressure should be regularly re-evaluated and response to diuretics should be assessed by monitoring urine output and fluid balance. Renal function and electrolytes should be closely monitored. Admission to an observation unit may be reasonable for patients who respond appropriately with ample diuresis and clinical improvement. In patients who have a poor response or those who develop renal insufficiency or hypotension, however, hospitalization is warranted. Once stabilized, patients can be transitioned to oral diuretic therapy, starting with the lowest effective dose. Some patients who have refractory signs of volume overload may require doses equivalent or similar to the daily IV requirement.

Vasodilators

Vasodilator therapy is widely used in the treatment of patients who have AHF with symptoms and signs of congestion and normal or elevated blood pressure. This class of agents includes a diverse group of drugs (eg, nitrates, nesiritide, nitroprusside) that produce multiple, similar hemodynamic changes in the failing circulatory system.

Nitroglycerin

Nitroglycerin is a potent venodilator and a mild arterial vasodilator at higher doses.[22] It mimics the effects of nitric oxide by stimulating guanylate cyclase and leading to smooth muscle relaxation in the vascular wall. It reduces left ventricular filling pressures, pulmonary congestion, wall stress, and myocardial oxygen consumption without compromising cardiac output.[23] At higher doses it may improve ischemia by inducing coronary artery dilation and increasing collateral blood flow. In addition to the IV form, it is also available in sublingual and topical preparations. The latter are frequently used in the ED but no clinical trial data exist describing their usefulness. The most common side effects are headache and hypotension. In addition, the potential benefit of nitroglycerin seems to be attenuated by a decreased vasodilatory response in patients who have heart failure, which is associated with neurohumoral activation and the early development of nitrate tolerance.[23,24] Consequently, careful titration and monitoring of nitroglycerin administration is imperative.

There is a paucity of controlled data concerning the use of nitrates in AHF. The dose-dependent improvement in hemodynamic function has been established by several small-scale studies,[23,25,26] whereas others have demonstrated the efficacy of high-dose IV nitroglycerin or isosorbide dinitrate in the management of AHF, with a low incidence of side effects.[19,27,28]

Recently a randomized placebo-controlled study showed a nonsignificant pulmonary capillary wedge pressure (PCWP) reduction with intravenous nitroglycerin.[29] Other improvements in hemodynamics, dyspnea, and global assessment were evident with nitroglycerin, although most did not reach statistical significance versus control.

Nesiritide

Nesiritide is a recombinant form of human brain natriuretic peptide with a balanced arterial, venous, and coronary vasodilatory effect and a modest natriuretic effect.[30] It has beneficial effects on hemodynamics (reduction in PCWP and increase in cardiac output) and symptoms.[31,32] The Vasodilation in the Acute Management of Congestive heart failure (VMAC) trial showed that compared with nitroglycerin, nesiritide produces a faster, greater, and more sustained reduction in PCWP with no significant difference in dyspnea, global clinical status, 30-day rehospitalization, and 6-month mortality rate[29] Hypotension is the most common side effect. Recently, concerns have emerged from two meta-analyses about the effect

of nesiritide on renal dysfunction and survival.[8,9] The results from meta-analyses should be cautiously interpreted, however, because nesiritide studies were not powered or designed to evaluate mortality or renal dysfunction.

Nitroprusside

Sodium nitroprusside is an arterial vasodilator that is mainly used in patients who have markedly increased afterload attributable to severe hypertension.[5] No randomized controlled mortality trials with nitroprusside in AHF have been conducted. It reduces systemic vascular resistance, increases stroke volume, and improves symptoms in AHF.[33,34] Trials evaluating patients who have myocardial infarction suggest an increased risk from nitroprusside use in patients who have associated AHF.[35] This increased risk is probably because high doses of the agent cause reflex tachycardia and may lead to "coronary steal," which may exacerbate myocardial ischemia; therefore, it is generally contraindicated in patients who have acute coronary syndrome and AHF.[5] Thiocyanate and cyanide levels increase in patients who have renal dysfunction and nitroprusside should be avoided in this population.

Clinical use of vasodilators

Vasodilator therapy is recommended as first-line therapy in patients who have AHF associated with an elevated SBP at presentation. These patients represent more than 50% of patients who have AHF in the ED.[2] Most are elderly women who have relatively preserved ejection fraction and they frequently have a SBP greater than 160 mm Hg.[2,3,7] Symptoms develop abruptly and severe dyspnea is the cardinal manifestation. Redistribution of fluids from systemic to pulmonary circulation leads to pulmonary rather than systemic congestion that is evident on examination and chest radiography. Accordingly, the clinical target is blood pressure control and response to therapy is relatively rapid in patients who are treated with early, aggressive vasodilation, more so than diuresis.[1,5,7]

Treatment of these patients is depicted in **Fig. 2**. Rapid sublingual administration of nitroglycerin spray or tablet either in the prehospital setting or in the ED dramatically improves the clinical status within minutes.[36] Intravenous vasodilator therapy (nitroglycerin or nesiritide) should then be started. The initial recommended dose of IV nitroglycerin is 10 to 20 µg/min, increased in increments of 5 to 10 µg/min every 3 to 5 minutes as needed. Nesiritide is given IV as a 2 µg/kg bolus followed by a 0.01 µg/kg/min infusion. Slow titration of IV vasodilators and frequent blood pressure measurement

Table 1
Pharmacologic options in the management of acute heart failure

Class	Drug	Dosage	Indications	Contraindications
Diuretics	Furosemide	Initial dosage 20–40 mg IV/po; may repeat every 6–8 h until desired effect Continuous infusion at 5–10 mg/h an alternative	Mild and moderate to severe fluid overload	Anuria Severe electrolyte depletion Hepatic coma
	Bumetanide	0.5–2 mg po 1–2 times daily 0.5–1 mg IV/IM Titrate until desired effect; do not exceed 10 mg/d		
	Torsemide	10–20 mg/d IV/po Titrate by doubling the dose until desired effect; do not exceed 200 mg/d		
Vasoactives	Nitroglycerin	Initial dosage 10–20 μg/kg/min IV infusion Titrate by 10 μg/kg/min increments until desired effect	AHF with symptoms of pulmonary congestion and adequate SBP	Hypotension Severe anemia Closed-angle glaucoma
	Sodium nitroprusside	Begin infusion at 0.3–0.5 μg/kg/min IV Titrate by 0.5 μg/kg/min increments to desired effect; average dose is 1–6 μg/kg/min Infusion rates of >10 μg/kg/min may cause cyanide toxicity	AHF associated with marked hypertension and increased afterload	Subaortic stenosis Decreased cerebral perfusion Arteriovenous shunt or coarctation of aorta (eg, compensatory hypertension)
	Nesiritide	2 μg/kg/IV bolus followed by IV infusion of 0.01 μg/kg/min	AHF with symptoms of pulmonary congestion and adequate SBP	Cardiogenic shock Hypotension
	Isosorbide dinitrate	Begin with 1 mg/h; Maximum dose 10 mg/h	AHF with symptoms of pulmonary congestion and adequate SBP	Hypotension
	Morphine	2–5 mg IV every 30–60 minutes	Anxiety due to dyspnea	Altered mental status Ventilatory depression Hypotension
	ACE inhibitors	Sublingual captopril 12.5–2.5 mg Enalaprilat 1 mg over 2 h	Limited data AHF with symptoms of pulmonary congestion and adequate SBP	Hypotension Renal impairment Angioedema

Inotropes	Dobutamine	0.5 µg/kg/min IV infusion Titrate to maintain adequate systolic BP and cardiac output	Low cardiac output Cardiogenic shock Milrinone preferred for patients already taking β-blocker	Idiopathic hypertrophic subaortic stenosis Atrial fibrillation or flutter Pheochromocytoma Ventricular fibrillation
	Dopamine	5 µg/kg/min IV infusion Titrate to maintain adequate systolic BP and cardiac output Do not exceed 20 µg/kg/min		
	Milrinone	50 µg/kg/min IV loading dose over 10 minutes; then 0.25–1.0 µg/kg/min infusion Titrate to maintain adequate systolic BP and cardiac output		Obstructive hypertrophic cardiomyopathy
	Levosimendan	0.05–0.2 µg/kg/min continuous IV infusion for 24 h without a loading dose	Acutely decompensated chronic heart failure especially on β-blocker and systolic BP>100 mm Hg	Severe hypotension Hepatic impairment Left ventricular outflow obstruction

Abbreviation: AHF, acute heart failure; BP, blood pressure; IM, intramuscular; IV, intravenous; SBP, systolic blood pressure.
Data from Kirk JD, Costanza MR. Managing patients with acute decompensated heart failure. Clin Courier 2006;23(56):1–14.

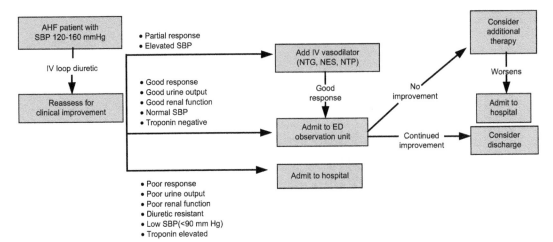

Fig. 1. Treatment algorithm for the patient who has AHF with normal systolic blood pressure at presentation. AHF, acute heart failure; ED, emergency department; IV, intravenous; NES, nesiritide; NTG, nitroglycerin; SBP, systolic blood pressure.

are recommended to avoid large decreases in blood pressure. Addition of an IV loop diuretic at the lowest possible effective dose may be reasonable if pulmonary congestion persists despite adequate blood pressure control or in the case of systemic volume overload. If the patient fails to respond, admission to the ICU is recommended. If the patient responds to initial therapy, admission to a monitored bed or observation unit is appropriate.

Vasodilators also have a role in the management of patients who have a more normal blood pressure at presentation, particularly those who are refractory to diuretic therapy. Careful titration of vasodilators in the ICU may be appropriate to maintain adequate perfusion. If at any point the patient becomes hypotensive, the dose of the

vasodilator should be reduced or discontinued if persistent. Evidence of hypoperfusion may warrant initiation of an intravenous inotrope, with guidance based on hemodynamic measurements.

Inotropes

Several clinical trials and registries have shown that 2% to 8% of patients who have AHF have severe left ventricular systolic dysfunction with reduced SBP ($\leq$90 mm Hg) and symptoms and signs of peripheral hypoperfusion and impaired renal function.[2,37] These patients exhibit a fourfold greater risk for adverse clinical outcomes in the next 6 months than those who have normal blood pressure and need emergent enhancement of cardiac contractility to achieve clinical stabilization

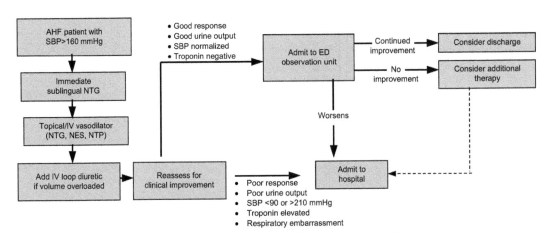

Fig. 2. Treatment algorithm for the patient who has AHF with elevated systolic blood pressure at presentation. AHF, acute heart failure; ED, emergency department; IV, intravenous; NES, nesiritide; NTG, nitroglycerin; NTP, nitroprusside; SBP, systolic blood pressure.

and symptomatic improvement.[38] The main targets of treatment in patients who have low output conditions are the attenuation of hypotension, improvement of peripheral tissue perfusion, protection of renal function, alleviation of congestion, and the prevention of new heart failure exacerbations.

The ideal inotropic agent would improve left ventricular systolic and diastolic function and reduce systemic and pulmonary vascular resistance, also causing a favorable or neutral effect on mortality, without increasing myocardial oxygen consumption and worsening metabolic status of cardiac muscle. Traditional inotropes, such as β-agonists and phosphodiesterase inhibitors, improve acutely the hemodynamic and clinical performance of patients who have AHF, but promote and accelerate detrimental biochemical pathways causing further myocardial injury and leading to increased short- and long-term mortality.[39,40] The investigational cardiac inodilator levosimendan may have better hemodynamic effects in patients who have AHF than traditional inotropes, and possesses some potential cardioprotective properties.[41,42] Despite its advantages, it failed to improve prognosis of patients who had AHF in recent multicenter randomized trials.[43,44]

Traditional inotropes

Classical inotropic agents (β-agonists, phosphodiesterase [PDE] inhibitors), such as dobutamine, dopamine, and milrinone, have been extensively used in the management of AHF exacerbations that are accompanied by low output state and marked hypoperfusion of peripheral tissues.[45,46] These drugs have been also used as a short-term bridge to other forms of destination therapy, such as cardiac transplantation, or as intermittent or prolonged infusions for the long-term treatment of patients who have stage D chronic heart failure resistant to conventional therapies.[45,46]

These agents enhance cardiac contractility through different biochemical pathways that increase the intracellular concentration of cyclic adenylate monophosphate (cAMP).[47] Beyond their positive inotropic properties, PDE inhibitors also have vasodilatory effects, because of inhibition of vascular smooth muscle cells. Moreover, because they exert their inotropic action distal to the β-adrenergic receptor, their effects are preserved even during concomitant administration of β-blockers.

Dopamine is an agent of particular interest, because it bears a dose-dependent mechanism of action. More specifically, at doses less than 2 mg/kg/min it acts on peripheral dopaminergic receptors, hence causing some peripheral vasodilation predominantly in the renal, splanchnic,

coronary, and cerebral vessels; at doses ranging between 2 to 5 mg/kg/min it acts as a β-adrenergic agonist, hence enhancing myocardial contractility, and at doses higher than 5 mg/kg/min it acts as an α-adrenergic receptor agonist, having peripheral vasoconstrictive effects.[48]

A retrospective analysis of 471 patients who had advanced heart failure who were treated with dobutamine (80 patients) or not showed that the dobutamine group had a higher occurrence of adverse outcomes, including worsening of heart failure, need for vasoactive medications, resuscitated cardiac arrest, and myocardial infarction, and a higher 6-month mortality rate.[49] In a trial of 203 patients who had low-output AHF, subjects were randomized to receive either levosimendan or dobutamine and examined hemodynamically before and after treatment. The proportion of patients who had hemodynamic improvement at 24 hours was significantly lower in the dobutamine arm, and this was accompanied by a higher mortality at 180 days.[50]

Another trial described patients who received milrinone for exacerbations of chronic heart failure and showed they had significantly higher rates of hypotensive episodes requiring intervention, new atrial arrhythmias, and higher rates of adverse clinical outcomes in the cases of heart failure secondary to ischemic cause than those who received placebo treatment.[51] Despite the short-term hemodynamic and symptomatic improvement, β-agonists and PDE inhibitors seem to increase long-term mortality in AHF, and their use must be exercised with caution.

Inodilators

Levosimendan is a pyridazinone-dinitrile derivative molecule that exerts positive inotropic effects by increasing the sensitivity of the cardiomyocyte contractile apparatus to intracellular calcium.[52,53] It is a powerful opener of ATP-sensitive potassium channels causing peripheral arterial and venous dilatation, leading to a reduction of peripheral vascular resistance and cardiac afterload. This process results in a significant increase of cardiac output through its combined positive inotropic and peripheral vasodilatory properties.[54–56]

Four large-scale randomized clinical trials have examined the effects of levosimendan administration on mortality in patients who had AHF. In the first, levosimendan caused a greater increase of cardiac index and decrease of PCWP in patients who had AHF than dobutamine (primary endpoint), with a higher overall survival at 180 days (secondary endpoint).[50] An investigation primarily of the safety of the drug also showed that a single IV levosimendan infusion was followed by significantly lower short-term and long-term mortality rates compared with placebo in patients who had post-myocardial infarction AHF.[57] More specifically, the risk for death or worsening of heart failure was significantly reduced during the 6 hours of infusion and during the first 24 hours in the levosimendan group. Moreover, mortality at 14 days and at 180 days posttreatment was also significantly lower compared with placebo.

Three recent trials showed that levosimendan was superior to placebo or dobutamine, respectively, in producing clinical improvement and beneficial neurohormonal modulation in patients who had AHF.[44,56,58] Levosimendan failed to lead to a greater reduction of 6-month mortality compared with placebo[58] or dobutamine[44] in these patients, however. Consequently, levosimendan remains an investigational drug in the United States but is currently used in several countries for the treatment of patients who have symptoms of low cardiac output AHF secondary to cardiac systolic dysfunction without severe hypotension.[5] More clinical data, deriving from specific sub-analyses of the existing trials or new clinical trials, are needed to identify clinical criteria of treatment response and the optimal and safest dosing and regimen of this agent.

Clinical use of inotropes

Patients who have marked systolic dysfunction and hypotension (SBP $\leq$ 90 mm Hg) and symptoms and signs of end-organ hypoperfusion require emergent augmentation of cardiac contractility to achieve clinical stabilization. Traditional IV inotropes are used as a first-line treatment in these patients. **Fig. 3** describes a proposed algorithm for the treatment of AHF with low SBP

($\leq$90 mmHg) or cardiogenic shock. These patients require management in the ICU and typically benefit from invasive hemodynamic monitoring to guide further therapy. The addition of a diuretic may be warranted by persistent evidence of pulmonary congestion and vasodilator therapy may be appropriate to address ongoing hemodynamic derangements, such as an elevated systemic vascular resistance and PCWP. In contrast, the addition of vasopressor therapy (norepinephrine) may be necessary if inotropic therapy fails to improve hypoperfusion despite an increase in cardiac output. These combinations of vasoactive agents should be used cautiously and only in the most critically ill patients under close supervision.

Patients who have a SBP between 90 and 120 mm Hg represent a hybrid group between normotensive and hypotensive AHF and close attention should be paid to detect any evidence of end-organ hypoperfusion. Typically, this is absent in most and most patients should be treated as normotensives, with IV diuretics as first-line therapy and vasodilators added as needed (see **Fig. 2**). If there is clinical worsening, such as persistent congestion, progressive renal dysfunction, or other signs of hypoperfusion under this therapeutic combination, inotropic support should be added and patients should be managed as described in **Fig. 3**.

Although inotropic therapy usually results in short-term symptomatic and hemodynamic improvement, and may stave off immediate death in gravely ill patients, the accumulating data suggest that it may lead to an adverse long-term prognosis. Consequently, there is an obvious need for novel inotropic agents that do not adversely affect patients' morbidity or mortality.

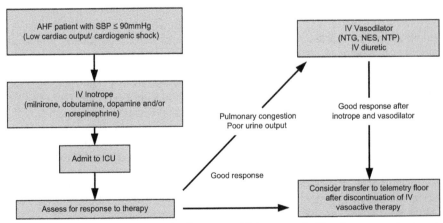

Fig. 3. Treatment algorithm for the patient who has AFH with low systolic blood pressure at presentation. AHF, acute heart failure; ICU, intensive care unit; IV, intravenous; NES, nesiritide; NTG, nitroglycerin; NTP, nitroprusside; SBP, systolic blood pressure.

Other Vasoactive Agents

Morphine

Morphine sulfate is a traditional therapy in AHF, despite the lack of much supporting data. Morphine reduces preload by producing mild venodilatation, relieves breathlessness, and exerts a calming effect. A recently published retrospective analysis of the Acute Decompensated Heart Failure National Registry showed that morphine is associated with a greater frequency of mechanical ventilation, prolonged hospitalization, more ICU admissions, and higher mortality.[59] Additional studies are needed to clarify these safety concerns.

Angiotensin converting enzyme inhibitors

ACE-I are considered standard of care in the management of chronic heart failure. Despite the plethora of data showing a substantial prognostic benefit when ACE-I are used in the chronic setting, only limited data are available for the acute setting.[60,61] Although a few studies have demonstrated hemodynamic improvement in AHF with ACE-I, their impact on clinical outcomes remains obscure. Their use is therefore not routinely recommended in the acute stabilization of AHF patients and additional research is needed.[5] Pre-existing therapy with ACE-I as a chronic heart failure medication should be continued during the AHF episode at the highest tolerated dose. Dosages should be reduced or discontinued altogether if the patient has symptomatic hypotension (SBP<100 mm Hg), any evidence of cardiogenic shock, elevated serum potassium (>5 mmol/L) or severe renal dysfunction (serum creatinine>2.5 mg/dL). Patients not currently being treated with ACE-I before admission should be started on this therapy during the hospitalization if none of the aforementioned contraindications exist.

Aldosterone antagonist

Persistent activation of aldosterone plays an important role in the pathophysiology of AHF; effective antagonism provides a substantial reduction in mortality, a reduction in AHF hospitalizations, and an improvement in functional class.[62] If serum potassium is less than 5 mmol/L and serum creatinine less than 2.5 mg/dL, an aldosterone antagonist (spironolactone 25 mg), should be added with repeat measurement of a chemistry panel and modification of drug dosing at 4 to 6 days later in-hospital or in outpatient heart failure clinic.

β-Blockers

Although data from randomized clinical trials are missing and the results from ongoing clinical trials in this area will be available in a few years, data from retrospective trials indicate that β-blockers should be continued during the AHF episode at the highest tolerated dose except for cases in which the patient has symptomatic hypotension or bradycardia, is hemodynamically unstable, or is in cardiogenic shock.[63]

SUMMARY

Effective use of diuretics, vasodilators, and inotropes to stabilize AHF relies on matching the most appropriately tailored therapy to specific clinical profiles. Some of the drugs may be harmful, and therefore the emphasis should be on patient safety and the attempt to minimize the deleterious effects of these therapies. Diuretics seem to be most beneficial in patients who have substantial volume overload, often seen in patients who have normal SBP. Vasodilator therapy seems to have its greatest usefulness in patients who have acute pulmonary edema associated with an elevated SBP and is recommended as first-line therapy in this group. Patients who have cardiogenic shock are at the highest risk and need emergent enhancement of cardiac contractility to achieve clinical stabilization. Inotropes are effective in restoring hemodynamic stability in this latter group but may lead to increased short- and long-term mortality. To date, successful treatment has been limited because no agent has been shown to reduce postdischarge mortality or readmission rates, and patients frequently remain symptomatic after treatment. Ongoing research is needed to further examine these agents and to develop novel therapies to address the unmet needs of the patient who has AHF.

ACKNOWLEDGMENT

The authors thank Dr. Lucas Pappas for his assistance in the preparation of this manuscript.

REFERENCES

1. Gheorghiade M, Zannad F, Sopko G, et al. International working group on acute heart failure syndromes. Acute heart failure syndromes: current state and framework for future research. Circulation 2005;112:3958–68.
2. Adams KF Jr, Fonarow GC, Emerman CL, et al. ADHERE scientific advisory committee and investigators. Characteristics and outcomes of patients hospitalized for heart failure in the United States: rationale, design, and preliminary observations from the first 100,000 cases in the Acute Decompensated Heart Failure National Registry (ADHERE). Am Heart J 2005;149:209–16.

3. Cleland JG, Swedberg K, Follath F, et al. Study group on diagnosis of the working group on heart failure of the European society of cardiology. The Euroheart failure survey programme—a survey on the quality of care among patients with heart failure in Europe. Part 1: patient characteristics and diagnosis. Eur Heart J 2003;24:442–63.

4. Heart Failure Society Of America. Executive summary: HFSA 2006 comprehensive heart failure practice guideline. J Card Fail 2006;12:10–38.

5. Nieminen MS, Böhm M, Cowie MR, et al. ESC committee for practice guideline (CPG). Executive summary of the guidelines on the diagnosis and treatment of acute heart failure: the task force on acute heart failure of the European society of cardiology. Eur Heart J 2005;26:384–416.

6. De Luca L, Fonarow GC, Mebazaa A, et al. Early pharmacological treatment of acute heart failure syndromes: a systematic review of clinical trials. Acute Card Care 2007;9:10–21.

7. Gheorghiade M, De Luca L, Fonarow GC, et al. Pathophysiologic targets in the early phase of acute heart failure syndromes. Am J Cardiol 2005;96(6A):11G–7G.

8. Sackner-Bernstein JD, Skopicki HA, Aaronson KD. Risk of worsening renal function with nesiritide in patients with acutely decompensated heart failure. Circulation 2005;111:1487–91.

9. Sackner-Bernstein JD, Kowalski M, Fox M, et al. Short-term risk of death after treatment with nesiritide for decompensated heart failure: a pooled analysis of randomized controlled trials. JAMA 2005;293:1900–5.

10. Zannad F, Mebazaa A, Juillière Y, et al. Clinical profile, contemporary management and one-year mortality in patients with severe acute heart failure syndromes: the EFICA study. Eur J Heart Fail 2006;8:697–705.

11. Gheorghiade M, Abraham WT, Albert NM, et al. Systolic blood pressure at admission, clinical characteristics, and outcomes in patients hospitalized with acute heart failure. JAMA 2006;296:2217–26.

12. Alla F, Zannad F, Filippatos G. Epidemiology of acute heart failure syndromes. Heart Fail Rev 2007;12:91–5.

13. Chatti R, Fradj NB, Trabelsi W, et al. Algorithm for therapeutic management of acute heart failure syndromes. Heart Fail Rev 2007;12:113–7.

14. Weinfeld MS, Chertow GM, Stevenson LW. Aggravated renal dysfunction during intensive therapy for advanced chronic heart failure. Am Heart J 1999;138:285–90.

15. Cooper HA, Dries DL, Davis CE, et al. Diuretics and risk of arrhythmic death in patients with left ventricular dysfunction. Circulation 1999;100:1311–5.

16. Jhund PS, McMurray J, Davie AP. The acute vascular effects of furosemide in heart failure. Br J Clin Pharmacol 2000;50:9–13.

17. Gottlieb SS, Brater DC, Thomas I, et al. BG9719 (CVT-124), an A1 adenosine receptor antagonist, protects against the decline in renal function observed with diuretic therapy. Circulation 2002;105:1348–53.

18. Cotter G, Weissgarten J, Metzkor E, et al. Increased toxicity of high-dose furosemide versus low-dose dopamine in the treatment of refractory congestive heart failure. Clin Pharmacol Ther 1997;62:187–93.

19. Cotter G, Metzkor E, Kaluski E, et al. Randomised trial of high-dose isosorbide dinitrate plus low-dose furosemide versus high-dose furosemide plus low-dose isosorbide dinitrate in severe pulmonary oedema. Lancet 1998;351:389–93.

20. Lahav M, Regev A, Ra'anani P, et al. Intermittent administration of furosemide vs continuous infusion preceded by a loading dose for congestive heart failure. Chest 1992;102:725–31.

21. Dormans TP, van Meyel JJ, Gerlag PG, et al. Diuretic efficacy of high dose furosemide in severe heart failure: bolus injection versus continuous infusion. J Am Coll Cardiol 1996;28:376–82.

22. Cohn PF, Gorlin R. Physiologic and clinical actions of nitroglycerin. Med Clin North Am 1974;58:407–15.

23. Elkayam U, Bitar F, Akhter MW, et al. Intravenous nitroglycerin in the treatment of decompensated heart failure: potential benefits and limitations. J Cardiovasc Pharmacol Ther 2004;9:227–41.

24. Katz SD, Biasucci L, Sabba C, et al. Impaired endothelium-mediated vasodilation in the peripheral vasculature of patients with congestive heart failure. J Am Coll Cardiol 1992;19:918–25.

25. Elkayam U, Roth A, Kumar A, et al. Hemodynamic and volumetric effects of venodilation with nitroglycerin in chronic mitral regurgitation. Am J Cardiol 1987;60:1106–11.

26. Loh E, Elkayam U, Cody R, et al. A randomized multicenter study comparing the efficacy and safety of intravenous milrinone and intravenous nitroglycerin in patients with advanced heart failure. J Card Fail 2001;7:114–21.

27. Nashed AH, Allegra JR. Intravenous nitroglycerin boluses in treating patients with cardiogenic pulmonary edema. Am J Emerg Med 1995;13:612–3.

28. Levy P, Compton S, Welch R, et al. Treatment of severe decompensated heart failure with high-dose intravenous nitroglycerin: a feasibility and outcome analysis. Ann Emerg Med 2007;50:144–52.

29. Publication Committee for the VMAC Investigators (Vasodilatation in the Management of Acute CHF) Intravenous nesiritide vs nitroglycerin for treatment of decompensated congestive heart failure: a randomized controlled trial. JAMA 2002;287:1531–40.

30. Levin ER, Gardner DG, Samson WK. Natriuretic peptides. N Engl J Med 1998;339:321–8.

31. Mills RM, LeJemtel TH, Horton DP, et al. Sustained hemodynamic effects of an infusion of nesiritide (human B-type natriuretic peptide) in heart failure: a randomized, double-blind, placebo-controlled clinical trial. Natrecor study group. J Am Coll Cardiol 1999;34:155–62.

32. Colucci WS, Elkayam U, Horton DP, et al. Intravenous nesiritide, a natriuretic peptide, in the treatment of decompensated congestive heart failure. Nesiritide study group. N Engl J Med 2000;343:246–53.

33. Guiha NH, Cohn JN, Mikulic E, et al. Treatment of refractory heart failure with infusion of nitroprusside. N Engl J Med 1974;291:587–92.

34. Khot UN, Novaro GM, Popović ZB, et al. Nitroprusside in critically ill patients with left ventricular dysfunction and aortic stenosis. N Engl J Med 2003;348:1756–63.

35. Cohn JN, Franciosa JA, Francis GS, et al. Effect of short-term infusion of sodium nitroprusside on mortality rate in acute myocardial infarction complicated by left ventricular failure: results of a Veterans Administration cooperative study. N Engl J Med 1982;306:1129–35.

36. Bussmann WD, Schupp D. Effect of sublingual nitroglycerin in emergency treatment of severe pulmonary edema. Am J Cardiol 1978;41:931–6.

37. Fonarow GC, Corday E. ADHERE scientific advisory committee. Overview of acutely decompensated congestive heart failure (ADHF): a report from the ADHERE registry. Heart Fail Rev 2004;9:179–85.

38. Milo-Cotter O, Adams KF, O'Connor CM, et al. Acute heart failure associated with high admission blood pressure—a distinct vascular disorder? Eur J Heart Fail 2007;9:178–83.

39. Thackray S, Easthaugh J, Freemantle N, et al. The effectiveness and relative effectiveness of intravenous inotropic drugs acting through the adrenergic pathway in patients with heart failure-a meta-regression analysis. Eur J Heart Fail 2002;4:515–29.

40. Packer M. The search for the ideal positive inotropic agent. N Engl J Med 1993;329:201–2.

41. Papp Z, Csapó K, Pollesello P, et al. Pharmacological mechanisms contributing to the clinical efficacy of levosimendan. Cardiovasc Drug Rev 2005;23:71–98.

42. Mebazaa A, Barraud D, Welschbillig S. Randomized clinical trials with levosimendan. Am J Cardiol 2005;96:74G–9G.

43. Cleland JG, Freemantle N, Coletta AP, et al. Clinical trials update from the American Heart Association: REPAIR-AMI, ASTAMI, JELIS, MEGA, REVIVE-II, SURVIVE, and PROACTIVE. Eur J Heart Fail 2006;8:105–10.

44. Mebazaa A, Nieminen MS, Packer M, et al. SURVIVE investigators. Levosimendan vs dobutamine for patients with acute decompensated heart failure: the SURVIVE randomized trial. JAMA 2007;297:1883–91.

45. Munger MA. Management of acute decompensated heart failure: treatment, controversy, and future directions. Pharmacotherapy 2006;26:131S–8S.

46. Zannad F, Adamopoulos C, Mebazaa A, et al. The challenge of acute decompensated heart failure. Heart Fail Rev 2006;11:135–9.

47. Felker GM, O'Connor CM. Inotropic therapy for heart failure: an evidence-based approach. Am Heart J 2001;142:393–401.

48. Parissis J, Farmakis D, Nieminen M. Classical inotropes and new cardiac enhancers. Heart Fail Rev 2007;12:149–56.

49. O'Connor CM, Gattis WA, Uretsky BF, et al. Continuous intravenous dobutamine is associated with an increased risk of death in patients with advanced heart failure: insights from the Flolan International Randomized Survival Trial (FIRST). Am Heart J 1999;138:78–86.

50. Follath F, Cleland JG, Just H, et al. Steering committee and investigators of the levosimendan infusion versus dobutamine (LIDO) study. Efficacy and safety of intravenous levosimendan compared with dobutamine in severe low-output heart failure (the LIDO study): a randomised double-blind trial. Lancet 2002;360:196–202.

51. Cuffe MS, Califf RM, Adams KF Jr, et al. Outcomes of a prospective trial of intravenous milrinone for exacerbations of chronic heart failure (OPTIME-CHF) investigators. Short-term intravenous milrinone for acute exacerbation of chronic heart failure: a randomized controlled trial. JAMA 2002;287:1541–7.

52. Figgit DP, Gilles PS, Goa KL. Levosimendan. Drugs 2001;61:613–27.

53. Perrone S, Kaplinsky EJ. Calcium sensitizer agents: a new class of inotropic agents in the treatment of decompensated heart failure. Int J Cardiol 2005;103:248–55.

54. Kivikko M, Lehtonen L. Levosimendan: a new inodilatory drug for the treatment of decompensated heart failure. Curr Pharm Des 2005;11:435–55.

55. Parissis J, Filippatos G, Farmakis D, et al. Levosimendan for the treatment of acute heart failure syndromes. Expert Opin Pharmacother 2005;6(15):2741–51.

56. DeLuca L, Colucci W, Nieminen M, et al. Evidence-based use of levosimendan in different clinical settings. Eur Heart J 2006;27:1908–20.

57. Moiseyev VS, Põder P, Andrejevs N, et al. Study investigators. Safety and efficacy of a novel calcium sensitizer, levosimendan, in patients with left ventricular failure due to an acute myocardial infarction. A randomized, placebo-controlled, double-blind study (RUSSLAN). Eur Heart J 2002;23:1422–32.

58. Packer M. The randomized multicenter evaluation of intravenous levosimendan efficacy-2 (REVIVE-2) trial. Late-breaking clinical trials. American Heart

Association. Presented at the Annual Scientific Session, Dallas (TX), 13–16 November 2005.

59. Peacock WF, Hollander JE, Diercks DB, et al. Morphine and outcomes in acute decompensated heart failure: an ADHERE analysis. Emerg Med J 2008;25: 205–9.

60. Swedberg K, Held P, Kjekshus J, et al. Effects of the early administration of enalapril on mortality in patients with acute myocardial infarction. Results of the cooperative new Scandinavian enalapril survival study II (CONSENSUS II). N Engl J Med 1992;327:678–84.

61. Annane D, Bellissant E, Pussard E, et al. Placebo-controlled, randomized, double-blind study of intravenous enalaprilat efficacy and safety in acute cardiogenic pulmonary edema. Circulation 1996; 94:1316–24.

62. Pitt B, Zannad F, Remme WJ, et al. For the randomized Aldactone evaluation study investigators. The effect of spironolactone on morbidity and mortality in patients with severe heart failure. N Engl J Med 1999;341:709–17.

63. Mebazaa A, Gheorghiade M, Piña IL, et al. Practical recommendations for prehospital and early in-hospital management of patients presenting with acute heart failure syndromes. Crit Care Med 2008;36: S129–39.

Circulatory Assist Devices in Heart Failure Patients

Brian C. Hiestand, MD, MPH, FACEP*

KEYWORDS

- Heart failure • Ventricular assist device
- Aortic balloon pump

Heart failure continues to increase in incidence and prevalence. Despite optimum medical therapy, overall survival from time of diagnosis has not increased appreciably. Heart transplantation is an option for a select subpopulation of patients who have heart failure; however, many patients have comorbidities that preclude transplantation or are too ill to survive the waiting period engendered by the scarcity of available donor hearts. Ventricular assist devices can be used to provide support to the failing heart, either as a bridge to planned eventual transplantation or as destination therapy to palliate symptoms and prolong life. In the acute setting, intra-aortic balloon pumps (IABPs) can temporize acute cardiogenic shock and are often used in the postinfarction window until stunned myocardium recovers, or as a transitional device to an implanted or percutaneous ventricular assist device. IABP support has also been described in the setting of beta-blocker and calcium-channel antagonist overdose.[1,2] In this section, we discuss the use of mechanical support for cardiogenic shock, ranging from the emergent setting to chronic indwelling device assistance.

INTRA-AORTIC BALLOON PUMPS

The IABP uses pressure-volume dynamics to optimize cardiac output and maximize coronary artery perfusion in the setting of acute left ventricular systolic dysfunction. Although frequently used in the perioperative setting during coronary artery bypass procedures, the IABP can be used to provide circulatory support for cardiogenic shock attributable to myocardial ischemia and infarction. IABPs are being increasingly used for postinfarction support,[3] and aeromedical transfer of patients who have balloon pumps is common.[4] The non-cardiologist physician should not only be familiar with this potential modality for the patient who has acute cardiogenic shock, but may be called on to assist with the management of a transfer patient who has a balloon pump already in place.

The American College of Cardiology/American Heart Association (ACC/AHA) guidelines for the management of ST segment elevation myocardial infarction (STEMI) strongly recommend IABP use in the setting of STEMI complicated by acute cardiogenic shock refractory to pharmacologic measures, with persistent low output states, or in patients refractory to medical management as a bridge to mechanical revascularization.[5] The recommendations are less robust in the setting of non–ST segment elevation myocardial infarction, but state that IABP therapy may be considered for persistent hypotension in this population also.[6] Balloon placement is contraindicated in the setting of aortic regurgitation, because the pressure wave generated by diastolic inflation simply bypasses the coronaries and enters the left ventricle, worsening valvular insufficiency. Balloon pump efficacy may also be compromised in the setting of irregular cardiac rhythms, because efficient inflation/deflation cycling depends on a fairly consistent interval between systolic contractions. Modern sensing algorithms are less prone to this error, however.

The IABP is typically placed through the femoral artery and advanced so that the cephalad end of the balloon is just distal to the takeoff of the

The Ohio State University, Columbus, OH, USA
* Department of Emergency Medicine, The Ohio State University, 149 Means Hall, 1654 Upham Drive, Columbus, OH 43210.
E-mail address: brian.hiestand@osumc.edu

Heart Failure Clin 5 (2009) 55–62
doi:10.1016/j.hfc.2008.08.002

subclavian artery. With a more distal placement coronary perfusion assistance is compromised; more proximal placement risks occlusion or damage to the subclavian artery. During systole, the balloon deflates, decreasing afterload and ventricular wall stress. During diastole, the balloon reinflates, increasing coronary perfusion pressure by way of retrograde pressure toward the aortic valve and coronary ostia. The IABP inflation/deflation cycle can be triggered by cardiac depolarization or pressure wave sensing, depending on the specific manufacturer and device settings. Generally, balloon pump augmentation is started at a ratio of two systolic contractions to one augmentation cycle; this can be increased to 1:1 if the patient's condition warrants, and weaned to longer intervals as the patient improves. **Fig. 1** demonstrates arterial waveforms using a 2:1 contraction/augmentation cycle and waveforms associated with common timing errors.

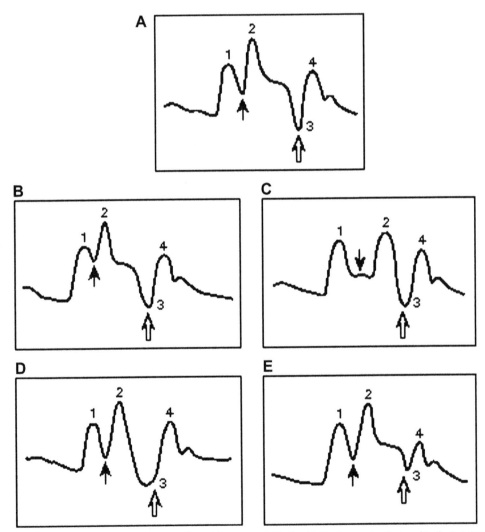

Fig. 1. Arterial waveforms seen in correct (A) and incorrect inflation/deflation cycle timing (B–E). A 1:2 ratio of assistance is shown. In (A), peak systolic pressure (1) is followed after systolic flow by balloon inflation (solid arrow), producing an augmented peak diastolic pressure (2). Balloon pressure drops, reaching a nadir (open arrow) that decreases the aortic end-diastolic pressure (3), decreasing afterload and subsequently the peak systolic pressure (4). In (B), the balloon inflates before the end of systole (solid arrow), producing a spiked, narrow diastolic augmentation (2) and resulting in a decrease in cardiac output. In (C), the inflation (solid arrow) begins late, providing a suboptimal augmented peak diastolic pressure. In (D), early deflation results in a "scooped" waveform, and afterload is not reduced, resulting in a peak systolic pressure (4) that remains elevated. Finally, (E) demonstrates late deflation with an elevated aortic end-diastolic pressure (3), resulting in compromised cardiac output. (Illustrations from Arrow Cardiac Care, provided courtesy of Teleflex Medical, Reading, PA.)

Complications due to IABP placement are not infrequent, with a wide range of reported rates (1%–47%) depending on how complications are defined.[7] Modern complication rates are much lower, with the incidence of most complications occurring in less than 1% of cases.[3] Ischemic complications, including impairment of distal limb, mesenteric, and splanchnic circulation, are known to occur.[7-10] Larger catheter size and increased duration of IABP use increase the risk for ischemia and arterial damage.[7,8] Complications caused by balloon thrombus emboli can be mitigated with anticoagulation, typically with heparin, but this also carries the risk for hemorrhagic consequences and is potentially contraindicated in postoperative patients.

Air embolism can occur because of balloon rupture, with helium and carbon dioxide as the most frequently used gases. Carbon dioxide has the advantage of being partially soluble in blood, potentially mitigating the consequences of balloon rupture. The use of helium allows for a smaller-diameter catheter for the balloon pump because of the fluid dynamic properties of helium, thus potentially decreasing the risk for complications directly associated with catheter placement.

Failure to improve hemodynamic parameters with the IABP is likely to be caused by poor timing of the inflation/deflation cycle, although malposition of the balloon should be considered. Most balloon pumps have the ability to sense and initiate the inflation cycle, based either on QRS signal or pressure waveform. Manual adjustment should be considered, however, if the patient fails to improve or deteriorates with the initiation of IABP support. Inflation should occur at the dicrotic notch on the pressure waveform displayed on the device monitor.[11,12] Deflation should be timed so that the nadir of the aortic pressure wave occurs just before the systolic contraction, minimizing afterload. With optimal timing, assisted peak diastolic pressure in the aorta should exceed systolic pressure, and assisted end-diastolic pressure in the aorta should be 5 to 10 mmHg less than unassisted end-diastolic pressure.

If there is mistiming of the inflation/deflation cycle, several untoward hemodynamic effects can occur. Early inflation induces premature closure of the aortic valve, decreasing stroke volume and cardiac output and increasing end-diastolic volume and left ventricular strain. Late inflation produces suboptimal diastolic augmentation and coronary support. Early deflation fails to provide a reduction in afterload at the time of systole, and late deflation substantially increases afterload, resulting in poor cardiac output.

IABP efficacy and outcomes in the acute setting have been predominantly established from post hoc analysis of trials and registry data. Secondary analysis of data from GUSTO I, which randomized patients who had STEMI to various fibrinolytic regimens, evaluated the outcomes of patients who had STEMI and shock, as categorized by IABP use.[13] Out of more than 40,000 patients, 310 met criteria for cardiogenic shock, with 62 receiving an IABP within the first day. Although immediate bleeding was increased and 30-day mortality was unaffected, 1-year mortality was improved in those patients who received IAPB within the first day of admission (57% versus 67%, $P = .04$).

In data published in 2000 from the SHOCK (Should we emergently revascularize Occluded Coronaries for cardiogenic shocK) registry, consisting of 884 patients who had acute myocardial infarction complicated by persistent hypotension and cardiogenic shock, IABP use (279 patients received IABP alone, and 160 patients received IABP and fibrinolytic therapy) was associated with a substantial reduction in mortality, both as a main effect and in conjunction with fibrinolytic therapy.[14] This finding was confounded, however, by the uneven distribution of subsequent percutaneous transluminal coronary angioplasty (PTCA) or coronary artery bypass grafting. Patients who had IABPs were more likely to undergo mechanical revascularization and to be transferred to tertiary referral centers,[15] which likely affected survival rates.

Data from the National Registry of Myocardial Infarction 2 provide the largest evidence base for the use of IABPs in cardiogenic shock and myocardial infarction. A comparison of 7268 patients who had IABPs and 15,912 who did not have IABPs[16] demonstrated that mortality decreased with fibrinolytic therapy plus IABP versus fibrinolytic therapy alone (49% versus 67%). The use of IABPs in patients receiving primary PTCA did not confer any survival advantage, however, and was associated with an increased risk for death (odds ratio 1.27, 95% confidence interval 1.07–1.50). The applicability of these data to current strategies in cardiac care may be somewhat limited, because 61% of patients received no reperfusion therapy in this cohort.

In summary, an IABP remains a valid short-term solution in patients who have profound and refractory cardiogenic shock. Physicians should be aware of this potential therapeutic option and the basic operating and physiologic principles the device uses to provide maximum benefit.

VENTRICULAR ASSIST DEVICES

Ventricular assist devices (VADs) supplant the circulatory function of one or both sides of the heart.

Intended for longer-term use than a balloon pump, general indications for VAD usage can include support for recovery of myocardial function, as a bridge to eventual transplantation, or as destination therapy for those patients whose hearts have suffered irreversible injury but are not candidates for cardiac transplantation.[17] The biomechanics of blood flow are relatively straightforward: an inflow cannula is connected to a pump, which is then connected to an outflow cannula. Circulatory support can be provided with a left ventricular assist device (LVAD), a right ventricular assist device (RVAD), or a biventricular assist device (BiVAD).

For left ventricular support, the inflow catheter is placed in either the left atrium or at the apex of the left ventricle. The outflow cannula is then surgically grafted into the aorta.[18] **Fig. 2** illustrates the Novacor Left Ventricular Assist System (WorldHeart, Ontario) as a typical LVAD configuration. For emergent, short-term use, a percutaneous LVAD can be placed, with the inflow catheter placed by venous cannulation into the right atrium, followed by perforation of the atrial septum into the left atrium. The outflow cannula is inserted into the femoral artery for systemic circulation. Percutaneous VAD placement can be accomplished in the cardiac catheterization laboratory. Placement of the inflow cannula into the left atrium, with either a percutaneous LVAD or surgically implanted LVAD, does carry an increased risk for

thromboembolism due to thrombus formation in the left ventricular cavity.[18] If extended cardiac support is required, transition from a percutaneous LVAD to a surgically implanted LVAD can occur when the patient is stable enough to consider an operation with the potential for cardiopulmonary bypass.

Right ventricular support is accomplished in much the same fashion. The inflow cannula can be placed in either the right atrium or right ventricle. The outflow cannula is then grafted into the pulmonary artery. Biventricular support requires two devices, one providing support to each side of the heart and inserted as above.

Blood flow is generated in either a pulsatile or continuous flow, depending on the specific device. Pulsatile flow can be generated by air bladder filling Abiomed BVS 5000, Abiomed BVS 5000 [Abiomed, Danvers, Massachusetts], Thoratec Percutaneous Ventricular Assist Device [PVAD], Thoratec Implantable Ventricular Assist Device [IVAD; Thoratec Corp., Pleasanton, California] or by a pusher plate that can be driven by either electric motor (Thoratec HeartMate XVE, Novacor Left Ventricular Assist System [LVAS; WorldHeart, Ontario]) or pneumatic system (Thoratec HeartMate IP). Continuous flow devices can be powered by centrifugal or rotary motors and are unique in that there are almost no detectable peripheral pulses when the devices are engaged despite adequate circulation. Although this absence of palpable pulse can be merely disconcerting to an unsuspecting health care provider in an awake, alert, responsive patient, it is conceivable that inappropriate cardiac resuscitation could be attempted on a patient rendered unconscious from noncardiac causes. With the exception of the DeBakey VAD Child Left Ventricular Assist System (MicroMed Technology, Houston, Texas), which carries a Humanitarian Device Exemption from the US Food and Drug Administration (FDA) as a bridge to transplant in pediatric patients, at the time of this writing all other continuous flow systems are considered investigational. Outpatient encounters can be anticipated to occur with patients enrolled in clinical trials of these devices, however.

Most VADs are FDA approved as a bridge to transplant or recovery from an acute insult. The FDA has approved the Thoratec HeartMate XVE, Thoratec IVAD, Thoratec PVAD, and the Novacor LVAS for outpatient use, and the Thoratec HeartMate XVE has been approved explicitly as long-term destination therapy for end-stage heart failure. There is increasing potential for the physician to care for a patient who has a VAD, either coincidentally or because of a device-related complication.

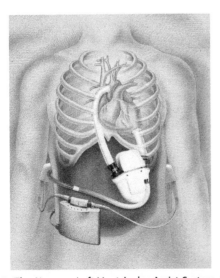

Fig. 2. The Novacor Left Ventricular Assist System. The intake conduit is attached to the apex of the left ventricle, with the outflow conduit grafted onto the aorta. The pump itself is implanted within the abdominal wall, with an external lead going to the controller console and power packs. (*Courtesy of* WorldHeart Inc., Ontario, Canada; with permission.)

The landmark trial establishing the usefulness of ventricular assist as destination therapy was the REMATCH (Randomized Evaluation of Mechanical Assistance for the Treatment of Congestive Heart failure) trial, which treated patients who had end-stage heart failure who did not qualify for transplantation with either optimal medical management or left ventricular support with the Thoratec HeartMate VE, an earlier generation of the Thoratec XVE.[19] Patients who had ventricular assistance had a 48% risk reduction in all-cause mortality compared with patients who had optimal medical management. Estimates of 1-year survival rates were 52% for the device group and 25% in the medical therapy group. Two-year survival rates were 29% for the device group and 13% for the medical therapy group.[20]

Similar results were seen in the recent INTrEPID (Investigation of NonTransplant-Eligible Patients who are Inotrope Dependent) trial, which compared two smaller cohorts of patients who received a Novacor LVAD with similar patients who declined LVAD implantation, had an artificial aortic valve, or who had "inadequate identifiable financial resources to cover the cost of device implantation and follow-up."[21] All patients had failed attempts to wean from inotropes before enrollment. The LVAD cohort had higher 6-month survival (46% versus 22%) and 1-year survival (27% versus 11%). Although not as methodologically rigorous as the REMATCH trial, the INTrEPID trial does demonstrate device efficacy in a very sick population of patients unable to be weaned from chronic inotrope support.

Of the four VADs currently approved for adult outpatient use, the Thoratec PVAD is the only one with the drive chamber located outside of the body. The other devices have the drive chamber placed internally with a driveline exiting through the abdominal wall to a control console providing operating control and power to the drive. The devices approved for outpatient use can be set to operate under fixed output conditions, or to sense physiologic demand and adjust the pump rate accordingly.

In the setting of malignant cardiac dysrhythmia, defibrillation or cardioversion can proceed as clinically indicated. Even though the pump may continue to run, blood flow depends on blood reaching the left atrium from the right heart. Rhythms such as ventricular fibrillation must therefore be defibrillated in patients who have an LVAD in place or no forward flow will occur. There are no specific recommendations for the Novacor LVAS or the Thoratec IVAD/PVAD,[22] but it is recommended that the driveline to the power supply/control console be transiently disconnected for the

Thoratec HeartMate XVE.[23] The Thoratec Heart-Mate XVE can be hand pumped by a pneumatic device that can be attached to the driveline in case of device failure or if the driveline has to be disconnected. Cardiopulmonary resuscitation (CPR) can lead to trauma to the intracardiac cannulae, device, and tissues in contact with the cannulae; thus hand pumping is preferred in the setting of cardiac arrest in a patient who has a Thoratec HeartMate XVE and an available hand pump.[23] If power can be immediately restored to the drive pump, systemic circulation will resume, albeit dependent on venous return to the heart (much like conventional CPR).

A substantial concern with artificial cardiac pumping devices relates to thrombosis attributable to contact of blood with nonnative vessel surfaces. The Novacor LVAS and Thoratec PVAD/IVAD systems require ongoing anticoagulation after insertion,[18] whereas the Thoratec Heart-Mate XVE does not require routine anticoagulation because of the engineered microstructure of the surfaces coming into contact with the bloodstream.[24] In the follow-up from the REMATCH trial, 10 cerebral infarctions and two hemorrhagic strokes occurred in the Thoratec HeartMate VE LVAD arm (16% occurrence rate) with a stroke rate of 0.19 events per patient year (compared with 0.052 per patient year in the medical management arm). A total of 42 "neurologic events," including metabolic encephalopathy, stroke, and transient ischemic attacks (TIAs), occurred in 30 of 68 patients who had LVADs versus 4 events in 4 of 61 medically managed patients.[25] In the INTrEPID study, patients who had the Novacor LVAD demonstrated a somewhat higher rate of cerebral embolic disease, with 62% of patients who had LVADs experiencing a stroke or TIA (20 patients had 30 strokes, and 10 patients experienced 15 TIAs) versus 11% of medically managed patients.[21] The patients who had LVADs in the INTrEPID study were routinely maintained on anticoagulation with warfarin, aspirin, and dipyridamole. No data were reported on whether septic emboli were the cause of any of these events, as opposed to purely thrombogenic embolization that could be ameliorated by modification (or routine initiation) of anticoagulation regimens. In nonneurologic embolic complications, the REMATCH trial reported an embolic event rate of 0.14 events per patient year. The INTrEPID trial did not report noncerebral thromboembolic events; however, the data submitted to the FDA for outpatient use approval documented a 14.7% rate of nonneurologic embolism.[24]

Infection is a constant risk for the device pocket itself and the blood-contacting surfaces within the

LVAD. Sepsis was the leading cause of death in the LVAD arm of the REMATCH trial, and the second leading cause of death in the LVAD arm of the INTrEPID study (17/41 deaths in 68 patients and 7/29 deaths in 37 patients, respectively).[19,21] Improvements in device engineering, such as a more flexible driveline that generates less torque on the surrounding tissue of the abdominal wall, have decreased the odds of bacterial invasion of the device pocket and other infectious complications.[26] Superficial infections can be managed with antibiotics and local wound care, including antibiotic-impregnated beads and even the use of tissue flaps for coverage;[27,28] infection of the blood-contacting surfaces should prompt immediate consideration of device change.[18]

Right ventricular failure is a known complication of artificial left ventricular support. Most cases occur in the immediate postoperative period; however, transition to biventricular support as late as 4 months after LVAD implantation has been required.[29] Right heart failure may also compromise pump output because of reduced filling of the LVAD. Women and patients who have smaller frames are more at risk for right heart failure; pulmonary vasodilators and inotropic support may be required while the possibility of biventricular support is considered.[29,30]

Device failures have become less common as engineering advances produce more durable components.[18] Although the Thoratec HeartMate XVE system does have a pneumatic hand pump backup, other systems have no immediate recourse in the case of operating system, power source, or drive pump failure other than replacement of external components. The Novacor LVAS does seem to have fewer mechanical device failures than other systems.[24] The Thoratec XVE system has undergone several engineering adjustments from the original VE system used in REMATCH that have significantly decreased the incidence of mechanical failure,[31] but there remains a need for long-term surveillance. Patient presentation with symptoms of acute decompensated heart failure should prompt an evaluation for VAD dysfunction by way of echocardiography[32] or cardiac catheterization.[33] Obvious signs of noncatastrophic pump dysfunction include audible grinding and expulsion of metal dust from the vent filter of the device.[32]

VADs represent an opportunity for catastrophically ill patients to regain function, mobility, and months to years of life. There are still substantial risks and costs associated with this therapy, estimated to be as high as $900,000 per quality-adjusted life year gained. New technologies are approaching the market, with many already in late-phase trials, and technical improvements on current technologies continue to improve reliability and decrease complications. At our own center, we have had patients refuse to return to the transplant list because of immense improvement in their condition with destination VAD implantation.

SUMMARY

Circulatory assist devices, although not without risk, may provide moderate to substantial improvement in cardiac function. Different devices can be considered based on the anticipated duration of need and the acuity of the cardiovascular failure being treated. A knowledge of indications, operation, and potential complications of these devices may allow the physician to optimize the care of catastrophically ill heart failure and cardiogenic shock patients.

REFERENCES

1. Salhanick SD, Wax PM. Treatment of atenolol overdose in a patient with renal failure using serial hemodialysis and hemoperfusion and associated echocardiographic findings. Vet Hum Toxicol 2000; 42(4):224–5.
2. Frierson J, Bailly D, Shultz T, et al. Refractory cardiogenic shock and complete heart block after unsuspected verapamil-SR and atenolol overdose. Clin Cardiol 1991;14(11):933–5.
3. Stone GW, Ohman EM, Miller MF, et al. Contemporary utilization and outcomes of intra-aortic balloon counterpulsation in acute myocardial infarction: the benchmark registry. J Am Coll Cardiol 2003;41(11): 1940–5.
4. MacDonald RD, Farquhar S. Transfer of intra-aortic balloon pump-dependent patients by paramedics. Prehosp Emerg Care 2005;9(4):449–53.
5. Antman EM, Anbe DT, Armstrong PW, et al. ACC/AHA guidelines for the management of patients with ST-elevation myocardial infarction: a report of the American College of Cardiology/American Heart Association task force on practice guidelines (committee to revise the 1999 guidelines for the management of patients with acute myocardial infarction). Circulation 2004;110(9):e82–292.
6. Anderson JL, Adams CD, Antman EM, et al. ACC/AHA 2007 guidelines for the management of patients with unstable angina/non-ST-elevation myocardial infarction: a report of the American College of Cardiology/American Heart Association task force on practice guidelines (writing committee to revise the 2002 guidelines for the management of patients with unstable angina/non-st-elevation myocardial infarction) developed in collaboration with the American College of Emergency Physicians,

the Society for Cardiovascular Angiography and Interventions, and the Society of Thoracic Surgeons endorsed by the American Association of Cardiovascular and Pulmonary Rehabilitation and the Society for Academic Emergency Medicine. J Am Coll Cardiol 2007;50(7):e1–157.

7. Scholz KH, Ragab S, von zur MF, et al. Complications of intra-aortic balloon counterpulsation. The role of catheter size and duration of support in a multivariate analysis of risk. Eur Heart J 1998; 19(3):458–65.

8. Meisel S, Shochat M, Sheikha SA, et al. Utilization of low-profile intra-aortic balloon catheters inserted by the sheathless technique in acute cardiac patients: clinical efficacy with a very low complication rate. Clin Cardiol 2004;27(11):600–4.

9. Arceo A, Urban P, Dorsaz PA, et al. In-hospital complications of percutaneous intraaortic balloon counterpulsation. Angiology 2003;54(5):577–85.

10. Shin H, Yozu R, Sumida T, et al. Acute ischemic hepatic failure resulting from intraaortic balloon pump malposition. Eur J Cardiothorac Surg 2000; 17(4):492–4.

11. Osentowski MK, Holt DW. Evaluating the efficacy of intra-aortic balloon pump timing using the auto-timing mode of operation with the datascope CS100. J Extra Corpor Technol 2007;39(2):87–90.

12. Santa-Cruz RA, Cohen MG, Ohman EM. Aortic counterpulsation: a review of the hemodynamic effects and indications for use. Catheter Cardiovasc Interv 2006;67(1):68–77.

13. Anderson RD, Ohman EM, Holmes DR Jr, et al. Use of intraaortic balloon counterpulsation in patients presenting with cardiogenic shock: observations from the Gusto-I study. global utilization of streptokinase and TPA for occluded coronary arteries. J Am Coll Cardiol 1997;30(3):708–15.

14. Hochman JS, Buller CE, Sleeper LA, et al. Cardiogenic shock complicating acute myocardial infarction–etiologies, management and outcome: a report from the shock trial registry. Should we emergently revascularize occluded coronaries for cardiogenic shock? J Am Coll Cardiol 2000; 36(3 Suppl A):1063–70.

15. Sanborn TA, Sleeper LA, Bates ER, et al. Impact of thrombolysis, intra-aortic balloon pump counterpulsation, and their combination in cardiogenic shock complicating acute myocardial infarction: a report from the shock trial registry. Should we emergently revascularize occluded coronaries for cardiogenic shock? J Am Coll Cardiol 2000;36(3 Suppl A): 1123–9.

16. Barron HV, Every NR, Parsons LS, et al. The use of intra-aortic balloon counterpulsation in patients with cardiogenic shock complicating acute myocardial infarction: data from the National Registry of Myocardial Infarction 2. Am Heart J 2001;141(6):933–9.

17. Sun BC. Indications for long-term assist device placement as bridge to transplantation. Cardiol Clin 2003;21(1):51–5.

18. Sun BC, Harter R, Gravlee GP. Devices for cardiac support and replacement. In: Hensley FA, Martin DE, Gravlee GP, editors. A practical approach to cardiac anesthesia. Philadelphia: Wolters Kluwer Health/Lippincott Williams & Wilkins; 2007. p. 587–603.

19. Rose EA, Gelijns AC, Moskowitz AJ, et al. Long-term mechanical left ventricular assistance for end-stage heart failure. N Engl J Med 2001; 345(20):1435–43.

20. Dembitsky WP, Tector AJ, Park S, et al. Left ventricular assist device performance with long-term circulatory support: lessons from the rematch trial. Ann Thorac Surg 2004;78(6):2123–9.

21. Rogers JG, Butler J, Lansman SL, et al. Chronic mechanical circulatory support for inotrope-dependent heart failure patients who are not transplant candidates: results of the intrepid trial. J Am Coll Cardiol 2007;50(8):741–7.

22. Madigan JD, Choudhri AF, Chen J, et al. Surgical management of the patient with an implanted cardiac device: implications of electromagnetic interference. Ann Surg 1999;230(5):639–47.

23. HeartMate Left Ventricular Assist System (LVAS) Community Living Manual. Pleasanton (CA): Thoratec Corporation; 2004.

24. Pasque MK, Rogers JG. Adverse events in the use of HeartMate vented electric and Novacor left ventricular assist devices: comparing apples and oranges. J Thorac Cardiovasc Surg 2002;124(6): 1063–7.

25. Lazar RM, Shapiro PA, Jaski BE, et al. Neurological events during long-term mechanical circulatory support for heart failure: the randomized evaluation of mechanical assistance for the treatment of congestive heart failure (rematch) experience. Circulation 2004;109(20):2423–7.

26. Long JW, Kfoury AG, Slaughter MS, et al. Long-term destination therapy with the HeartMate XVE left ventricular assist device: improved outcomes since the rematch study. Congest Heart Fail 2005;11(3): 133–8.

27. McKellar SH, Allred BD, Marks JD, et al. Treatment of infected left ventricular assist device using antibiotic-impregnated beads. Ann Thorac Surg 1999; 67(2):554–5.

28. Sajjadian A, Valerio IL, Acurturk O, et al. Omental transposition flap for salvage of ventricular assist devices. Plast Reconstr Surg 2006;118(4):919–26.

29. Ochiai Y, McCarthy PM, Smedira NG, et al. Predictors of severe right ventricular failure after implantable left ventricular assist device insertion: analysis of 245 patients. Circulation 2002;106(12 Suppl 1): I198–202.

30. Dang NC, Topkara VK, Mercando M, et al. Right heart failure after left ventricular assist device implantation in patients with chronic congestive heart failure. J Heart Lung Transplant 2006;25(1):1–6.

31. Pagani FD, Long JW, Dembitsky WP, et al. Improved mechanical reliability of the HeartMate XVE left ventricular assist system. Ann Thorac Surg 2006; 82(4):1413–8.

32. Myers TJ, Palanichamy N, La Francesca S, et al. Management of multiple left ventricular assist device failures in a patient. J Heart Lung Transplant 2007; 26(1):98–100.

33. Horton SC, Khodaverdian R, Powers A, et al. Left ventricular assist device malfunction: a systematic approach to diagnosis. J Am Coll Cardiol 2004; 43(9):1574–83.

Cardiac Devices in Emergency Department Heart Failure Patients

James F. Neuenschwander II, MD, FACEP*

KEYWORDS

- Heart failure • Cardiac arrhythmias
- Cardiac pacing • Ultrafiltration • Pacemaker
- Internal cardioverter defibrillator

Noncardiologists frequently provide care for patients with cardiac devices in the event that a cardiologist is not available or the patient is too ill to wait for a scheduled office appointment. As these devices are quite sophisticated, this article attempts to provide a basic understanding of the indications for these therapies, how to diagnose a potential problem, and whom to contact if a malfunction has occurred. The article also discusses the information obtainable from these devices and how it can be incorporated into the clinical approach to help guide management.

IMPLANTABLE PACEMAKERS AND INTERNAL CARDIAC DEFIBRILLATORS
History and Background

With an aging United States population, the prevalence of heart disease continues to increase. Patients who previously would have died from complications of their diseases now survive to present to the hospital in acute distress. Furthermore, an increasing population of at-risk patients provides a greater number of patients who can derive benefit from devices to improve their cardiac function.

The first pacemaker was implanted in 1958 and the first defibrillator was placed at the Johns Hopkins Hospital in 1980. When key studies demonstrated increased survival in patients with the implantation of an internal cardioverter defibrillator (ICD),[1-3] the number of patients with such devices increased dramatically. More than 100,000 such devices are implanted annually in the United States alone, and the noncardiologist can expect to encounter an increasing number of patients with these devices.[4] Several studies have shown the cost effectiveness of ICDs in patients at high risk for ventricular tachycardia/ventricular fibrillation (VT/VF) when compared with antiarrhythmic drug therapy.[5] ICDs have been shown to benefit patients with documented VT/VF (secondary prevention) and patients at risk for VT/VF with a lower ejection fraction but no prior VT/VF (primary prevention) when compared with antiarrhythmic therapy.[6]

An ICD consists of a pulse generator, a lead system, and electrodes capable of sensing and shocking. The size of the devices has decreased and they can be implanted subcutaneously or in the area of the pectoral muscle. Some of these devices are capable of defibrillation, cardioversion, and pacing both bradycardic and tachycardic rhythms. The monitoring of these devices has also become sophisticated enough that physiologic data can be tracked in the patient's home through telemetry and can provide reporting to medical providers on a daily basis. Although an ICD can only be programmed by highly trained and qualified personnel, the interrogation of such devices is straight forward, requiring only the

The author has received funding support from Medtronic for Research Grant Speakers Bureau: Medtronic, St. Jude, Boston Scientific.
The Ohio State University, Columbus, OH, USA
* Department of Emergency Medicine, The Ohio State University, 376 West 10th Avenue, Columbus, OH 43210-1252.
E-mail address: james.neuenschwander@osumc.edu

Heart Failure Clin 5 (2009) 63–73
doi:10.1016/j.hfc.2008.08.012

> **Box 1**
> **Class I/II recommendations for pacemaker/internal cardiac defibrillator defribrillator implantation**
>
> *Pacemaker indications*
>
> Sinus node dysfunction
>
> Atrioventricular (AV) node conduction abnormality
>
> Type II second-degree block
>
> Third-degree block
>
> Cardiomyopathy
>
> Autonomic nervous system disorder
>
> Atrial fibrillation with sinus node dysfunction
>
> *ICD indications*
>
> Cardiac arrest because of ventricular fibrillation or ventricular tachycardia
>
> Ventricular tachycardia in association with structural heart disease
>
> Syncope of undetermined origin with clinically relevant, hemodynamically significant sustained ventricular tachycardia
>
> Nonsustained ventricular tachycardia in patients with coronary disease, prior myocardial infarction,
>
> *Left ventricular (LV) dysfunction*
>
> Spontaneous sustained ventricular tachycardia in patients without structural heart disease not amenable to other treatments
>
> Patients with LV ejection fraction less than 30% at least 1 month after myocardial infarction and 3 months after coronary artery revascularization surgery
>
> Cardiac arrest presumed to be due to ventricular fibrillation when electrophysiology testing is precluded by other medical conditions
>
> Symptoms (eg, syncope) attributable to ventricular tachyarrhythmias in cardiac transplant candidates
>
> Familial or inherited conditions with a high risk for life-threatening ventricular tachyarrhythmias
>
> Long QT syndrome or hypertrophic cardiomyopathy
>
> Nonsustained ventricular tachycardia with coronary artery disease, prior myocardial infarction, LV dysfunction, and inducible sustained ventricular tachycardia or fibrillation at electrophysiology study
>
> Recurrent syncope of undetermined origin in the presence of ventricular dysfunction and inducible ventricular arrhythmias at electrophysiology study
>
> Syncope of unexplained origin or family history of unexplained sudden cardiac death in association with typical or atypical right bundle-branch block and ST-segment elevations (Brugada syndrome)
>
> Syncope in patients with advanced structural heart disease in whom thorough invasive and noninvasive investigations have failed to define a cause
>
> *Data from* Gregoratos G, Abrams J, Epstein AE, et al. ACC/AHA/NASPE 2002 guideline update for implantation of cardiac pacemakers and antiarrhythmia devices: summary article: a report of the American College of Cardiology/American Heart Association Task Force on Practice Guidelines (ACC/AHA/NASPE Committee to Update the 1998 Pacemaker Guidelines). Circulation 2002;106(16)2145–61; and McMullan J, Valento M, Attari M, et al. Care of the pacemaker/implantable cardioverter defibrillator patient in the ED. Am J Emerg Med 2007;25(7)812–22.

proper equipment and the education to interpret the results.[7]

Indications for pacemakers/ICDs are expanding and are important for physicians to understand (**Box 1**).[8,9] As patients in the United States medical system are frequently discharged from the hospital as soon as possible, physicians may want to take a more active role in making early consultations to cardiologists for evaluation of device implantation. Early consultation may promote the likelihood of a referral if a device is warranted. It should be noted that not all patients benefit from ICD implantation. Current guidelines recommend against ICD implantation in patients with the occurrence of VT/VF while the patient is in the acute phase of ST elevation myocardial infarction, noncardiac terminal illness that is expected to result in death within 6 months or less, those with New York Heart Association (NYHA) congestive heart failure that is class IV, and correctable causes of arrhythmias, such as acute myocardial infarction, electrolyte imbalance, or drug toxicity.[9]

The functionality of the pacemaker and ICD is described by a five position code established by the North American Society of Pacing and Electrophysiology and the British Pacing and Electrophysiology Group (**Table 1**).[9,10] For example, a pacemaker may be described as DVI, indicating that both chambers (D for Dual) atrial and ventricular are paced. The second letter V indicates that the ventricle is (third letter, I) inhibited by native ventricular activity but the atrium is not (see **Box 1** and **Table 1**).[8–11]

Patients may present to the Emergency Department (ED) with a variety of complications following pacemaker or ICD implantation, including heart failure, acute myocardial infarction, infection, vascular injury, hemorrhage, arrhythmias, and thromboembolism.[11,12] Inadvertent shocks, component failure, lead fracture, pacemaker interference,

Table 1
Pacemaker terminology as adopted by the North American Society of Pacing and Electrophysiology and the British Pacing and Electrophysiology Group

Position 1	Position 2	Position 3	Position 4	Position 5
Chamber paced	Chamber sensed	Response to sensed event	Programmability and rate response	Anti-tachycardia function
V = Ventricle	V =Ventricle	I = Inhibited	O = Not programmable	O = None
A = Atrium	A = Atrium	T = Triggered or tracking	P = Simple programming	P = Pacing
D = Dual	D = Dual	D = Dual	M = Multiprogrammable	S = Shock
O = No pacing	O = No sensing	O = No response	C = Communicating (M & telemetry) R = Rate responsive	D = Dual (shock and pacing)

From McMullan J, Valento M, Attari M, et al. Care of the pacemaker/implantable cardioverter defibrillator patient in the ED. Am J Emerg Med 2007;25(7):812–22; with permission.

a false sensation of being shocked or "phantom shock," and psychologic disorders are other potential complications with which patients may present.[12,13]

Presentation and Evaluation of the Patient with an Internal Cardioverter Defribrillator or Pacemaker

Patients may present with ICD or pacemaker issues for a number of different reasons. The history should include their specific complaint and the timing and issues surrounding their presentation. The physical examination should be done with careful attention paid to hemodynamic status, the implantation site, and overall cardiovascular status. Cardiac tamponade can occur following a device being inserted, so the classic triad of muffled heart sounds, hypotension, and distended neck veins must be sought out in a patient with recent device placement. Evidence of infection, such as erythema, edema, tenderness, and fluctuance over the pacemaker pocket should be noted.

Ancillary testing should include an electrocardiograph (EKG) to evaluate rhythm, conduction, and other potential cardiac abnormalities. A chest radiograph looking for lead fracture or lead displacement can be useful. Cardiac markers can be added when an ischemic event may have precipitated the presentation. It should be noted that cardiac markers may remain briefly elevated after implantation because of manipulation of the myocardium. Electrolytes may be helpful in evaluating the etiology of an arrhythmia and levels of any significant medications should be checked.

Pacemaker or Internal Cardioverter Defribrillator Interrogation

Patients presenting with possible cardiac symptoms, such as lightheadedness, syncope, ICD discharge, or palpitations should have an interrogation of their pacemaker or ICD. While it may be that minor modifications to the pacemaker or ICD are all that are required to avert a hospitalization, the diagnostic evaluation and medical interventions should proceed while waiting for an interrogation. Once a representative of the pacemaker manufacturer or other trained specialist has been identified, the interrogation can proceed. The process occurs by radiofrequency transmission after a "wand" is placed over the device. The interrogation can provide information including, but not limited to, the date it was implanted, the physician that implanted it, model, type, battery status, lead integrity, programmed rate, mode, atrial fibrillation load, episodes of VT/VF, and in some cases, parameters to evaluate heart failure. Most pacemakers and ICDs will retain information for up to a year concerning the amount of time spent in pacing, heart rate ranges, high rate atrial and ventricular episodes, and specifics of the type and time of therapies, such as shocks or overdrive pacing. Some devices contain the ability to determine how many hours a patient has been active, their heart rate variability, and the amount of internal thoracic impendence.

When patients present with the complaint of being shocked, the interrogation can determine if the shock actually occurred or not. The appropriateness of the shock can also be distinguished, as supraventricular tachycardia may occasionally trigger a shock. Electromagnetic interference with the device can sometimes produce symptoms and will be discussed in the subsection titled "Other pacemaker issues." Arrhythmias can produce dizziness or syncope and evaluating the pacemaker can help in the evaluation of the patient.

The patient with a pacemaker or ICD is supposed to carry a card with information including manufacturer, model number, therapeutic options, and lead system. Each device can only be interrogated by the manufacturer's programmer or reader. A representative of the device (pacemaker or ICD) company or other electrophysiology nurse or technician can be contacted to interrogate the equipment. The Appendix lists company names and contact numbers for the majority of devices used currently. If the patient does not have a card, a search of the medical records for the operation note will likely provide the make and model of the implantable device. In addition, device manufacturers maintain registries with the patient's identification to assist with correctly matching a patient to their device.

Using Device Data in Heart Failure Management

Some devices possess data that may be useful in diagnosing the presence or absence of heart failure. Impedance cardiography (ICG) has been shown to be a noninvasive measurement of cardiac output, cardiac index, and thoracic fluid content.[14,15] Electrical impedance is the resistance to flow of an electrical current. Blood and fluids are good conductors and therefore have low impedance, while bone and tissue have higher impedance because of their poor conductivity.[16] These devices have been shown to provide information that is helpful in determining a diagnosis in the ED, identifying patients at increased near-term risk of recurrent decompensation, or predict hospitalization. ICG monitors can be used at the bedside by applying four pairs of electrodes to the neck and thorax. As the flow of fluid changes, the electrical impedance changes proportionally. The machine can then calculate a number of hemodynamic parameters, including systemic vascular resistance, stroke volume, cardiac output, and an index of thoracic fluid. The increased fluid in the thorax that occurs in a heart failure exacerbation decreases overall average impedance and can suggest a fluid overloaded state.[14–16]

Some ICDs have the capability of monitoring intrathoracic impedance.[17–19] Selected Medtronic ICDs have this capability in the form of Optivol, which has shown an inverse correlation between intrathoracic impedance and intracardiac filling pressure in the NYHA class III and IV patients.[18]

In a study by Wang, the device recorded 64 measurements between noon and 5 PM and averaged them for a single data point per day. Impedance measurement decreased with increased thoracic fluid an average of about 2 weeks before symptom onset and hospitalization, suggesting that physicians may be able to intervene before symptom onset. A default setting for Optivol had a 76.9% sensitivity for predicting hospitalization.[19] Less encouraging results were reported in another study, which demonstrated a sensitivity of 60% to detect heart failure decompensation but had a 40% false-positive rate.[20] These devices show promise in preliminary data, yet larger trials are needed in the acute care setting.

Some manufacturers of pacemakers and ICDs, such as Boston Scientific, provide home monitoring of device functions, blood pressure, and weight measurements. This information has the potential to be very helpful to a physician managing the patient. The amount of time a patient spends in daily activity can be tracked and used to help determine the likelihood of heart failure. Heart rate variability and atrial fibrillation burden can also be incorporated into determining the presence or absence of heart failure.[21]

Surgical Complications of Pacemakers and Internal Cardioverter Defribrillators

Surgical complications stemming from pacemaker or ICD implantation are numerous and can be encountered in the ED. Arterial or venous bleeding because of dissection of fascial planes can cause a hematoma at the implantation site. Up to 1% to 2% of all large palpable hematomas will require surgical evacuation.[22] Surgical intervention is recommended and needle aspiration should be avoided because of its ineffectiveness and risk of introducing infection.[23]

Infections with ICDs can be classified as early (less than 60 days) after implantation or late. Up to 8% of patients will be affected by infection of their device.[9] The early infections present as typical skin infections with erythema, edema, and tenderness at the wound site. Late infections have a more indolent presentation and pain can be the only complaint. *Staphylococcus aureus* and *epidermidis* are cited as being responsible for about 70% to 95% of all pacemaker and ICD infections and current recommendations state vancomycin should be started in the ED.[24,25] A complete blood count, blood cultures, and empiric antibiotics should be started when an infection is suspected. Aspiration of the device pocket can be useful and is best left to a physician experienced with this procedure because of the potential of damaging a lead or other complications. A noncontrast CT of the chest can help in determining how extensive the infection has become. As with any infected hardware, definitive treatment is to remove any or all of the affected equipment.[22,23,26,27] A rare complication of pacemaker or ICD implantation is wound dehiscence, which can occur postoperatively and is attributed to stress on the suture lines. Surgical intervention for this problem is required.[23]

Lead Complications of Pacemakers and Internal Cardioverter Defribrillator

Lead placement and interface abnormalities at the electrode/myocardium junction can give rise to complications in patients with a pacemaker or ICD. Pneumothorax is estimated to occur in about 1.6% to 2.6% of all cases.[28] The patient will typically complain of shortness of breath and present within the first 24 to 48 hours after the procedure. Local standards will dictate management, but most physicians will consider treating a 10% or greater pneumothorax with tube thoracostomy.

Air embolism can occur during a pacemaker or ICD implantation and should be considered in the patient presenting with dyspnea. This complication is usually well tolerated because the emboli are usually small and absorbed into the lung parenchyma. In the case of large emboli that cause hemodynamic compromise or hemodynamic instability, inotropic support, 100% oxygen, and hyperbaric oxygen may be needed.[23,29]

Venous thromboembolism can occur because of a damaged endothelium during lead placement. When the clot occurs in the subclavian or brachiocephalic vein, the patient can present with swelling and pain in the arm of the affected side. Superior vena cava syndrome can also occur, but is rare and can be diagnosed with duplex ultrasound. Treatment is anticoagulation. Lead removal is rarely indicated in this setting and in some cases may even lead to extension of the thrombus.[23,30]

Infection is a serious complication. Bacterial growth along the lead and its insulation are usually caused by staphylococci. Vegetations can be visualized with transesophageal echocardiography and blood cultures may be helpful in identifying the causative agent. Endocarditis can present acutely with fever and signs of sepsis. Fevers, chills, wasting, and pulmonary involvement can characterize chronic infections in the patient that is two or more years from implantation.[31] Lead infection is an absolute indication for lead removal and empiric antibiotics.[23]

A lead can dislodge and migrate from the myocardium interface and is commonly seen in the first 1 to 2 days after a pacemaker is implanted. Late dislodgement is rare, owing to fibrinous adherence of the lead that occurs secondary to the inflammatory response. A chest radiograph will demonstrate the leads in the coronary sinus, left ventricle, or in the inferior or superior vena cava. The leads can also migrate to the pulmonary artery or the atrium outside of the appendage. Hiccups and pectoral spasm can be encountered in the event of a lead migration or dislodgement.[9,27] This occurs secondary to diaphragmatic irritation and can be diagnosed on chest radiograph. Treatment is lead replacement and the patient can be kept comfortable by deactivating the ICD if external monitoring and defibrillation are available.

Separation of the lead can present as pacemaker malfunction with either failure to capture or undersensing (see "Pacemaker malfunctions and terms").[30] Coronary sinus lead dislodgement alternatively can lead to atrial oversensing and ventricular inhibition. Patients may present in a number of ways but their symptoms will most likely stem from their pacemaker not functioning. They may feel tired or present in heart failure or atrial fibrillation. Myocardial perforation, dysrhythmias, and pulmonary vein thrombosis can also result from lead dislodgement.[23] If a patient is having a lead complication and is unable to pace as a result, external or transvenous pacing should be instituted, especially if the patient is hemodynamically compromised.

A perforation of the myocardium can occur during lead placement and can be difficult to diagnose. The electrode can penetrate the myocardium and stimulate the surrounding structures, including the diaphragm, causing hiccups. The more concerning complication is a pericardial effusion, which may be diagnosed with a bedside ultrasound. An emergent pericardiocentesis may be indicated in the setting of cardiac tamponade.[4,32]

Pacemaker Malfunctions and Terms

"Failure to pace" is the abnormal absence of an artifact of stimulation from the pacemaker and is characterized by the absence on EKG of pacing spikes after an escape interval.[32] Patients may have symptoms such as fatigue or heart failure. This can occur secondary to lack of pacemaker output or failure to capture. Output failures can occur with intrinsic pacemaker problems, such as battery malfunction, lead fracture, or connection issues. Trauma can damage the pacemaker or generator, which will necessitate temporary external pacing.

"Failure to capture" is defined as the inability of an appropriately discharged pacing spike to depolarize nonrefractory tissue.[32] Failure to capture can be visualized on EKG as a pacer spike that does not produce an effective pacing stimulus. Multiple causes, including battery failure, lead fracture or dislodgement, faulty connections, and cardiac perforations can cause failure to capture. Electrolyte derangements can lead to this problem, as well as antidysrhythmic drugs at supratherapeutic levels and even flecainide at therapeutic levels.[9]

"Oversensing" is the unintended detection of electrical complexes by the pacemaker and is characterized on EKG by inhibition of the pacemaker and by the absence of pacing spikes after an exceeded escape interval.[32] Oversensing can occur when the pacemaker senses the ventricle is in its native rhythm by accidentally interpreting a skeletal muscle contraction as ventricular. Electromagnetic interference, lithotripsy, cellular telephones, and lead fractures can lead to this complication.

"Undersensing" is defined as failure of the pacemaker to detect an electrical complex demonstrated on EKG by pacing spikes that are preceded by intrinsic P waves or QRS complexes. This can occur with lead fracture, lead positioning, inappropriate program sensitivity, myocardial infarction, myocardial fibrosis, electrolyte disturbances, battery failure, antiarrhythmic medications, and component failure.[32]

To manage these patients, physicians should first consider external pacing in symptomatic pacemaker-dependent patients while the source of the problem is sought. A chest radiograph can be helpful in identifying a lead fracture or migration. Correctable causes, such as hyperkalemia or acidosis or alkalosis should be addressed quickly, as they can lead to failure to capture. Antidysrhythmic medication levels need evaluation and treatment in appropriate patients. An electrophysiologist should be consulted early in all these processes for input and updates.

Pacemaker-Induced Tachycardias

Pacemaker-mediated tachycardia (PMT) can occur when a re-entry dysrhythmia is triggered by a premature ventricular complex. When a retrograde signal is transmitted through the AV node, the atria are depolarized and the atrial sensor then stimulates the ventricle to contract, thus creating a nonstop loop. The rate is limited by the programmed limit so the tachycardia may not be pronounced, but in some instances ischemia can develop. PMT can be treated by placing a magnet over the pacer that places it into an asynchronous mode. Another treatment option is adenosine, which effectively blocks retrograde AV conduction.[24] Most pacemakers on the market today have algorithms to prevent and terminate PMT.

Runaway pacemaker occurs because of generator malfunction owing to external damage, battery failure, or some other cause. A tachycardia up to 400 beats per minute can occur, which can trigger other arrhythmias such as VT/VF.[24] The emergency physician can place a magnet over the pacer to slow the rate, but definitive treatment, such as reprogramming or generator removal, is often necessary. In severe cases, severing the leads may be warranted.[33] Most modern pacemakers are programmed not to discharge above an upper limit, so encountering this situation is very unlikely.

Other Pacemaker Issues

Pacemaker syndrome can occur when suboptimal pacing modes or programming lead to a loss of AV synchrony. This situation is encountered most frequently in single chamber ventricular-paced systems, but can occur in dual chamber systems as well. Typically, the patient will present with symptoms of decreased perfusion, such as fatigue, headache, confusion, dyspnea, and even syncope. Symptoms are because of the decrease in preload, which is lost when the atrial contribution is negated and the pressure in the atria increases. Eventually cardiac output will fall and blood pressure can decrease, leading to alteration in baroreceptors, which can lead to increased vagal tone. Acute heart failure can develop with this syndrome as well. The management of pacemaker syndrome is to restore AV synchrony through a mechanism, such as switching from a single chamber to dual-chamber pacing system.

Acute coronary syndrome is difficult to diagnose in pacemaker patients with ventricular pacing because of their baseline left bundle branch pattern on EKG. Sgarbossa and colleagues[34] developed criteria that include looking for ST elevation of 5 mm or more that are discordant with (in the opposite direction from) the QRS complex, concordant ST elevation of 1 mm or greater, and ST depression of 1 mm or greater in leads V1, V2, or V3, which may be of some utility. In patients who are not pacemaker-dependent, the rate can be slowed and the native rhythm may demonstrate an injury current.

Interference with pacemakers is possible with some forms of external electromagnetic interference (EMI), such as cell phones. Pacemaker settings, such as mode, sensitivity, polarity, and refractory period, can be affected. Although permanent damage is unlikely form most forms of

EMI, high-energy sources, such as external defibrillation, must be used with caution. If external defibrillator paddles are used, they should be placed in the anterior/posterior position and away from the device as much as possible to avoid damaging the circuit. MRI is contraindicated in patients with pacemakers and ICDs, although some case reports have shown success.[35] Complications, such as reprogramming devices, inappropriate therapies, high-rate pacing, burns, and other injuries have been reported in patients undergoing an MRI. Efforts to manufacture an MRI-safe device are underway but have not been completely successful thus far.[4,26] Lithotripsy, which is used in the treatment of nephrolithiasis, can also cause complications, but specific measures to increase safety can be taken. Cell phones rarely cause more than temporary complaints of palpitations and can be eliminated as the distance between the pacemaker and cell phone is widened.

Evaluation of the Patient Presenting for an Internal Cardioverter Defribrillator Shock or Shocks

Most cardiologists do not encourage their patients to go to the ED after a single shock unless they experienced specific symptoms, such as chest pain or syncope. But the firing of an ICD can be concerning to the patient and their loved ones and often prompts an ED visit. Once in the ED a careful history concerning the timing and events surrounding the shock should be gathered. Cardiology consultation is warranted. Often an interrogation will be done and reassurance can be given to the patient. If more concerning symptoms surrounding the shock are present, such as syncope, chest pain, palpitations, and dyspnea, a more extensive work-up is recommended.

When a patient presents for multiple shocks, the situation is more concerning. The evaluation in the ED should begin by placing the patient on a cardiac monitor and having external defibrillation immediately available. Interrogation of the device should be arranged while the work-up for correctable causes, such as metabolic and electrolyte disturbances, commences. An EKG and chest radiograph are useful sources of information in the process.

Acute coronary syndrome leading to arrhythmias can cause ICD intervention. EKG evaluation may show transient ST elevation or depression in the after-shock state, even in the absence of cardiac ischemia. The EKG should return to normal state within 15 minutes of a shock if no ischemia is occurring. If the EKG does not return to its baseline within that time, new coronary artery ischemia is likely. Elevated cardiac biomarkers are common after a shock and make the diagnosis even more difficult. One third of patients will have elevated troponin T, and about 16% will have elevated troponin I up to 24 hours after an ICD fires.[26,36]

Patients may have a brief bradycardic episode following an ICD shock and dependent pacing is not uncommon. The amount of time the patient needs the pacing varies, but it usually begins within 5 seconds after the shock. Most ICDs have this feature, although future subcutaneous models may not.[27,37]

"Electrical storm" refers to high numbers of successive shocks in a short period.[30] Definitions vary on this phenomenon but the occurrence of three or more distinct episodes of arrhythmia requiring intervention in a 24-hour period is often cited.[38–40] It is estimated that up to 30% of all patients with ICDs will experience a "storm" at some point. The distinction between appropriate and inappropriate shocks must be determined, but device malfunction can be a common cause for this problem. Because recurrent VT is prevalent in this situation, aggressive management is warranted.[40] Use of the magnet to stop further shocks is only warranted when the therapy is clearly inappropriate, as in the alert and stable patient with atrial fibrillation and rapid ventricular response. If the rhythm causing the shocks is malignant, therapy should be directed at terminating the arrhythmia. External cardioversion may be necessary if internal cardioversion is unsuccessful and drugs like amiodarone should be considered.[26,40] Patients with electrical storm should be admitted to the intensive care unit for aggressive monitoring and an electrophysiologist should be consulted as soon as possible for possible catheter ablation of an arrhythmogenic foci to quiet the storm.[23]

Inappropriate shocks are most commonly the result of supraventricular tachycardias, including atrial fibrillation and atrial flutter.[4,27] Although these rhythms are rarely lethal, they frequently require interventions, such as rate control, anticoagulation, and ICD-sensing threshold adjustments. Complexes that can sometimes be mistakenly interpreted as ventricular tachycardia are a new left bundle branch block or unusually prominent P, T, or U waves.[4,23] Any patient presenting with a new pathologic rhythm should receive the same standard care regardless of the presence of an ICD.

Malfunction of device components, such as lead fractures, insulation damage, and loose connections frequently lead to ED visits because of ICD discharges.[27] The diagnosis may be evident on chest radiograph, but device interrogation is needed for confirmation. Hospitalization is recommended for a device failure until the repair or replacement is complete.

A multitude of electromagnetic interference sources causing shocks have been named, including cell phones, television remote controls, large speakers, metal detectors, slot machines, electric razors, and antitheft detection devices.[27] Although exposure to these sources may be identified in some instances, work-up for other correctable sources of pacemaker malfunction is warranted.

The use of magnets to disable inappropriate ICD therapies is necessary in some instances and can be done without altering the back-up bradycardia-pacing function.[26,27] Some ICDs will not restart their therapies after the magnet is removed; thus, all devices will need interrogation after a magnet is used. External pacing and defibrillation may be needed. In some instances a patient's body habitus may render a single magnet ineffective and the use of two magnets in "stacked" fashion has been reported.[23]

Cardiac arrest in the patient with an ICD raises certain questions in health care providers but does not need to be treated much differently than usual. Advanced cardiac life-support protocols are recommended with the paddles being placed in anterior-posterior pattern to avoid damaging the device.[4,26,32] An unpleasant tingle has been described by resuscitation providers during an ICD discharge; no injury to providers has been reported and can be avoided by wearing gloves.[4,41]

An ICD may fail to rescue a patient in up to one-third of all cardiac deaths, even if the rhythm is appropriate for shock therapy.[42] Failure of these devices to meet expectations has prompted researchers, clinicians, government agencies, and industry to work to improve the effectiveness of these instruments. Many ICDs will only deliver five successive shocks, to conserve battery life and to avoid the risk of damaging heart muscle and the heart's conduction system.[27,41] Additionally, lidocaine and amiodarone can increase the defibrillation threshold, making ICD therapy ineffective.[26,27] If a patient is successfully resuscitated, the ICD will need to be interrogated to insure proper functioning before external monitoring and therapies are stopped.[43]

Ethical issues around the end of life can occur with patients who have ICDs. The patient may ask a physician to discontinue the ICD therapy because the shocks are painful and they have decided to reject further treatment. This is ethically equivalent to withdrawing specific therapies, such as hemodialysis, and is therefore appropriate because of the firmly established right of informed patients to be free of unwanted medical intervention.[44] Certainly conversations with the patient, the family, their primary care physician, and other concerned parties can be entered with the hope of finding a solution that best fits each situation.

Central venous catheter placement can be affected if an ICD is present. Thrombosis along the lead system is common, with complete occlusion approaching 20% at 2 years[22] and subclavian stenosis is common too.[27] Because of these factors, accessing the ipsilateral subclavian vein of a device is complicated. Additionally, contacting the lead system with a metal wire can cause an inappropriate shock, but can be avoided by temporarily deactivating the ICD or not using a metal guidewire. Pulmonary artery catheters offer unique challenges and are probably best inserted with the assistance of fluoroscopy.[4] Femoral vein catheters may be the safest option, but the contralateral subclavian or internal jugular can be accessed with caution.[43]

Electrocautery can be mistaken as an arrhythmia and lead to an ICD shock. Suggestions to disable the device before surgery have been made[4,26] when using unipolar devices, although bipolar devices (ie, Bovie) are generally considered safe. Radiation therapy can be damaging to ICDs and should be considered as a source of problems for patients undergoing that type of therapy for cancer. The device can be safely shielded to prevent malfunction.[27]

Occasionally patients will present to the ED with a beeping device. This can signal any number of internal dysfunctions, such as lead fracture, software failure, battery depletion or other issues with the ICD.[4,27] Interrogation is indicated while the patient is safely monitored with external defibrillation and pacing immediately available.

New onset right heart failure can be encountered when ICDs damage valve leaflets and precipitate severe tricuspid valve regurgitation. The mechanism of damage can be from adhesion, perforation, or primary impairment of valve leaflets.[45] Echocardiography can confirm the diagnosis and lead replacement and valvular repair are urgently indicated.

Industry recalls and safety alerts can affect up to 43% of all ICD patients.[8,46,47] This has garnered a fair amount of anxiety and distrust among patients and can make encounters somewhat difficult. Little help, other than monitoring and supportive care, can be offered by the physician. Information concerning what device or equipment is under recall can be obtained from the manufacturer (see Appendix) and distributed to the patient to discuss with their cardiologist.

Succinylcholine can cause muscle fasciculations and can lead to inappropriate shocks associated with oversensing.[48] Nondepolarizing agents can be used as an alternative, or the emergency physician can use a "defasciculating" dose before administering succinylcholine.

ULTRAFILTRATION

Ultrafiltration has become a therapy option for patients with an element of "diuretic resistance" that are volume overloaded. Hydrostatic pressures draw off fluid across a semipermeable membrane, thus eliminating excess fluids. Small swings in electrolyte balances have been experienced even when large volumes are removed. The patient also seems to experience fewer hemodynamic imbalances in comparison to hemodialysis, even when 500 or more milliliters an hour have been taken off.[49,50] Using peripheral access points has made this modality possible in a multitude of clinical sites including the ED.[51] More studies are to be undertaken to assess the future role of ultrafiltration in the management of heart failure.

SUMMARY

Patients with pacemakers and internal cardioverter defibrillators can experience a number of benefits and complications related to their devices. Physicians must be aware of the internal workings and potential complications associated with this technology. The number of patients with these devices is likely to increase and so is their level of sophistication, so consistent attention is necessary to stay up to date with patient management. Along with the evolving pacemaker and ICD therapy available, ultrafiltration has the promise to improve patient care.

APPENDIX: 24-HOUR CONTACT NUMBERS FOR INDUSTRY REPRESENTATIVES OF PACEMAKERS AND INTERNAL CARDIOVERTER DEFRIBRILLATORS

Biotronik: 800-284-6689
Boston Scientific (formerly Guidant):
  800-227-3422
Medtronic: 800-633-8766
St.Jude Medical: 800-722-3774

REFERENCES

1. Moss AJ, Hall WJ, Cannom DS, et al. Improved survival with an implanted defibrillator in patients with coronary disease at high risk for ventricular arrhythmia. Multicenter Automatic Defibrillator Implantation Trial investigators. N Engl J Med 1996;335(26): 1933–40.
2. Moss AJ, Zareba W, Hall WJ, et al. Prophylactic implantation of a defibrillator in patients with myocardial infarction and reduced ejection fraction. N Engl J Med 2002;346(12):877–83.
3. Bardy GH, Lee KL, Mark DB, et al. Amiodarone or an implantable cardioverter-defibrillator for congestive heart failure. N Engl J Med 2005;352(3):225–37.
4. Stevenson WG, Chaitman BR, Ellenbogen KA, et al. Clinical assessment and management of patients with implanted cardioverter-defibrillators presenting to non-electrophysiologists. Circulation 2004;110(25):3866–9.
5. Lynd LD, O'Brien BJ. Cost-effectiveness of the implantable cardioverter defibrillator: a review of current evidence. J Cardiovasc Electrophysiol 2003; 14(Suppl 9):S99–103.
6. Bhatia A, Cooley R, Berger M, et al. The implantable cardioverter defibrillator: technology, indications, and impact on cardiovascular survival. Curr Probl Cardiol 2004;29(6):303–56.
7. Neuenschwander J, Hiestand BC, Sondrup L, et al. The benefit of interrogating defibrillators by emergency department personnel [abstract]. Presented at the American College of Emergency Physicians.
8. Gregoratos G, Abrams J, Epstein AE, et al. ACC/ AHA/NASPE 2002 guideline update for implantation of cardiac pacemakers and antiarrhythmia devices: summary article: a report of the American College of Cardiology/American Heart Association Task Force on Practice Guidelines (ACC/AHA/NASPE Committee to Update the 1998 Pacemaker Guidelines). Circulation 2002;106(16):2145–61.
9. McMullan J, Valento M, Attari M, et al. Care of the pacemaker/implantable cardioverter defibrillator patient in the ED. Am J Emerg Med 2007;25(7):812–22.
10. Bernstein AD, Daubert JC, Fletcher RD, et al. The revised NASPE/BPEG generic code for antibradycardia, adaptive-rate, and multisite pacing. North American Society of Pacing and Electrophysiology/ British Pacing and Electrophysiology Group. Pacing Clin Electrophysiol 2002;25(2):260–4.
11. Greene HL. Antiarrhythmic drugs versus implantable defibrillators: the need for a randomized controlled study. Am Heart J 1994;127(4 Pt 2):1171–8.
12. Spratt KA, Blumberg EA, Wood CA, et al. Infections of implantable cardioverter defibrillators: approach to management. Clin Infect Dis 1993;17(4):679–85.
13. Herrmann C, von Zur MF, Schaumann A, et al. Standardized assessment of psychological well-being and quality-of-life in patients with implanted defibrillators. Pacing Clin Electrophysiol 1997;20(1 Pt 1):95–103.
14. Packer M, Abraham WT, Mehra MR, et al. Utility of impedance cardiography for the identification of short-term risk of clinical decompensation in stable patients with chronic heart failure. J Am Coll Cardiol 2006;47(11):2245–52.

15. Peacock WF, Summers RL, Vogel J, et al. Impact of impedance cardiography on diagnosis and therapy of emergent dyspnea: the ED-IMPACT trial. Acad Emerg Med 2006;13(4):365–71.

16. Wong GC, Ayas NT. Clinical approaches to the diagnosis of acute heart failure. Curr Opin Cardiol 2007; 22(3):207–13.

17. Yamokoski LM, Haas GJ, Gans B, et al. Optivol fluid status monitoring with an implantable cardiac device: a heart failure management system. Expert Rev Med Devices 2007;4(6):775–80.

18. Yu CM, Wang L, Chau E, et al. Intrathoracic impedance monitoring in patients with heart failure: correlation with fluid status and feasibility of early warning preceding hospitalization. Circulation 2005;112(6):841–8.

19. Wang L. Fundamentals of intrathoracic impedance monitoring in heart failure. Am J Cardiol 2007; 99(10A):3G–10G.

20. Vollmann D, Nagele H, Schauerte P, et al. Clinical utility of intrathoracic impedance monitoring to alert patients with an implanted device of deteriorating chronic heart failure. Eur Heart J 2007;28(15):1835–40.

21. Jensen SB, Galvin CA, Thompson B, et al. Optimizing therapy for heart failure patients: cardiac resynchronization and defibrillator therapy. J Cardiovasc Nurs 2007;22(2):118–24.

22. Pavia S, Wilkoff B. The management of surgical complications of pacemaker and implantable cardioverter-defibrillators. Curr Opin Cardiol 2001;16(1): 66–71.

23. Trohman RG, Kim MH, Pinski SL. Cardiac pacing: the state of the art. Lancet 2004;364(9446):1701–19.

24. Cardall TY, Brady WJ, Chan TC, et al. Permanent cardiac pacemakers: issues relevant to the emergency physician, part II. J Emerg Med 1999;17(4): 697–709.

25. Chambers ST. Diagnosis and management of staphylococcal infections of pacemakers and cardiac defibrillators. Intern Med J 2005;35(Suppl 2):S63–71.

26. Pinski SL. Emergencies related to implantable cardioverter-defibrillators. Crit Care Med 2000; 28(Suppl 10):N174–80.

27. Glikson M, Friedman PA. The implantable cardioverter defibrillator. Lancet 2001;357(9262): 1107–17.

28. Burney K, Burchard F, Papouchado M, et al. Cardiac pacing systems and implantable cardiac defibrillators (ICDs): a radiological perspective of equipment, anatomy and complications. Clin Radiol 2004;59(8): 699–708.

29. Benson J, Adkinson C, Collier R. Hyperbaric oxygen therapy of iatrogenic cerebral arterial gas embolism. Undersea Hyperb Med 2003;30(2):117–26.

30. Byrd CL. Management of implant complications. In: Ellenbogen KA, Kay GN, Wilkoff B, editors. Clinical cardiac pacing. Philadelphia: W.B. Saunders Company; 1995. p. 491–522.

31. Klug D, Lacroix D, Savoye C, et al. Systemic infection related to endocarditis on pacemaker leads: clinical presentation and management. Circulation 1997;95(8):2098–107.

32. Morales TY, Falcon Chevere JL. Implantable electrical devices for dysrhythmia: what every emergency physician must know. Bol Assoc Med P R 2004; 96(3):161–8.

33. Sarko JA, Tiffany BR. Cardiac pacemakers: evaluation and management of malfunctions. Am J Emerg Med 2000;18(4):435–40.

34. Sgarbossa EB, Pinski SL, Barbagelata A, et al. Electrocardiographic diagnosis of evolving acute myocardial infarction in the presence of left bundle-branch block. GUSTO-1 (Global Utilization of Streptokinase and Tissue Plasminogen Activator for Occluded Coronary Arteries) Investigators. N Engl J Med 1996;334(8):481–7.

35. Naehle CP, Sommer T, Meyer C, et al. Strategy for safe performance of magnetic resonance imaging on a patient with implantable cardioverter defibrillator. Pacing Clin Electrophysiol 2006;29(1):113–6.

36. Hurst TM, Hinrichs M, Breidenbach C, et al. Detection of myocardial injury during transvenous implantation of automatic cardioverter-defibrillators. J Am Coll Cardiol 1999;34(2):402–8.

37. Eysmann SB, Marchlinski FE, Buxton AE, et al. Electrocardiographic changes after cardioversion of ventricular arrhythmias. Circulation 1986;73(1):73–81.

38. Arya A, Haghjoo M, Dehghani MR, et al. Prevalence and predictors of electrical storm in patients with implantable cardioverter-defibrillator. Am J Cardiol 2006;97(3):389–92.

39. Credner SC, Klingenheben T, Mauss O, et al. Electrical storm in patients with transvenous implantable cardioverter-defibrillators: incidence, management and prognostic implications. J Am Coll Cardiol 1998;32(7):1909–15.

40. Exner DV, Pinski SL, Wyse DG, et al. Electrical storm presages nonsudden death: the antiarrhythmics versus implantable defibrillators (AVID) trial. Circulation 2001;103(16):2066–71.

41. Calle PA, Buylaert W. When an AED meets an ICD. Automated external defibrillator. Implantable cardioverter defibrillator. Resuscitation 1998;38(3): 177–83.

42. Anderson KP. Sudden cardiac death unresponsive to implantable defibrillator therapy: an urgent target for clinicians, industry and government. J Interv Card Electrophysiol 2005;14(2):71–8.

43. McPherson CA, Manthous C. Permanent pacemakers and implantable defibrillators: considerations for intensivists. Am J Respir Crit Care Med 2004;170(9):933–40.

44. Manganello TD. Disabling the pacemaker: the heart-rending decision every competent patient has a right to make. Health Care Law Mon 2000;3–15.

45. Lin G, Nishimura RA, Connolly HM, et al. Severe symptomatic tricuspid valve regurgitation due to permanent pacemaker or implantable cardioverter-defibrillator leads. J Am Coll Cardiol 2005;45(10): 1672–5.

46. Hauser RG, Kallinen L. Deaths associated with implantable cardioverter defibrillator failure and deactivation reported in the United States Food and Drug Administration Manufacturer and User Facility Device Experience Database. Heart Rhythm 2004; 1(4):399–405.

47. Maisel WH. Physician management of pacemaker and implantable cardioverter defibrillator advisories. Pacing Clin Electrophysiol 2004;27(4):437–42.

48. Stone KR, McPherson CA. Assessment and management of patients with pacemakers and implantable cardioverter defibrillators. Crit Care Med 2004;32(Suppl 4):S155–65.

49. Agostoni PG, Marenzi GC, Pepi M, et al. Isolated ultrafiltration in moderate congestive heart failure. J Am Coll Cardiol 1993;21(2):424–31.

50. DiLeo M, Pacitti A, Bergerone S, et al. Ultrafiltration in the treatment of refractory congestive heart failure. Clin Cardiol 1988;11(7):449–52.

51. Jaski BE, Ha J, Denys BG, et al. Peripherally inserted veno-venous ultrafiltration for rapid treatment of volume overloaded patients. J Card Fail 2003;9(3):227–31.

Acute Heart Failure Risk Stratification: Can We Define Low Risk?

Sean P. Collins, MD, MSc[a],*, Alan B. Storrow, MD[b]

KEYWORDS

- Acute heart failure • Risk-stratification
- Emergency department

The emergency department (ED) evaluation and management of patients who have potential acute heart failure syndromes (AHFS) has remained a significant challenge for decades. Unlike advances in the assessment and treatment of patients who have acute coronary syndrome (**Table 1**), the emergency physician's diagnostic tools for heart failure have remained limited, and the complexity of the syndrome itself has led to risk-averse practice styles with extremely high admission rates.

Moreover, the prevalence of AHFS continues to increase as a result of an aging population, improved survival from acute myocardial infarction, and better management of chronic heart failure. As a direct result, ED visits for AHFS are expected to continue to increase. Despite the development of new diagnostic and prognostic tools, patients who have AHFS continue to have poorly defined treatment end points and a high rate of critical care admissions.[1–3] Previous studies of risk stratification have identified markers of high risk in AHFS, but identification of the "safe for ED discharge" patient at low risk remains elusive. Unfortunately, the lack of high-risk features does not necessarily equate with low risk. Recently, new diagnostic markers and technology have become promising and even commonplace to assist emergency physicians in risk prediction for patients who have AHFS. Familiarity with these approaches is essential for improved care for patients who have heart failure and for resource use. This article reviews the available literature and describes patient features that need to be accounted for in disposition decision-making.

IMPACT OF ACUTE HEART FAILURE SYNDROMES

In 2005, more than 1 million hospital discharges had a primary diagnosis of acute heart failure and consumed 3% of the total national health care budget.[4–6] The high incidence of adverse events in patients who have AHFS has not changed in decades: in-hospital mortality is 4% to 7%; 60-day mortality and recidivism rates are approximately 10% and 25%, respectively.[7–10] There is significant unpredictability about the natural course of AHFS and uncertainty regarding acute clinical stability. Largely as a result of this uncertainty, more than 80% of ED presentations for AHFS are admitted to the hospital. Patients who have AHFS largely rely on EDs and emergency physicians for acute management, because 80% of AHFS admissions originate in an ED. Patients admitted and treated in an inpatient bed for heart failure account for the majority of hospital expenditures.[1,2,11] Based on American College of Cardiology/American Heart Association (ACC/AHA) or Agency for Healthcare Research and Quality guidelines, however, it has been suggested that up to 50% of admitted patients are at low risk and may be candidates for outpatient therapy, with a potential savings of $2.5 billion.[3,12]

Previous Guideline Recommendations for Acute Heart Failure Syndromes

Poor ED risk stratification, particularly overestimation of disease severity, is the fundamental cause

a University of Cincinnati School of Medicine, Cincinnati, OH, USA
b Vanderbilt University School of Medicine, Nashville, TN, USA
* Corresponding author. Department of Emergency Medicine, University of Cincinnati, Medical Sciences Building, Room 6109, 231 Albert Sabin Way, Cincinnati, OH 45267.
E-mail address: sean.collins@uc.edu (S.P. Collins).

Heart Failure Clin 5 (2009) 75–83
doi:10.1016/j.hfc.2008.08.010

Table 1
Characteristics of acute myocardial infarction and acute heart failure syndromes resulting in hospitalization in the United States

Characteristic	Acute Myocardial Infarction	Acute Heart Failure Syndromes
Incidence	1 million/year	1 million/year
Mortality		
Prehospital	High	?
In-hospital	3%–4%	3%–4%
60–90 day	2%	10%
Targets	Clearly defined (thrombosis)	Uncertain
Interventions in clinical trials	Beneficial	Minimal/no benefit/harmful
ACC/AHA recommendations	Level A	None

From Gheorghiade M, Zannad F, Sopko G, et al. Acute heart failure syndromes: current state and framework for future research. Circulation 2005;112(25):3959; with permission.

of the overuse of limited in-hospital resources for this rapidly growing patient population.[2,13] Improving the ability of the emergency physician to decide on the most appropriate disposition of patients who have acute heart failure is critical to maximize the allocation of in-hospital resources.

A review shows that current guidelines for ED disposition are based on little evidence or are provided without any evidence whatsoever.[14–17] The 1995 ACC/AHA guidelines limit their disposition recommendations (class I and II) to hospital admission for new-onset heart failure, chronic heart failure with mild to moderate decompensation, or chronic heart failure complicated by acutely threatening events or clinical situations. Criteria for these conditions are not specifically defined, however. The 2005 ACC/AHA guidelines addressed the evaluation and management of chronic heart failure.[16] The Heart Failure Society of America published detailed guidelines on heart failure management but did not address ED disposition.[14] The European Society of Cardiology addressed diagnosis and treatment of acute heart failure but did not give recommendations on risk stratification or ED disposition.[18] The American College of Emergency Physicians recently published guidelines describing four topics for the emergency physician but, like their predecessors did not provide guidance for risk stratification or disposition.[19]

Defining Heart Failure for the Emergency Department: A New Paradigm

Heart failure can be simplistically defined as a clinical syndrome resulting from any structural or functional cardiac disorder that impairs the ability of the ventricle to fill with or eject blood.[16] The cardinal manifestations are dyspnea and fatigue (exercise intolerance), as well as fluid retention (pulmonary congestion and peripheral edema). A better ED or acute care term would be acute heart failure syndrome (AHFS), defined as a gradual or rapid change in heart failure signs and symptoms, resulting in a need for urgent therapy.[20] These signs and symptoms are primarily due to pulmonary congestion from elevated LV filling pressures and can occur in patients who have preserved or reduced ejection fraction. The term *diastolic dysfunction* refers to an abnormality of LV filling or relaxation; with the addition of effort intolerance and dyspnea, it is called "diastolic heart failure or" "acute heart failure with preserved ejection fraction."[21–23] Acute heart failure syndrome admissions are about 50% female; approximately 75% will have known heart failure, and nearly 50% will have preserved EF.[7,8] For a substantial proportion, the causes in the western world are coronary artery disease, hypertension, and dilated cardiomyopathy.

HIGH-RISK FEATURES THAT CAN BE DETERMINED AT EMERGENCY DEPARTMENT PRESENTATION

During the last 2 decades, many studies of AHFS risk stratification have been conducted and have identified variables predicting early events in patients who have AHFS (**Table 2**). Selker and colleagues[24] developed a model to predict acute hospital mortality from data available to the ED physician within the first 10 minutes of presentation (patients' age, systolic blood pressure and findings, and ECG abnormalities). The model was validated prospectively for mortality, but its validity for morbidity and other acute sequelae is unknown. Additionally, the ability of the model to identify a low-risk patient who can be discharged home safely has not been assessed. Thus, because the model was developed to identify the high-risk patient, and the absence of high-risk features does not define low risk, the usefulness of this model in identifying the low-risk patient is unclear.

Chin and Goldman[25,26] developed a risk model using a larger number of variables (vital signs, co-morbidities, ECG findings, and laboratory data). The model is successful in predicting morbidity as well as mortality, but it cannot delineate the low-risk patient. Katz[27] developed a model that could predict 81% of complications. This model was based on ED information but included a 4-hour diuresis measure, making it less helpful as a decision-making tool early in the emergency setting. Delaying such decision-making can result in a potentially life-threatening therapeutic delay. Additionally, the model missed 19% of cardiopulmonary complications, making it unsuitable for safe implementation.

In one of the largest studies to date, classification and regression tree methodology was used on 45 variables in 65,275 patients who had heart failure to predict in-hospital mortality.[28] Three variables were used to differentiate high-risk patients from low-risk patients: blood urea nitrogen (BUN), systolic blood pressure (SBP), and creatinine. Patients who had a BUN level greater than 43 mg/dL, a SBP less than 115 mm Hg, and a creatinine level over 2.75 mg/dL had a 22% in-hospital mortality rate. Further, the odds ratio for mortality between patients identified as being at high or low risk was 12.9 (95% confidence interval [CI], 10.4–15.9). Although this model is perhaps the most elegant available to date, it remains highly limited because only 39 of more than 100 variables available to the ED physician were considered, and the model was designed only to predict inpatient mortality. Further, patients defined as being at low risk had an inpatient mortality rate of 2.1%, a number exceedingly high to be considered "low-risk" in the ED.

Several recent retrospective analyses of clinical trials and registries reaffirm these findings.[29,30] Hyponatremia (<135 mmol/L) on hospital admission has been associated with increased in-hospital and postdischarge mortality and with increased rates of readmission.[30] Patients who had systolic blood pressure lower than 120 mm Hg on admission had an almost threefold greater risk of in-hospital mortality than patients who had systolic blood pressure higher than 140 mm Hg (7.2% vs. 2.5%, $P < .001$).[29] Finally, renal dysfunction (elevated BUN or creatinine levels) on hospital admission also has been associated with increased rates of in-hospital and postdischarge mortality.[31–33]

In summary, several markers are associated with poor clinical outcomes: an elevated BUN or creatinine level, a low SBP, hyponatremia, ischemic ECG changes, and elevated cardiac biomarkers. Not clear, however, is whether the absence of high-risk physiologic variables can indicate that a patient is at low risk of early events.

LOW-RISK FEATURES THAT CAN BE DETERMINED AT EMERGENCY DEPARTMENT PRESENTATION

Conversely, little has been published to guide the emergency physician in identifying patients who may be categorized as low-risk and possibly discharged after a brief ED stay. A retrospective analysis of a statewide database was performed to identify variables predictive of a low risk of inpatient death or serious complications.[34] Recursive partitioning classified 17.2% of patients as low risk (0.3% mortality, 1.0% inpatient complications). The resultant model was somewhat cumbersome but also identified serum sodium, SBP, and creatinine as differentiators between patients at low and high risk. This model subsequently was validated in more than 8300 admitted patients from a similar database. The authors found that 19% of patients could be classified as low risk, defined as having a 1% to 3% risk of serious complications or death within 30 days of hospitalization.[35] Diercks[36] studied a prospective convenience sample of patients who had AHFS to identify a low-risk cohort of patients who had AHFS suitable for observation unit management. Patients who had a systolic blood pressure over 160 mm Hg at ED presentation and a normal initial cardiac troponin I level were significantly more likely to be discharged from the observation unit and not experience any 30-day adverse events (death, readmission, myocardial infarction, or arrhythmias).

NATRIURETIC PEPTIDES AND RISK STRATIFICATION

Several investigations have evaluated the prognostic ability of natriuretic peptides.[37–43] A study of 325 patients in the ED demonstrated the ability of serum natriuretic peptide (BNP) to predict future cardiac events.[38] Patients presenting to the ED with dyspnea had BNP levels drawn and were followed for 6 months for the combined end points of death (both cardiac and noncardiac), hospital admission with a cardiac diagnosis, and repeat ED visits for heart failure. The area under the receiver operating characteristic curve was 0.87 (95% CI,

Table 2
Previous modeling studies with reported outcomes and variables found to be significant risk indicators

Author/Year	N	Subject Type	Study Type	Outcome[a]	Significant Variables
Filippatos/2007	302	I	R	60-day death/readmission	BUN > 40 mg/dL
Gheorghiade/2007	48,612	I	R	In-hospital and 30-day mortality	Na^{2+} < 135 mmol/L
Formiga/2007	414	I	R	In-hospital mortality	Barthel index, creatinine, edema
Diercks/2006[b]	499	E	P	Length of stay <24 h, 30-day events	SBP, troponin I
Rohde/2006					
Gheorghiade/2006	48,612	I	R	In-hospital and 30-day mortality	SBP < 120
Barsheshet/2006	1122	I	R	In-hospital mortality	Age, glucose, female sex, creatinine, low SBP, NYHA class III/IV
Burkhardt/2005	385	I	R	Observation unit discharge	BUN
Auble/2005[b]	33,533	I	R	Inpatient complications and mortality	Na^{2+}, SBP, white blood cell count, pH, creatinine
Fonarow/2005	65,275	I	R	Inpatient mortality	BUN, creatinine, SBP
Klein/2005	949	I	R	Days hospitalized over 2 months	Na^{2+}
Felker/2004	949	I	R	60-day mortality/readmission	Age, SBP, BUN, Na^{2+}, Hgb, # past admissions, class IV symptoms
Lee/2003	4031	I	R	30-day and 1-year mortality	Age, SBP, RR, BUN, Na^{2+}
Harjai/2001	434	I	R	30-day readmission	Sex; COPD; prior admissions
Butler/1998	120	I	R	Inpatient complications	O_2 saturation; creatinine; pulmonary edema
Villacorta/1998	57	I	R	Inpatient/6-month death	Na^{2+}; sex
Chin/1997	257	I	R, S	60-day readmission/death	Marital status; comorbidity index; SBP on admission; No ST-T changes

Chin/1996	435	I	R	Inpatient complications	Initial SBP; RR; Na^{2+}; ST-T changes
Selker/1994	401	I	PA, R	Inpatient mortality	Age; SBP; T-wave flattening; heart rate
Brophy/1993	153	E	P	Length of stay and 6-month mortality	Left atrial size; cardiac ischemia; diuresis
Esdaile/1992	191	I	PA, R	Inpatient mortality	Age; chest pain; cardiac ischemia; valvular disease; arrhythmia; new onset; poor response
Katz/1988	216	E	R	2-day complications	4-hour diuresis; history of pulmonary edema; T-wave abnormalities; jugular vein distension
Plotnick/1982	55	I	PA, R	Inpatient and 1-year mortality	SBP on admission; dyspnea; peak creatinine phosphokinase

Abbreviations: COPD, chronic obstructive pulmonary disease; E, emergency department patients; Hgb, hemoglobin; I, inpatients; NYHA, New York Heart Association; PA, patient assessment; R, retrospective chart review; RR, respiratory rate; S, survey.
a Complications include mortality.
b Identified markers of low risk.

0.83–0.92) for BNP's ability to predict a combined end point. The cumulative probability of a heart-failure event within 6 months was 51% in the 67 patients who had a BNP level higher than 480 pg/mL, compared with 2.5% in the 205 patients who had BNP values less than 230 pg/mL. BNP also has been shown to predict adverse events and to determine a disposition strategy more accurately than a physician's assessment based on level of severity.[43] Finally, a retrospective analysis of 77,467 patients from the Acute Decompensated Heart Failure National Registry found a nearly linear relationship between BNP quartiles and in-hospital mortality.[40] Similar findings have been reported for N-terminal proBNP (NT-proBNP).[41,44–46] In a pooled analysis of 1256 patients, NT-proBNP was a significant predictor of subsequent adverse events.[41] An NT-proBNP concentration greater than 5180 pg/mL was strongly predictive of death by 76 days (odds ratio, 5.2; 95% CI, 2.2–8.1; $P < .001$).

PROMISING NEW TECHNOLOGIES AND TECHNIQUES

An S3 cardiac gallop is indicative of heart failure, and studies have demonstrated it has excellent specificity but poor sensitivity.[47] Although the presence of an S3 gallop can be normal in adolescents and young adults, its detection in patients older than 40 years is considered abnormal.[48–51] Further, it has been suggested that patients who have a detectable S3 gallop have an increased risk of hospitalization and death compared with patients without a detectable S3 gallop.[52–54]

Identification of an S3 gallop is difficult. In the aforementioned studies that suggest a low incidence of S3 detection in heart failure, the physicians may have been unable to detect a sound that in fact was present. Technology has been developed that may assist the clinician in detecting an S3 gallop at the bedside by measuring heart sound energy using an electronic stethoscope or another means of recording heart tones. Using a sophisticated software algorithm, information on the

presence of an S3 gallop, and potentially its intensity, is available. With continued development of such technology, the ability to detect extra heart sounds should improve significantly. Early results have shown promising specificity, improved ED physicians' diagnostic confidence, and provided additive, independent prognostic information.[55–59]

Finally, T-wave alternans has been investigated as a potential risk-stratification tool in AHFS. T-wave alternans describes beat-to-beat fluctuations in T-wave morphology that have been associated anecdotally with the onset of ventricular fibrillation. Microvolt T-wave alternans recording now can be performed during submaximal exercise. A series of beats are recorded at a stable heart rate, and the T-wave amplitude is plotted with respect to the QRS complex. These data then undergo spectral analysis to determine if there are sufficient T-wave fluctuations to call the test "positive."[60] Some studies have suggested an increased rate of long-term death and malignant arrhythmias in patients who have abnormal T-wave alternans.[61,62] Yet to be determined is the ability to perform this test in real time in the ED and whether abnormal results carry an increased risk of near-term events.

SUMMARY

A change in the conservative decision paradigm for patients who have heart failure will require a novel approach; even with the development of new diagnostic and prognostic tools, poor ED risk stratification and the high rate of critical care admissions for patients who have heart failure have not changed in decades.[1–3] The traditional history and physical examination have serious limitations. The current literature suggests that serum BUN, creatinine, sodium, cardiac biomarkers, and natriuretic peptides are helpful for initial risk stratification (**Table 3**).

A decision tool based on a validated ED risk model could improve assessment and initial disposition decisions. In other disease processes, such as acute coronary syndromes[63–65] and community-acquired pneumonia,[66–68] such

Table 3 Potential modifiable risk markers in acute heart failure	
Source	Marker
Past medical history	Coronary artery disease
Physical examination	Systolic blood pressure, respiratory rate, oxygen saturation
Laboratory findings	BUN, creatinine, sodium, natriuretic peptide levels
Ancillary studies	Ischemic ECG changes suggesting coronary artery disease

approaches have proven effective in safely decreasing admissions for low-risk patients. The process of risk stratification in patients who have heart failure lags decades behind the processes in place for these other conditions. A prospectively derived, multicenter, useful, ED risk-stratification model for patients who have signs and symptoms of heart failure is needed and is the focus of an ongoing National Heart, Lung, and Blood Institute grant.[69]

REFERENCES

1. Polanczyk CA, Rohde LE, Philbin EA, et al. A new casemix adjustment index for hospital mortality among patients with congestive heart failure. Med Care 1998;36(10):1489–99.

2. Smith WR, Poses RM, McClish DK, et al. Prognostic judgments and triage decisions for patients with acute congestive heart failure. Chest 2002;121(5):1610–7.

3. Graff L, Orledge J, Radford MJ, et al. Correlation of the agency for health care policy and research congestive heart failure admission guideline with mortality: peer review organization voluntary hospital association initiative to decrease events (PROVIDE) for congestive heart failure. Ann Emerg Med 1999; 34(4 Pt 1):429–37.

4. O'Connell JB, Bristow M. Economic impact of heart failure in the United States: a time for a different approach. J Heart Lung Transplant 1994;13:S107–12.

5. Stevenson LW, Braunwald E. Recognition and management of patients with heart failure. In: Goldman L, Braunwald E, editors. Primary cardiology. Philadelphia: WB Saunders; 1998. p. 310–29.

6. American Heart Association. Heart disease and stroke statistics–2006 update. Dallas (TX): American Heart Association 2005.

7. Adams KF Jr, Fonarow GC, Emerman CL, et al. Characteristics and outcomes of patients hospitalized for heart failure in the United States: rationale, design, and preliminary observations from the first 100,000 cases in the Acute Decompensated Heart Failure National Registry (ADHERE). Am Heart J 2005;149(2):209–16.

8. Cleland JG, Swedberg K, Follath F, et al. The Euro heart failure survey programme—a survey on the quality of care among patients with heart failure in Europe. Part 1: patient characteristics and diagnosis. Eur Heart J 2003;24(5):442–63.

9. Cuffe MS, Califf RM, Adams KF Jr, et al. Short-term intravenous milrinone for acute exacerbation of chronic heart failure: a randomized controlled trial. JAMA 2002;287(12):1541–7.

10. VMAC Investigators. Intravenous nesiritide vs nitroglycerin for treatment of decompensated congestive heart failure: a randomized controlled trial. JAMA 2002;287(12):1531–40.

11. Institute NHLaB. Morbidity and mortality: 2002 chart book on cardiovascular, lung, and blood diseases. Bethesda (MD): National Institutes of Health; 2002.

12. Butler J, Hanumanthu S, Chomsky D, et al. Frequency of low-risk hospital admissions for heart failure. Am J Cardiol 1998;81(1):41–4.

13. Poses RM, Smith WR, McClish DK, et al. Physicians' survival predictions for patients with acute congestive heart failure. Arch Intern Med 1997;157(9): 1001–7.

14. Heart Failure Society of America. HFSA 2006 comprehensive heart failure practice guideline. J Card Fail 2006;12(1):e1–2.

15. Hsieh M, Auble TE, Yealy DM. Evidence-based emergency medicine. Predicting the future: can this patient with acute congestive heart failure be safely discharged from the emergency department? Ann Emerg Med 2002;39(2):181–9.

16. Hunt SA, Abraham WT, Chin MH, et al. ACC/AHA 2005 guideline update for the diagnosis and management of chronic heart failure in the adult—summary article: a report of the American College of Cardiology/American Heart Association task force on practice guidelines (writing committee to update the 2001 guidelines for the evaluation and management of heart failure). J Am Coll Cardiol 2005;46(6):1116–43.

17. Konstam M, Dracup K, Baker D. Clinical practice guidelines No 11: heart failure: evaluation and care of patients with left-ventricular systolic dysfunction. Agency for Health Care Policy and Research 1994;94(0612).

18. Nieminen MS, Bohm M, Cowie MR, et al. Executive summary of the guidelines on the diagnosis and treatment of acute heart failure: the task force on acute heart failure of the European Society of Cardiology. Eur Heart J 2005;26(4):384–416.

19. Silvers SM, Howell JM, Kosowsky JM, et al. Clinical policy: critical issues in the evaluation and management of adult patients presenting to the emergency department with acute heart failure syndromes. Ann Emerg Med 2007;49(5):627–69.

20. Gheorghiade M, Zannad F, Sopko G, et al. Acute heart failure syndromes: current state and framework for future research. Circulation 2005;112(25): 3958–68.

21. Aurigemma GP, Gaasch WH. Clinical practice. Diastolic heart failure. N Engl J Med 2004;351(11): 1097–105.

22. Bhatia RS, Tu JV, Lee DS, et al. Outcome of heart failure with preserved ejection fraction in a population-based study. N Engl J Med 2006;355(3):260–9.

23. Owan TE, Hodge DO, Herges RM, et al. Trends in prevalence and outcome of heart failure with preserved ejection fraction. N Engl J Med 2006; 355(3):251–9.

24. Selker HP, Griffith JL, D'Agostino RB. A time-insensitive predictive instrument for acute hospital mortality

due to congestive heart failure: development, testing, and use for comparing hospitals: a multicenter study. Med Care;32(10):1040–52.

25. Chin MH, Goldman L. Correlates of major complications or death in patients admitted to the hospital with congestive heart failure. Arch Intern Med 1996;156(16):1814–20.

26. Chin MH, Goldman L. Correlates of early hospital readmission or death in patients with congestive heart failure. Am J Cardiol 1997;79(12):1640–4.

27. Katz MH, Nicholson PW, Singer DE, et al. The triage decision in pulmonary edema. J Gen Intern Med 1988;3(6):533–9.

28. Fonarow GC, Adams KF Jr, Abraham WT, et al. Risk stratification for in-hospital mortality in acutely decompensated heart failure: classification and regression tree analysis. JAMA 2005;293(5):572–80.

29. Gheorghiade M, Abraham WT, Albert NM, et al. Systolic blood pressure at admission, clinical characteristics, and outcomes in patients hospitalized with acute heart failure. JAMA 2006;296(18):2217–26.

30. Gheorghiade M, Rossi JS, Cotts W, et al. Characterization and prognostic value of persistent hyponatremia in patients with severe heart failure in the ESCAPE Trial. Arch Intern Med 2007;167(18):1998–2005.

31. Damman K, Navis G, Voors AA, et al. Worsening renal function and prognosis in heart failure: systematic review and meta-analysis. J Card Fail 2007;13(8):599–608.

32. Krumholz HM, Chen YT, Vaccarino V, et al. Correlates and impact on outcomes of worsening renal function in patients > or = 65 years of age with heart failure. Am J Cardiol 2000;85(9):1110–3.

33. Smith GL, Vaccarino V, Kosiborod M, et al. Worsening renal function: what is a clinically meaningful change in creatinine during hospitalization with heart failure? J Card Fail 2003;9(1):13–25.

34. Auble TE, Hsieh M, Gardner W, et al. A prediction rule to identify low-risk patients with heart failure. Acad Emerg Med 2005;12(6):514–21.

35. Hsieh M, Auble TE, Yealy DM. Validation of the acute heart failure index. Ann Emerg Med 2008;51(1):37–44.

36. Diercks DB, Peacock WF, Kirk JD, et al. ED patients with heart failure: identification of an observational unit-appropriate cohort. Am J Emerg Med 2006;24(3):319–24.

37. Bayes-Genis A, Lopez L, Zapico E, et al. NT-ProBNP reduction percentage during admission for acutely decompensated heart failure predicts long-term cardiovascular mortality. J Card Fail 2005;11(Suppl. 5):S3–8.

38. Harrison A, Morrison LK, Krishnaswamy P, et al. B-type natriuretic peptide predicts future cardiac events in patients presenting to the emergency department with dyspnea. Ann Emerg Med 2002;39(2):131–8.

39. Cheng V, Kazanagra R, Garcia A, et al. A rapid bedside test for B-type peptide predicts treatment outcomes in patients admitted for decompensated heart failure: a pilot study. J Am Coll Cardiol 2001;37(2):386–91.

40. Fonarow GC, Peacock WF, Phillips CO, et al. Admission B-type natriuretic peptide levels and in-hospital mortality in acute decompensated heart failure. J Am Coll Cardiol 2007;49(19):1943–50.

41. Januzzi JL, van Kimmenade R, Lainchbury J, et al. NT-proBNP testing for diagnosis and short-term prognosis in acute destabilized heart failure: an international pooled analysis of 1256 patients: the International Collaborative of NT-proBNP study. Eur Heart J 2006;27(3):330–7.

42. Yu CM, Sanderson JE. Plasma brain natriuretic peptide—an independent predictor of cardiovascular mortality in acute heart failure. Eur J Heart Fail 1999;1(1):59–65.

43. Maisel A, Hollander JE, Guss D, et al. Primary results of the rapid emergency department heart failure outpatient trial (REDHOT). A multicenter study of B-type natriuretic peptide levels, emergency department decision making, and outcomes in patients presenting with shortness of breath. J Am Coll Cardiol 2004;44(6):1328–33.

44. Kirk V, Bay M, Parner J, et al. N-terminal proBNP and mortality in hospitalised patients with heart failure and preserved vs. reduced systolic function: data from the prospective Copenhagen Hospital Heart Failure study (CHHF). Eur J Heart Fail 2004;6(3):335–41.

45. Januzzi JL Jr, Sakhuja R, O'Donoghue M, et al. Utility of amino-terminal pro-brain natriuretic peptide testing for prediction of 1-year mortality in patients with dyspnea treated in the emergency department. Arch Intern Med 2006;166(3):315–20.

46. Chen AA, Wood MJ, Krauser DG, et al. NT-proBNP levels, echocardiographic findings, and outcomes in breathless patients: results from the ProBNP Investigation of Dyspnoea in the Emergency Department (PRIDE) echocardiographic substudy. Eur Heart J 2006;27(7):839–45.

47. Wang CS, FitzGerald JM, Schulzer M, et al. Does this dyspneic patient in the emergency department have congestive heart failure? JAMA 2005;294(15):1944–56.

48. Evans W. The use of phonocardiography in clinical medicine. Lancet 1951;1:1083–5.

49. Reddy PS. The third heart sound. Int J Cardiol 1985;7(3):213–21.

50. Reddy PS, Salerni R, Shaver JA. Normal and abnormal heart sounds in cardiac diagnosis: part II. diastolic sounds. Curr Probl Cardiol 1985;10(4):1–55.

51. Sloan A. Cardiac gallop rhythm. Medicine 1958;37:197–215.

52. Drazner MH, Rame JE, Stevenson LW, et al. Prognostic importance of elevated jugular venous pressure and a third heart sound in patients with heart failure. N Engl J Med 2001;345(8):574–81.

53. Glover DR, Littler WA. Factors influencing survival and mode of death in severe chronic ischaemic cardiac failure. Br Heart J 1987;57(2):125–32.

54. Rame JE, Dries DL, Drazner MH. The prognostic value of the physical examination in patients with chronic heart failure. Congest Heart Fail 2003;9(3): 170–5, 178.

55. Collins SP, Kontos M, Diercks D, et al. Heart failure and audicor technology for rapid diagnosis and initial treatment of ED patients with suspected heart failure (HEARD-IT). Presented at the meeting of the Society of Academic Emergency Medicine. Chicago, 2007.

56. Collins SP, Lindsell CJ, Peacock WF, et al. The combined utility of an S3 heart sound and B-type natriuretic peptide levels in emergency department patients with dyspnea. J Card Fail 2006;12(4):286–92.

57. Collins SP, Lindsell CJ, Peacock WF, et al. Prevalence of S3 and S4 in ED patients with decompensated heart failure. Presented at the meeting of the American College of Emergency Physicians. San Francisco, October 2004.

58. Collins SP, Lindsell CJ, Peacock WF, et al. Prevalence of electronically detected abnormal heart sounds in acute decompensated heart failure before and after treatment. Presented at the meeting of the American College of Cardiology. Orlando (FL), 2005.

59. Storrow A, Sp C, Wf P, et al. Length of stay and charges are increased in patients with digitally detected third heart sounds. Paper presented at Society for Academic Emergency Medicine. New York, 2005.

60. Myles RC, Jackson CE, Tsorlalis I, et al. Is microvolt T-wave alternans the answer to risk stratification in heart failure? Circulation 2007;116(25):2984–91.

61. Salerno-Uriarte JA, De Ferrari GM, Klersy C, et al. Prognostic value of T-wave alternans in patients with heart failure due to nonischemic cardiomyopathy: results of the ALPHA Study. J Am Coll Cardiol 2007;50(19):1896–904.

62. Baravelli M, Salerno-Uriarte D, Guzzetti D, et al. Predictive significance for sudden death of microvolt-level T wave alternans in New York Heart Association class II congestive heart failure patients: a prospective study. Int J Cardiol 2005;105(1):53–7.

63. Tatum JL, Jesse RL, Kontos MC, et al. Comprehensive strategy for the evaluation and triage of the chest pain patient. Ann Emerg Med 1997;29(1): 116–25.

64. Gibler WB, Runyon JP, Levy RC, et al. A rapid diagnostic and treatment center for patients with chest pain in the emergency department. Ann Emerg Med 1995;25(1):1–8.

65. Storrow AB, Gibler WB. Chest pain centers: diagnosis of acute coronary syndromes. Ann Emerg Med 2000;35(5):449–61.

66. Yealy DM, Auble TE, Stone RA, et al. The emergency department community-acquired pneumonia trial: methodology of a quality improvement intervention. Ann Emerg Med 2004;43(6):770–82.

67. Marrie TJ, Lau CY, Wheeler SL, et al. A controlled trial of a critical pathway for treatment of community-acquired pneumonia. CAPITAL study investigators. Community-acquired pneumonia intervention trial assessing levofloxacin. JAMA 2000;283(6): 749–55.

68. Fine MJ, Auble TE, Yealy DM, et al. A prediction rule to identify low-risk patients with community-acquired pneumonia. N Engl J Med 1997;336(4):243–50.

69. Storrow AB, Collins S, Disalvo T, et al. Improving heart failure risk stratification in the ED: stratify 1r01hl088459-01. Vanderbilt University. NHLBI; 2007.

Observation Unit Management of Acute Decompensated Heart Failure

Jon W. Schrock, MD*, Charles L. Emerman, MD

KEYWORDS
- Heart failure - Observation medicine

Emergency department (ED) presentations for acute decompensated heart failure (ADHF) have increased at a dramatic rate. In the 1990s, ADHF presentations accounted for between 1% and 3% of all ED visits and increased at an average rate of more than 18,000 visits annually.[1,2] Providing care for these large numbers of patients has significant societal implications because heart failure is the leading diagnosis for Medicare patients older than 65 years and accounts for more bills more than any other disease.[3] Hospital charges for 1 week of inpatient treatment of ADHF averaged approximately $10,000 in the 1990s, and is even higher today.[4] Costs for the treatment of ADHF vary on a daily basis, with nearly 75% of ADHF-related costs occurring in the first 48 hours.[5]

The costs of ADHF are not just an ED problem but begin at its front door. Of patients who have a primary diagnosis of ADHF discharged from the hospital, nearly 80% arrive through the ED.[6,7] On a national level, the direct and indirect costs for treating ADHF were projected to reach more than $34.8 billion dollars in 2008.[8] The financial impact of ADHF is not stagnant; as the baby boomer generation continues to age, the burden of heart failure on society will continue to increase.[9,10]

To prepare for this growth, government and hospital administrators are looking for more effective and less costly methods to deliver care to these patients. ED observation units (OU) have been found to be one of the most cost-effective ways to manage patients who have mild to moderately ill presentations of asthma, chest pain, and heart failure.[11–18] These units have been associated with a high degree of patient satisfaction and increased diagnostic accuracy.[19–23] When evidence-based protocols are used in observation care for ADHF, return ED visits and readmissions decrease significantly.[12]

OU treatment of ADHF is cost-effective for several rather distinct reasons. OUs are able to provide rapid and focused treatment for patients who have ADHF through specific treatment protocols that follow current American Heart Association (AHA) guidelines and can be implemented immediately. The several-hour delay in care often seen when patients are transferred from the ED to the hospital floor is greatly shortened because observation unit beds are often more available due to greater turnover. The use of protocols can help reduce the number and severity of complications seen with patients who have ADHF.[24] Medical therapies are started earlier in OUs than with typical inpatient admission on a hospital floor. A significant secondary benefit is the decrease in ED diversion and delays in care for future patients, because the ED beds are no longer occupied.[25,26]

The establishment of OUs for the extended care of patients in the ED has evolved over the past 3 decades. Observation medicine initially began as a method to contain costs for conditions with uncertain clinical courses or diagnoses. The most common admissions to the initial OUs were for alcohol intoxication or withdrawal and

MetroHealth Medical Center, Cleveland, OH, USA
* Corresponding author. Department of Emergency Medicine, MetroHealth Medical Center, Case Western Reserve University School of Medicine, 2500 MetroHealth Drive, BG353, Cleveland, OH 44109-1998.
E-mail address: jschrock@metrohealth.org (J. W. Schrock).

Heart Failure Clin 5 (2009) 85–100
doi:10.1016/j.hfc.2008.08.015
1551-7136/08/$ – see front matter. Published by Elsevier Inc.

overdoses.[27,28] With little regulation and guidance, more than a decade passed before the idea of observational care caught on. Once the benefits of OUs became more obvious, the model blossomed into a branch of emergency medicine with unique features and goals.

In 1987, more than 10 years after the inception of the OU, the American College of Emergency Physicians Practice Management Committee published a list of features it deemed important in managing observation patients. The committee stated that the goal was "to improve the delivery and quality of medical care to all patients."[29] Recommendations included clearly designating is the individuals responsible for observation patients at all times, locating units within or adjacent to the ED, and creating protocols for transferring patients in and out of the units.

OU beds are designed for short-term care of mild to moderately ill patients, typically 24 hours and, except in extreme cases, less than 48 hours.[30] The physical placement of OUs can vary depending on the needs and restraints of the institutions developing them. Most OUs are in dedicated areas within the ED using existing beds,[31] allowing proximity for physicians and nurses and avoiding the financial expense of building and running a separate facility. Using beds within the ED can contribute to overcrowding, which has become an ever-increasing problem.

As EDs grow and invest in the infrastructure, many will create a separate adjacent clinical area for an OU. The advantages of this include a stable location for patient care and a stable nursing pool composed of staff working solely in the OU. A separate clinical area allows centralization of physical resources required to run an OU and eases education of staff caring for patients in the unit. Physicians caring for these patients are close if emergencies arise, but patients are shielded from the volume and commotion often seen in many EDs.

Some departments may place patients in a virtual observation unit with set protocols but no permanent physical space. This model allows OU beds to be located literally on any floor in a hospital, assuming that the level of care for these patients remains constant. The disadvantages of this type of OU include difficulty maintaining appropriate training and certification of nursing staff caring for patients in the unit, potentially large distances between patients and physicians caring for them, and lack of familiarity of other staff with OU protocols and practice.

The Joint Commission, formerly The Joint Commission on the Accreditation of Healthcare Organizations, requires that OU staffing approximates nurse-to-patient ratios of a hospital floor caring for similar patients. This directive often leads to a nursing-to-patient ratio of 1:4 or 1:5 for the typical OU. Nursing staffing levels can be adjusted throughout the day as the number of patients requiring care in the OU changes, but should not exceed predetermined nurse-to-patient ratios determined by that institution.

CENTERS FOR MEDICARE & MEDICAID SERVICES: CODING

Observation unit stays are billed differently from ED visits or hospitalized in-patient stays. The Centers for Medicare and Medicaid Services (CMS) considers OU visits outpatient observation services to be billed under revenue code 762. The observation period determines whether further inpatient treatment is needed, therefore allowing for its outpatient status. Observation services begin when the nurse notes the arrival of the patient in observation status, because observation is not a physical location. Patients could be accepted into observation status in the ED or any location within the hospital. Observation care continues until physicians order the patients discharged or admitted to the hospital.

Much like ED reimbursement from CMS, rates of professional billing are related to the level of medical complexity of the case and the documentation supporting that complexity. Observational billing is unique in that two separate sets of codes are used, depending on whether the patient is admitted and discharged on the same calendar day. Codes 99234 through 99236 are used for same-day discharges and codes 99217 through 99220 are used for patients undergoing care for two or more calendar days. CMS allows for professional and technical billing for OU care.

CMS allows billable observation services for up to 48 hours for the technical fee but allows exceptions if patients stay longer than 48 hours. However, these extensions cannot be preauthorized. For patients who stay longer than 48 hours and are admitted to a hospital floor, the technical portion of the OU bill often will be bundled into the technical portion of the hospital bill, not allowing for separate collection by the hospital and OU. The professional fee does not change in this scenario.

Until recently, CMS allowed a separate ambulatory payment classification (APC) group payment for technical charges for only three diseases: heart failure, asthma, and chest pain. This rule is changing in 2008 with the adoption of a composite APC, which will provide payment for observation services of all diagnoses. The codes include 8002, which will cover observation care for patients admitted directly to an OU from a clinic or outpatient setting, and 8003, which will reimburse observation patients admitted after a high-level ED visit signified by documentation supporting a level 4 or 5 ED visit (current procedural terminology [CPT] codes 99284 and 99285). The requirements to meet these codes include a minimum of 8 hours of observational care, a qualifying ED visit, and the absence of any surgical intervention requiring placement in observational care. Patients who have a stay of less than 8 hours can be paid under APC 0604.[32]

As part of this plan, CMS will bundle technical charges from the ED visit with the observational visit. Although this procedure seems to be an effort to streamline the billing process and improve efficiency, how this change will affect overall reimbursement for institutions is unclear.

STAGES OF OBSERVATION UNIT CARE

Patients presenting with ADHF must be correctly assessed and stabilized in the ED before any disposition decision is made. Although this statement is easy to make in clinical practice, the diagnosis of ADHF can be much more challenging. Using clinical judgment alone to diagnose ADHF resulted in an accuracy rate of 74%. The physicians caring for these patients had a 27% rate of diagnostic uncertainty.[33]

Using markers such as B-type natriuretic peptide (BNP) and N-terminal pro-BNP increases the diagnostic accuracy of clinicians treating patients who have possible ADHF.[34–37] Accurate diagnosis in the ED can be important, because subsequent providers may follow the same care plan until another diagnosis becomes obvious. Other conditions, such as pulmonary embolism, acute coronary syndrome, chronic obstructive pulmonary disease, and pulmonary hypertension, should be considered before patients are placed in the OU. A prominent problem with ADHF is its recidivism; the most common historical finding in a patient admitted for ADHF is a prior history of heart failure.[38]

After diagnosis, stabilization can begin in the ED. Several medications may be used for initial stabilization. Primary ED medications for ADHF include afterload reducers, such as nitroglycerin, nitroprusside, nesiritide, or hydralazine. These medications can quickly reduce afterload, because approximately 50% of patients present with elevated systolic blood pressure.[39,40] Diuretics are common first-line agents used in the acute management of ADHF. Reports have suggested they are used in approximately 70% to 90% of patients who have ADHF.[40,41]

Other medications used in the ED to treat ADHF include angiotensin-converting enzyme (ACE) inhibitors that block the renin-angiotensin-aldosterone system (RAAS), which is often elevated in patients presenting in acute heart failure. ACE inhibitors can cause hypotension, and therefore should be used carefully or withheld in patients who have borderline hypotension or are also being treated with vasoactive agents, such as nitroglycerin or nesiritide. For patients intolerant of ACE inhibitors because of cough or angioedema, angiotensin receptor blockers (ARBs) can be used. These medications block the RAAS through inhibiting the angiotensin II receptor, and can also cause hypotension.

Another nonpharmaceutical modalities for treatment of ADHF in the ED is noninvasive positive pressure ventilation (NPPV). This means of respiratory assistance is useful in patients who are dyspneic but alert and cooperative and do not have a large oxygen requirement. Forms of NPPV include continuous positive airway pressure and bilevel positive airway pressure. These noninvasive means of ventilatory assistance are used as a bridge to avoid intubation until concurrent medical therapy, such as preload reduction, afterload reduction, and diuretics, has time to work. Rotating tourniquets are not a usual means of modern care, although they were used previously for initial stabilization.

CHOOSING PATIENTS FOR OBSERVATIONAL CARE

When treating patients who have ADHF in an ED that has an OU, deciding which patients are appropriate for observational care is important. Experts have suggested that ED physicians often overestimate the severity of illness in patients who have ADHF and that this has led to excess expense and unnecessary use of critical care hospital beds.[42,43] Although this line of thought has some truth, it is difficult to criticize the treatment rendered by ADHF because no good risk stratification tools exist for this patient population.

The absence of a useful risk stratification tool is certainly not cause by a lack of trying. Attempts by emergency physicians and cardiologists have had limited success. Multiple ED and inpatient studies have attempted to risk-stratify patients who have ADHF.[44–50] Unfortunately, most of these studies use mortality or complications, including ventricular fibrillation, defibrillation, cardiopulmonary resuscitation (CPR), and intubation, as end points. Other clinically relevant end points for an OU population, such as dyspnea, return visits, length of stay, have not been studied prospectively. These studies have attempted to identify the high-risk population and assume that the patients not positive for high-risk features are a low-risk population.

Only one study by Auble and colleagues[51] has evaluated multiple decision rules in a head-to-head fashion. In this study, the investigators compared four decision rules, including two by Fonarrow and colleagues,[47] using the Acute Decompensated Heart Failure National Registry, a rule developed by Lee and colleagues[48] from the Enhanced Feedback for Effective Cardiology Treatment trial, and the Brigham and Women's hospital rule.[52] The rules varied from a rather simple decision tree, to more complex point systems, to a rather complicated multivariate logistic regression model using blood urea nitrogen levels, vital signs, and age. Outcomes included death and lifesaving interventions, such as defibrillation, CPR, intubation, and coronary artery bypass graft surgery.

Rates of inpatient death or complications among the low-risk population groups ranged from 6.7% to 9.2%, and rates of 30-day mortality were between 4% and 6%. Most ED physicians would find these rates unacceptably high for admitting a population to an OU.

More recently, a study published by Hsieh and colleagues[53] attempted to validate the acute heart failure index in a retrospective population of more than 8000 patients. In this decision tree, patients who had prior diagnosis of heart failure and no evidence of acute myocardial infarction or ischemia were evaluated for low-risk features. Nineteen other variables, including medical history, laboratory values, vital signs, EKG, and chest radiograph results, were used in a complex decision tree with a total of 14 possible low-risk end points.

The acute heart failure index classified 19.2% of patients as low-risk. Among these patients, death at 30 days occurred in 2.9% (95% CI, 2.1%–3.7%), and 1.7% (95% CI, 1.1%–2.4%) experienced serious complications. These results seem to show a significant improvement over the prior decision rules. The complexity of this rule is problematic and would realistically only allow its use if incorporated into a computerized algorithm as part of an electronic charting program or a program incorporated on a handheld computer. This algorithm, as part of a functional program using "yes" or "no" answers to determine morbidity and mortality risk, can be found at http://www.pitt.edu/~hfpr/. This decision rule still requires prospective validation in multiple geographic regions before it can be supported for widespread use.

Because few singularly useful low-risk characteristics exist, one must know which features may represent a high risk for morbidity and mortality for patients presenting with ADHF. Burkhardt and colleagues[45] retrospectively evaluated 385 patients OU and found that only an elevated blood urea nitrogen (BUN) of greater than 30 mg/dL was associated with OU treatment failure. Elevated serum creatinine levels and hyponatremia were associated with nonsignificant trends toward OU treatment failure.

Dierks and colleagues[44] evaluated 499 patients who had ADHF treated in an ED to determine which characteristics were suitable for OU treatment. Patients were enrolled prospectively and followed up for 30 days. Outcomes included death, myocardial infarction, arrhythmia, and rehospitalization. An initial ED systolic blood pressure of greater than 160 mm Hg and negative troponin I serum value were found to predict successful OU treatment. Other laboratory values associated with a poor prognosis in ADHF include anemia, elevated serum creatinine, and hyponatremia.[46,47,54,55]

Diuretic resistance was also proven to be a powerful predictor of worse prognosis in patients who have ADHF.[56–58] Patients who have recently noticed decreased efficacy of their diuretics or are taking exceedingly high doses of diuretics may be considered poor OU candidates.

Previously, patients who had a low ejection fraction (EF) were often considered to have a worse prognosis[59–61] However, more recent data evaluating patients who had newly diagnosed ADHF suggests that the current rates of mortality at 30 days and 1 year are not affected by the EF.[62] Because no prospective studies have evaluated EF as a risk factor for OU treatment failure, establishing an absolute EF value below which patients would not be considered for OU treatment would be imprudent.

Another pragmatic feature to help determine a patient's viability for OU treatment is average length of recent hospital admissions. If a patient's previous four admissions each resulted in a week-long hospital stay, that individual may not be the best candidate for OU treatment. Patients who have other active comorbid conditions that may complicate ADHF treatment, such as renal insufficiency or active pulmonary disease, may more strongly considered for inpatient admission. These decisions should be made on an individual basis, and should include the patient's primary care physician or cardiologist.

TREATMENT IN THE OBSERVATION UNIT

Using processes of care, an effective, evidence-based treatment standard can be created for patients who have ADHF admitted to an OU. As with most effective protocols, this process begins long before any patient is admitted. ED physicians must meet with the hospital's cardiology group or groups to discuss which population of patients who have heart failure would best benefit from treatment in an OU setting. Requests for unique exclusions can be discussed and enacted if deemed reasonable.

For example, when creating the ADHF protocol, cardiologists at Metro Health Medical Center requested that all patients who had newly diagnosed ADHF be admitted directly to cardiology. This practice was based on the expectation that patient evaluation would require several days of hospitalization. This process may not be required in all institutions, such as those in which an appropriate rapid workup may still occur for patients who have newly diagnosed heart failure.

OU treatment of ADHF consists largely of afterload reduction and diuretic therapy. Other therapies can be offered, such as nesiritide infusion or ultrafiltration. More nursing-intensive therapies, including inotrope infusions or nitroglycerin drips, often require more care than an OU can provide, and patients taking these medications have a low likelihood of discharge home in 48 hours. The mainstay of treatment is diuretic therapy, which is started in the ED and continued in the OU. Afterload reduction and treatment of the hyperstimulated renin angiotensin system includes ACE inhibitors or ARBs, which could be given in the ED or OU. Second-line agents include vasodilator therapy, such as nesiritide or long-acting nitrates. For patients who have known diuretic resistance, ultrafiltration therapy is a reasonable treatment if available.

Unfortunately, despite optimal medical treatment, some patients may decompensate, requiring additional higher-intensity care. Some signs of deterioration in patients who have ADHF that may be monitored in the OU setting include hypotension; worsening hypoxia; chest pain or symptoms suggesting acute coronary syndrome; anuria or oliguria; and acute dysrhythmias, such as ventricular tachycardia or atrial fibrillation with rapid ventricular response. Orders should include parameters for unstable vital signs to signal physician notification when patients experience clinical deterioration.

Most patients for whom OU treatment of ADHF fails can be admitted safely to a hospital floor for continued treatment. Patients who have symptoms of acute coronary syndrome or dysrhythmias may require cardiac monitoring. Patients who have hypotension may require inotrope therapy and a higher level of nursing care. Systems should be in place to make these transitions as effortless as possible well before patients are admitted to an OU.

Having a realistic idea of the total number of patients who have ADHF who will be admitted to an OU is ideal. This projection will provide the administration with a reasonable estimate of the number of patients who will be placed in the OU. Recent studies have suggested that approximately 30% of patients presenting to the ED with ADHF would be suitable for OU care.[44,45]

Creating protocols to ease admission and create uniform treatment is ideal in an environment in which physician care may be transferred two or three times a day and dedicated unit coverage may be limited to 8 hours per day. **Fig. 1** provides an example of the heart failure admission protocol used at MetroHealth Medical Center. The orders were created with assistance from cardiologists and were designed to be filled out completely and allow for no ambiguity. Patients should be weighed on arrival to allow comparison when they return in ADHF. Strict monitoring of oral consumption and urinary output is essential to determine the efficacy of diuretic therapy. Parameters for physician contact should be included, because the physician caring for these patients will often not be in the immediate vicinity. Low-salt and diabetic diets should be available. Fluid restriction may be required if the patient is fluid overloaded and unable to comply with dietary demands.

Laboratory tests should include a complete blood cell count to check for anemia and a basic metabolic panel to assess electrolyte status. BNP should be measured at admission and can be followed serially to assess ventricular wall stress response to therapy. In patients treated with nesiritide, a recombinant form of BNP will be measured along with native BNP, and this measurement should be performed 2 hours after the nesiritide infusion is discontinued.

Liver function tests (LFTs) should be measured to determine if cholestatic hepatic dysfunction is occurring as a result of poor perfusion, because more than 40% of patients in ADHF will present with abnormal LFTs.[63] Thyroid function should be evaluated but may be withheld if performed in the previous year and the patient is not currently taking thyroid replacement therapy.

Cardiac markers may be ordered at the physician's discretion for patients presenting with symptoms of acute coronary syndrome and ADHF. For patients who have no prior history of congestive heart failure, cardiac markers should be ordered to rule out myocardial ischemia as a cause of the ADHF episode.

Use of cardiac markers in patients who have known congestive heart failure is more controversial. Although many institutions, including MetroHealth Medical Center, often admit patients who

MetroHealth Medical Center

PHYSICIAN'S ORDER SHEET

ALL ORDERS MUST BE WRITTEN IN THE METRIC SYSTEM
USING GENERIC NAMES AND INCLUDE DATE, TIME, AND
PHYSICIAN'S SIGNATURE.
  ANOTHER BRAND OF DRUG IDENTICAL IN FORM AND
CONTENT MAY BE DISPENSED.

USE BALL POINT PEN

ALLERGY?   ☐ YES   ☐ NO
IF SO, WHAT:_____
WEIGHT _____kg   HEIGHT_____IN/CM

DATE	HOUR	ORDERS	NURSE'S NOTATION	DATE	HOUR	NURSE'S SIGNATURE
		Admit to Clinical Decision Unit				
		Diagnosis: Congestive Heart Failure Exacerbation *(Page 1 of 2)*				
		Condition: Stable				
		Vitals: ☐ Every 2 hours X 2 then every 4 hours				
		☐ Notify physician for HR greater than 110 or less than 60 RR greater than				
		25 or less than 10				
		☐ SBP greater than 180 or less than 90 or DBP greater than 110				
		or less than 40				
		Activity: ☐ Bed rest ☐ Bathroom privileges ☐ As tolerated				
		Allergies: ☐ NKDA				
		☐ Other:_____				
		Nursing: ☐ Call MD for worsening dyspnea or increasing O2 requirement				
		☐ cardiac monitor ☐ continuous pulse oximetry				
		☐ Measure fluid input and output, patient weight at admission				
		☐ Monitor release for testing				
		IVF ☐ Saline lock				
		Diet: ☐ Regular ☐ Low Salt ☐ Diabetic ☐ NPO				
		☐ **Consult Social Work for**				
		Laboratory:				
		☐ CBC				
		☐ BMP				
		☐ B type natriuretic peptide				
		☐ LFTs				
		☐ Cardiac markers (troponin, CKMB) at 0, 4, and 8 hrs				
		☐ TSH if not obtained within last year.				
		☐ Repeat B type natriuretic 2 hrs after nesiritide is discontinued				
		Attending: _____ **PIN#:**_____				
		CHF CDUProtocol.doc				
		SO-CDU CHF 05/05				

MH1868-1
05/05

Fig. 1. The heart failure admission protocol for MetroHealth Medical Center. (*Courtesy of* MetroHealth Medical Center, Cleveland, OH.)

MetroHealth Medical Center

PHYSICIAN'S ORDER SHEET

ALL ORDERS MUST BE WRITTEN IN THE METRIC SYSTEM USING GENERIC NAMES AND INCLUDE DATE, TIME, AND PHYSICIAN'S SIGNATURE.

ANOTHER BRAND OF DRUG IDENTICAL IN FORM AND CONTENT MAY BE DISPENSED.

USE BALL POINT PEN

ALLERGY? ☐ YES ☐ NO

IF SO, WHAT:_____

WEIGHT _____kg HEIGHT_____IN/CM

DATE	HOUR	ORDERS	NURSE'S NOTATION	DATE	HOUR	NURSE'S SIGNATURE
		Admit to Clinical Decision Unit				
		Diagnosis: Congestive Heart Failure Exacerbation *(Page 2 of 2)*				
		Imaging: Indication				
		☐ Chest X-ray				
		☐ PA/Lat				
		☐ ECG at admission and 12 hrs				
		Medications: *Please review allergy list prior to administration*				
		List Patient Weight: _____				
		☐ O2 via nasal cannula at ___ L/min				
		☐ Wean O2 as tolerated without dyspnea and O2 saturation greater than 92%				
		☐ Albuterol aerosol 2.5mg/3mL PO EVERY 2 hrs- if no wheezing hold and				
		contact MD				
		☐ Furosemide ____mg IV X 1 (max 180mg)				
		☐ Furosemide continuous infusion _____mg/hr IV (5-10mg/hr: max 40mg/hr)				
		Notify physician when diuresis reaches 3 Liters				
		☐ Nesiritide 2mcg/Kg bolus- _____ mcg IV bolus				
		Then Nesiritide 0.01 mcg/Kg/min gtt IV _____ mcg/min				
		Hold Nesiritide for SBP less than 110 or DBP less than 40				
		☐ Nitroglycerin at _____ mcg/minute IV				
		Hold Nitroglycerinfor SBP less than 110 or DBP less than 40				
		☐ Nitropaste ___ inches topical every 8 hours (Do not administer if				
		patient is on Nesiritide)				
		☐ Enalapril ____ mg IV X 1				
		☐ Acetaminophen 650 mg tab, PO every 4 hours PRN mild pain				
		☐ Zolpidem 10mg PO QHS				
		Home medications:				
		Attending: _____ **PIN#:**_____				
MH1868-2 05/05		CHF CDUProtocol.doc				

SO-CDU CHF 05/05

Fig. 1. *(continued)*

have known ADHF to hospital floors without a "rule–out" period in a telemetry bed, whether this is an optimal practice is unknown. The current AHA guidelines for management of ADHF do not even mention cardiac markers or troponin.[64]

What is known is that the rate of positive cardiac markers in patients who have ADHF approaches 20%.[65] A positive troponin test is an independent risk factor for death if seen in the ED presentation,[66] which has led some authors to propose testing cardiac markers on all patients presenting with ADHF.[67] The rate of coronary artery disease in patients who have known heart failure is more than 50%. Baseline elevations in troponin I do not differ between patients who have idiopathic and ischemic cardiomyopathy.[68,69]

Echocardiography is recommended in the 2005 AHA guidelines on the management of chronic heart failure.[64] However, whether this study must be repeated in subsequent admissions is unclear. The authors' practice is to obtain an echocardiography study if the patient has not been evaluated in the prior year, or if new findings on physical examination suggest structural cardiac changes that may influence outcome, such as mitral regurgitation or aortic stenosis not previously noted or worse than prior examinations.

Medical treatment of ADHF in the OU should continue the treatment plan begun in the ED. For patients placed on diuretics, two approaches are available. Many patients receive intravenous boluses of furosemide to encourage fluid loss. If the initial dose is not completely effective, a second or third dose may be given. Several studies have suggested that continuous intravenous infusions of furosemide result in greater diuresis and less ototoxicity, particularly if begun early in the hospitalization.[70–73] Continuous infusion medications present a risk for excessive diuresis, and therefore stop-gap measures should appear in the OU orders instructing the nursing staff to discontinue the medication once a desired level of diuresis is reached. Electrolytes should be monitored and replaced as needed when aggressive diuresis is being performed.

B-blockers have become a mainstay of heart failure treatment because they have been shown to decrease morbidity and mortality.[74–77] Patients who have known heart failure should take a daily β-blocker. Currently approved formulations include metoprolol, bisoprolol, or carvedilol. B-blockers help decrease the heart's exposure to chronic adrenergic stimulation and decrease ventricular remodeling.

Because most patients who have heart failure are currently undergoing this therapy, the question arises of what to do if they are currently in ADHF and being admitted to an OU; should the β-blocker be held? Prior dogma has instructed physicians to stop β-blockers in ADHF episodes. Although β-blockers can depress cardiac contraction, suddenly stopping them may expose the heart to increased endogenous catecholamines, which could produce tachydysrhythmias and myocardial ischemia.

Experts have suggested that patients in mild to moderate ADHF and who were not hypotensive should be maintained on β-blockers.[78–80] Evidence supports that patients who have acute myocardial infarction experiencing ADHF benefit from β-blocker treatment.[81] More recent studies have determined an increase in morbidity and mortality and increased length of stay may be associated with decreasing or stopping β-blocker therapy for patients in ADHF.[82,83] The most recent published American College of Cardiology (ACC) guidelines suggest that patients who have been taking β-blockers long-term decrease or stop them only if evidence of hypoperfusion is present.[64] **Table 1** lists the starting dosages of β-blockers approved for use in the treatment of heart failure. Doses may be adjusted if bradycardia or hypotension develops.

Like β-blockers, ACE inhibitors and ARBs have shown direct long-term mortality benefits to patients who have heart failure.[84–87] Patients diagnosed with systolic heart failure and no contraindication should be placed on an ACE inhibitor or ARB. These medications should be started at low doses and gradually titrated upward. Patients who have a history of renal insufficiency or hyperkalemia should avoid these medications unless closely follow by their physician. For patients being started on them, serum potassium levels should be checked at 3 days and 1 week initially to check for hyperkalemia. If the patient seems unreliable or unable to return for blood draws, it may be more prudent for the primary care physician to begin this medication. **Table 1** lists the starting doses for ACE inhibitors and ARBs.

Digitalis is a cardiac glycoside that has been used in the treatment of ADHF for more than 2 centuries. Digitalis blocks myocardial sodium potassium adenosine triphosphatase (Na-K-ATPase). Enzymatic blockade in the kidney causes natriuresis, which increases sodium excretion, and decreases renin release. Although once a mainstay of heart failure treatment, digitalis has been relegated to a second-line therapy by some groups and was changed from class I to class IIa classification in the most recent AHA update.[64,88,89] Other studies have suggested that it may still be useful but only at a lower serum concentration than used previously.[90,91] Digitalis is still recommended for patients who have persistent heart failure symptoms who have not responded to treatment with β-blockers, diuretics, or ACE inhibitors (or ARBs). It is not indicated as a medication to stabilize an ADHF episode. Therefore, its usefulness in the OU setting is limited, and it may be best newly prescribed under the guidance of a consulting cardiologist.

Long-acting nitrates, such as isosorbide dinitrate, have been recommended for select patients

Table 1
Acute decompensated heart failure medications used in the observation setting

Drug	Initial Dose	Target Dose	Half-Life (h)	Approximate Cost for 30-day Prescription[a]	Adverse Reactions (Comments)
ACE inhibitors					
Lisinopril	5 mg qd	20 mg qd	12	$12.99	Hypotension, hyperkalemia, angioedema, cough, renal insufficiency (need to monitor potassium, check 1–2 wk after initiating therapy, monitor creatinine with impaired renal function)
Captopril	6.25 mg TID	50 mg tid	1.9	$9.99	
Angiotensin receptor blockers					
Losartan	50 mg qd	100 mg qd	2	$85.51	Hypotension, hyperkalemia, angioedema, cough, and rarely rhabdomyolysis (need to monitor potassium, check 1–2 wk after initiating therapy, monitor creatinine with impaired renal function)
Valsartan	20 mg bid	40 mg bid	6	$114.36	
Loop diuretics					
Furosemide	10 mg qd	Variable	2	$2.85	Hypotension, hypokalemia, hypomagnesemia, hyponatremia, hyperlipidemia, ototoxicity, myelosuppression (patients may require electrolyte supplementation)
Bumetanide	0.5 mg qd	Variable	1.5	$23.52	
Thiazide diuretics					
Hydrochlorothiazide	25 mg qd	Variable	6–15	$2.39	Dizziness, headaches, muscle cramps, hypotension, hypokalemia, hypomagnesemia, hyponatremia, hypercalcemia (start at lowest dose, may require electrolyte monitoring)
Metolazone	0.5 mg qd	Variable	14	$37.37	
Beta-blockers					
Carvedilol	3.125 mg bid	25mg bid	7–10	$31.98	Hyperglycemia, hypotension, bradycardia, dizziness, fatigue (avoid stopping drug abruptly)
Metoprolol XL	12.5 mg qd	Variable	7	$35.99	
Bisoprolol	2.5 mg qd	Variable	9–12	$31.00	
Digitalis					
Digoxin	0.125 mg qd	Variable	40	$12.99	Anorexia, vomiting, diarrhea, and dizziness (avoid in patients who have atrioventricular block, such as Wolff-Parkinson-White syndrome, and those who have hypokalemia)
Nitrates					
Isosorbide dinitrate	20 mg qd	Variable	1	$5.65	Hypotension, headache, syncope (often used in combination with hydralazine, not to be used with impotence medications)
Combination medications					
Isosorbide dinitrate/ hydrochlorothiazide	20–37.5 mg tid	Variable	1–15	$191.97	Hypotension, headache, syncope, hypokalemia, hypomagnesemia, hyponatremia, hypercalcemia (not to be used with impotence medications)

a Prices listed assume 1-month supply. (*Data from* Drugstore.com. Accessed February 1, 2008.)

who have ADHF.[64] These patients include those who are symptomatic on maximal therapy and those who have exertional or nocturnal dyspnea. Long-acting nitrates have been shown to offer better survival than placebo but not ACE inhibitors and therefore should not be given in their place.[92] Side effects include headache and hypotension. Tolerance is common with extended use, and therefore they are not prescribed around the clock. Because these are second-line agents for heart failure, cardiology guidance may be useful in choosing to which patients oral nitrates should be prescribed.

Hydralazine is a direct vascular smooth muscle relaxant used often in combination with long-acting nitrates. It is not as effective as ACE inhibitors in reducing mortality in patients who have heart failure but may be used in those intolerant of ACE inhibitors and ARBs.[93] When used in combination with long-acting nitrates and ACE inhibitors or β-blockers, hydralazine was found to be particularly effective at reducing mortality in African Americans.[94] The results of this research led to the creation of BiDil, a combination medication containing isosorbide dinitrate and hydralazine. This medication was the first to receive approval from the U.S. Food and Drug Administration (FDA) for treating disease in a specific race. Current guidelines do not suggest this combination as a first-line agent in African Americans who can tolerate ACE inhibitors and β-blockers.[64]

Nitroglycerin is a potent vasodilator with both venous and arteriole vasodilator properties. It is effective at reducing preload and afterload rapidly in patients presenting in ADHF. The half-life of intravenous nitroglycerin is 1 to 4 minutes, requiring that it be given in a continuous intravenous drip or topical form. The intravenous form is often used for flash pulmonary edema or ADHF presentations with elevated blood pressure. However, because this form requires frequent titration, it is not ideal for OU use. A sublingual tablet and spray forms are also available, with physiologic affects lasting from 1 to 6 hours after administration.[95] The tablet and topical forms can be used in an OU setting but should not supplant other more effective therapies, such as ACE inhibitors. Nitrates should be avoided in patients taking medications for erectile dysfunction, such as sildenafil, because the combination can cause severe hypotension.

Nesiritide is a recombinant form of BNP that is given intravenously and produces both natriuresis and vasodilation.[96] Nesiritide has distinct advantages over other intravenous vasodilators, including nitroglycerin and nitroprusside, because it does not require intravenous titration or invasive hemodynamic monitoring, making it more practical for OU use. Studies suggest that it provides more rapid improvement of symptoms and decreases mortality and hospital admissions compared with dobutamine, and facilitates more rapid decrease in pulmonary capillary wedge pressure compared with nitroglycerin.[41,97]

Nesiritide is given intravenously with an initial loading dose and then a maintenance infusion. It can cause hypotension, which may be potentiated by the use of other medications affecting pressure, and therefore ACE inhibitors are typically withheld. In the OU setting, nesiritide was shown to decrease the duration of hospitalization by 4 days and showed nonsignificant trends in decreased hospitalization after OU treatment and 30-day hospital readmission.[18]

Although nesiritide was becoming widely used for the treatment of ADHF in ED and OU areas, this practice changed after two published meta-analyses suggested that it may worsen renal function and increase mortality.[98,99] These findings led to a rapid decrease in the use of nesiritide for ADHF.[100] Multiple editorials have supported and refuted the use of nesiritide in ADHF.[101–103] More recent studies have suggested that nesiritide does not affect renal function or that it may be a dose-related phenomonon.[104,105] A large-scale prospective study is currently addressing the safety and efficacy of nesiritide in ADHF. Information from this and other prospective studies will be needed to determine the usefulness of nesiritide and which patients it would benefit most. Currently, nesiritide remains a second-line agent for the treatment of ADHF.

Inotropes, including dobutamine, dopamine, milrinone, and amrinone, may be used to increase cardiac output and renal blood flow. They are often reserved for patients who have severely depressed cardiac output not responding to afterload reduction and are administered to fewer than 15% of patients who have ADHF.[106] Inotropes are administered as a constant infusion and are not used in OU care because they are often given over several days.

Ultrafiltration recently became a treatment option for patients in ADHF. Ultrafiltration is a type of membrane filtration using hydrostatic pressure to force liquid and small solutes through a semipermeable membrane. One company has received FDA approval for use of an ultrafiltration device in ADHF. The Aquadex Flexflow requires two 18-gauge or larger peripheral intravenous catheters or a double-lumen central venous catheter to draw off blood and return blood, minus the filtered portion, to the patient. The patient must be anticoagulated with heparin before use to prevent clotting of the filter. Patients who have contraindications to anticoagulation would not be candidates for this therapy. The device can remove up to 500 mL/h of ultrafiltrate, which consists of water and sodium. The rate of fluid removal is improved with the use of larger-gauge intravenous lines or catheters. Patients may be maintained on ACE inhibitors, β-blockers, and even diuretics, but intravenous vasodilators should be avoided.

The device seems to be effective in treating patients resistant to diuretics who are fluid overloaded. One study showed an average fluid removal of more than 8 L with no change in sodium, potassium, creatinine, or BUN.[107] The Ultrafiltration versus Intravenous Diuretics for Patients Hospitalized for Acute Decompensated Congestive Heart Failure trial compared ultrafiltration with standard care for ADHF in hospitalized patients and showed a greater amount of weight and net fluid loss in the ultrafiltration group. Even more impressive was the 50% reduction in rehospitalizations for heart failure and return ED or clinic visits within 90 days of discharge.[108]

Although this new technology seems promising, particularly for patients resistant to diuretics, its usefulness in the OU setting is unclear. The need for larger venous access and anticoagulation make it less desirable for patients familiar with diuretic treatment. Further studies are needed to determine the usefulness of ultrafiltration in the OU population.

The long-term risk for sudden cardiac death in patients who have severe systolic dysfunction is significant, with one third to one half of patients who have heart failure dying unexpectedly.[109,110] Several trials have shown survival benefit for patients who have ischemic heart failure and ejection fractions less than 35%.[111–114] Placement of implantable cardiac defibrillators (ICD) has now become standard care, largely replacing antiarrhythmic therapy, and the cost of placement is currently covered by Medicare for patients who meet eligibility requirements. These criteria include EF of 35% or less, New York Heart Association class II or III disease for greater than 9 months, and inducible or sustained ventricular tachycardia.

Patients who seem eligible for ICD placement or ho have a history of ventricular tachycardia should be referred to a cardiologist for electrophysiologic study. Patients who have a history of palpitations, syncope, or near-syncope may be referred for outpatient continuous cardiac monitoring, such as a Holter or event monitor, to determine if significant arrhythmias are occurring.

Some medications should likely be avoided or at least not started while patients are being treated for ADHF, including nonsteroidal anti-inflammatory agents, calcium channel blockers, and diabetic agents, such as metformin, thiazolidinedione, and cisapride.

Criteria for determining discharge are often based on a patient's clinical presentation after a period of treatment. Several authors have provided more explicit discharge criteria for patients in the OU treated for ADHF.[115–117] Most of these recommendations have not been prospectively studied but are pragmatic assessments of the patient's clinical status. Evidence suggests that urine output less than 1 L after treatment predicts treatment failure.[118] Some findings that may suggest that the patient has not improved include the presence of a third heart sound, increased BUN, hypotension, hypoxia, and dyspnea at rest or with minimal exertion. Having patients ambulate through the department is often prudent to show that they will be able to do so if discharged. Some suggested discharge criteria include:

> Clinically improved dyspnea
> Ability to ambulate back to baseline
> Urine output greater than 1 L
> Resting heart rate less than 100 beats/min and systolic blood pressure greater than 80 mm Hg
> Pulse oximetry greater than 91% if not normally on supplemental oxygen
> No clinical or EKG evidence of cardiac ischemia
> No significant increase in serum BUN or creatinine
> No new or significant dysrhythmias

The most recent AHA/ACC guidelines for the treatment of ADHF do not provide discharge criteria but recommend that patients be euvolemic before discharge.[64]

It is extremely important to start recommended heart failure medications and provide prescriptions to patients discharged after OU therapy, because studies have shown that providing appropriate long-term heart failure medications, such as β-blockers and ACE inhibitors, reduces mortality.[119]

Discharge education is an important aspect of care that is often overlooked but can have a large beneficial effect if administered properly. Education concerning smoking and medication and dietary compliance can reduce recidivism and decrease medical expenses for these patients.[120–123]

The importance of smoking cessation education and therapy deserves additional mention. Simply by quitting smoking, patients can reduce their mortality by 30% within 2 years. This mortality benefit is similar to that seen with the use of β-blockers or ACE inhibitors in the treatment of heart failure.[124,125] Having patients receive the advice directly from the treating physician is very influential and can increase rates of smoking cessation greater than 60%.[126]

If resources are available, a multidisciplinary team, including cardiologist dietitians, social workers, and heart failure educators such as nurse practitioners, would be ideal to provide patient information on the importance of medication and dietary compliance, exercise, smoking cessation, and following up with future tests and appointments. Other areas for patient education include monitoring dyspnea symptoms and weight and notifying the physician for worsening conditions. The AHA Get with the Guidelines program offers Internet-based educational tools to educate patients who have heart failure who are being discharged. Ensuring that patients are taking appropriate medications, such as β-blockers and ACE inhibitors, is extremely important. Patients who leave with prescriptions for cardiac medications are more likely to adhere to that medication regimen.[127]

SUMMARY

ADHF is a common illness presenting to the ED that is amenable to OU treatment. As the number of baby boomers continues to grow and the incidence of heart failure increases, the financial implications of ADHF treatment will become more prominent. Obtaining institutional support and developing a good working relationship with cardiology colleagues is vital to creating workable ADHF protocols for whichever type of OU an institution decides to use.

REFERENCES

1. Hugli O, Braun JE, Kim S, et al. United States emergency department visits for acute decompensated heart failure, 1992 to 2001. Am J Cardiol 2005; 96(11):1537–42.
2. Burt CW, Schappert SM. Ambulatory care visits to physician offices, hospital outpatient departments, and emergency departments: United States, 1999–2000. Vital Health Stat 2004;13(157):1–70.
3. Massie BM, Shah NB. Evolving trends in the epidemiologic factors of heart failure: rationale for preventive strategies and comprehensive disease management. Am Heart J 1997;133(6):703–12.
4. O'Connell JB, Bristow MR. Economic impact of heart failure in the United States: time for a different approach. J Heart Lung Transplant 1994;13(4): S107–12.
5. O'Connell JB. The economic burden of heart failure. Clin Cardiol 2000;23(Suppl.3):III6–10.
6. Graff L, Orledge J, Radford MJ, et al. Correlation of the agency for health care policy and research congestive heart failure admission guideline with mortality: peer review organization voluntary hospital association initiative to decrease events (provide) for congestive heart failure. Ann Emerg Med 1999;34(4 Pt 1):429–37.
7. Polanczyk CA, Rohde LE, Philbin EA, et al. A new casemix adjustment index for hospital mortality among patients with congestive heart failure. Med Care 1998;36(10):1489–99.
8. Rosamond W, Flegal K, Furie K, et al. Heart disease and stroke statistics–2008 update: a report from the American Heart Association Statistics Committee and Stroke Statistics Subcommittee. Circulation 2008;117(4):e25–146.
9. Stewart S, MacIntyre K, Capewell S, et al. Heart failure and the aging population: an increasing burden in the 21st century? Heart 2003;89(1): 49–53.
10. Ansari M, Massie BM. Heart failure: how big is the problem? Who are the patients? What does the future hold? Am Heart J 2003;146(1):1–4.
11. Storrow AB, Collins SP, Lyons MS, et al. Emergency department observation of heart failure: preliminary analysis of safety and cost. Congest Heart Fail 2005;11(2):68–72.
12. Peacock WF, Remer EE, Aponte J, et al. Effective observation unit treatment of decompensated heart failure. Congest Heart Fail 2002;8(2):68–73.
13. Ross MA, Compton S, Medado P, et al. An emergency department diagnostic protocol for patients with transient ischemic attack: a randomized controlled trial. Ann Emerg Med 2007;50(2):109–19.
14. Trommald M, Aaserud M, Bjorndal A. [Observational units–same good service to lower costs?]. Tidsskr Nor Laegeforen 2000;120(25):3029–34 [in Norwegian].
15. Goodacre S, Nicholl J, Dixon S, et al. Randomised controlled trial and economic evaluation of a chest pain observation unit compared with routine care. BMJ 2004;328(7434):1–6.
16. Roberts RR, Zalenski RJ, Mensah EK, et al. Costs of an emergency department-based accelerated diagnostic protocol vs hospitalization in patients with chest pain: a randomized controlled trial. JAMA 1997;278(20):1670–6.
17. Gaspoz JM, Lee TH, Weinstein MC, et al. Cost-effectiveness of a new short-stay unit to "rule out" acute myocardial infarction in low risk patients. J Am Coll Cardiol 1994;24(5):1249–59.
18. Peacock WFt, Holland R, Gyarmathy R, et al. Observation unit treatment of heart failure with nesiritide: results from the proaction trial. J Emerg Med 2005;29(3):243–52.
19. McDermott MF, Murphy DG, Zalenski RJ, et al. A comparison between emergency diagnostic and treatment unit and inpatient care in the

management of acute asthma. Arch Intern Med 1997;157(18):2055–62.

20. Rydman RJ, Zalenski RJ, Roberts RR, et al. Patient satisfaction with an emergency department chest pain observation unit. Ann Emerg Med 1997;29(1):109–15.

21. Henneman PL, Marx JA, Cantrill SC, et al. The use of an emergency department observation unit in the management of abdominal trauma. Ann Emerg Med 1989;18(6):647–50.

22. Shen WK, Decker WW, Smars PA, et al. Syncope evaluation in the emergency department study (seeds): a multidisciplinary approach to syncope management. Circulation 2004;110(24):3636–45.

23. Graff L, Radford MJ, Werne C. Probability of appendicitis before and after observation. Ann Emerg Med 1991;20(5):503–7.

24. Aghababian RV. Acutely decompensated heart failure: opportunities to improve care and outcomes in the emergency department. Rev Cardiovasc Med 2002;4(Suppl. 3):S3–9.

25. Kelen GD, Scheulen JJ, Hill PM. Effect of an emergency department (ed) managed acute care unit on ED overcrowding and emergency medical services diversion. Acad Emerg Med 2001;8(11):1095–100.

26. Ross MA, Wilson AG, McPherson M. The impact of an ED observation unit bed on inpatient bed availability. Acad Emerg Med 2001;8(5):576.

27. Diamond NJ, Schofferman JA, Elliot JW. Evaluation of an emergency department observation ward. JACEP 1976;5(1):29–31.

28. Landers Fa WJ, McNbney WK. Observation ward utilization. JACEP 1975;4:123–5.

29. Emergency department observation units. American college of emergency physicians. Ann Emerg Med 1988;17(1):95–6.

30. Centers for Medicare & Medicaid Services. CMS manual system. Department of Health & Human Services. Pub 100–04 Medicare claims processing. Available at: http://www.cms.hhs.gov/transmittals/downloads/R1430CPTXT.pdf. Accessed September 15, 2008.

31. Yealy DM, De Hart DA, Ellis G, et al. A survey of observation units in the United States. Am J Emerg Med 1989;7(6):576–80.

32. Department of Health and Human Services. Medicare and Medicaid Programs. Interim and Final Rule. Federal Register. Available at: http://www.cms.hhs.gov/HospitalOutpatientPPS/Downloads/cms1392fc.pdf. Accessed December 13, 2007.

33. McCullough PA, Nowak RM, McCord J, et al. B-type natriuretic peptide and clinical judgment in emergency diagnosis of heart failure: analysis from breathing not properly (BNP) multinational study. Circulation 2002;106(4):416–22.

34. Clerico A, Fontana M, Zyw L, et al. Comparison of the diagnostic accuracy of brain natriuretic peptide (BNP) and the n-terminal part of the propeptide of BNP immunoassays in chronic and acute heart failure: a systematic review. Clin Chem 2007;53(5):813–22.

35. Dokainish H, Zoghbi WA, Lakkis NM, et al. Comparative accuracy of B-type natriuretic peptide and tissue Doppler echocardiography in the diagnosis of congestive heart failure. Am J Cardiol 2004;93(9):1130–5.

36. Latour-Perez J, Coves-Orts FJ, Abad-Terrado C, et al. Accuracy of B-type natriuretic peptide levels in the diagnosis of left ventricular dysfunction and heart failure: a systematic review. Eur J Heart Fail. 2006;8(4):390–9.

37. Mueller T, Gegenhuber A, Poelz W, et al. Diagnostic accuracy of B type natriuretic peptide and amino terminal proBNP in the emergency diagnosis of heart failure. Heart 2005;91(5):606–12.

38. Wang CS, FitzGerald JM, Schulzer M, et al. Does this dyspneic patient in the emergency department have congestive heart failure? JAMA 2005;294(15):1944–56.

39. Benjamin EJ, Levy D, Vaziri SM, et al. Independent risk factors for atrial fibrillation in a population-based cohort. The Framingham Heart Study. JAMA 1994;271(11):840–4.

40. Adams KF Jr, Fonarow GC, Emerman CL, et al. Characteristics and outcomes of patients hospitalized for heart failure in the United States: rationale, design, and preliminary observations from the first 100,000 cases in the acute decompensated heart failure national registry (ADHERE). Am Heart J 2005;149(2):209–16.

41. VMAC Investigators. Intravenous nesiritide vs nitroglycerin for treatment of decompensated congestive heart failure: a randomized controlled trial. JAMA 2002;287(12):1531–40.

42. Smith WR, Poses RM, McClish DK, et al. Prognostic judgments and triage decisions for patients with acute congestive heart failure. Chest 2002;121(5):1610–7.

43. Butler J, Hanumanthu S, Chomsky D, et al. Frequency of low-risk hospital admissions for heart failure. Am J Cardiol 1998;81(1):41–4.

44. Diercks DB, Peacock WF, Kirk JD, et al. ED patients with heart failure: identification of an observational unit-appropriate cohort. Am J Emerg Med 2006;24(3):319–24.

45. Burkhardt J, Peacock WF, Emerman CL. Predictors of emergency department observation unit outcomes. Acad Emerg Med 2005;12(9):869–74.

46. Auble TE, Hsieh M, Gardner W, et al. A prediction rule to identify low-risk patients with heart failure. Acad Emerg Med 2005;12(6):514–21.

47. Fonarow GC, Adams KF Jr, Abraham WT, et al. Risk stratification for in-hospital mortality in acutely decompensated heart failure: classification and

regression tree analysis. JAMA 2005;293(5): 572–80.

48. Lee DS, Austin PC, Rouleau JL, et al. Predicting mortality among patients hospitalized for heart failure: derivation and validation of a clinical model. JAMA 2003;290(19):2581–7.

49. Brophy JM, Deslauriers G, Rouleau JL. Long-term prognosis of patients presenting to the emergency room with decompensated congestive heart failure. Can J Cardiol 1994;10(5):543–7.

50. Brophy JM, Deslauriers G, Boucher B, et al. The hospital course and short term prognosis of patients presenting to the emergency room with decompensated congestive heart failure. Can J Cardiol 1993;9(3):219–24.

51. Auble TE, Hsieh M, McCausland JB, et al. Comparison of four clinical prediction rules for estimating risk in heart failure. Ann Emerg Med 2007;50(2): 127–35.

52. Chin MH, Goldman L. Correlates of major complications or death in patients admitted to the hospital with congestive heart failure. Arch Intern Med 1996;156(16):1814–20.

53. Hsieh M, Auble TE, Yealy DM. Validation of the acute heart failure index. Ann Emerg Med 2008; 51(1):37–44.

54. Gheorghiade M, Rossi JS, Cotts W, et al. Characterization and prognostic value of persistent hyponatremia in patients with severe heart failure in the ESCAPE trial. Arch Intern Med 2007;167(18): 1998–2005.

55. Felker GM, Adams KF Jr, Gattis WA, et al. Anemia as a risk factor and therapeutic target in heart failure. J Am Coll Cardiol 2004;44(5):959–66.

56. Butler J, Forman DE, Abraham WT, et al. Relationship between heart failure treatment and development of worsening renal function among hospitalized patients. Am Heart J 2004;147(2):331–8.

57. Kramer BK, Schweda F, Riegger GA. Diuretic treatment and diuretic resistance in heart failure. Am J Med 1999;106(1):90–6.

58. Neuberg GW, Miller AB, O'Connor CM, et al. Diuretic resistance predicts mortality in patients with advanced heart failure. Am Heart J 2002; 144(1):31–8.

59. Redfield MM, Jacobsen SJ, Burnett JC Jr, et al. Burden of systolic and diastolic ventricular dysfunction in the community: appreciating the scope of the heart failure epidemic. JAMA 2003;289(2): 194–202.

60. Smith GL, Masoudi FA, Vaccarino V, et al. Outcomes in heart failure patients with preserved ejection fraction: mortality, readmission, and functional decline. J Am Coll Cardiol 2003;41(9):1510–8.

61. Vasan RS, Larson MG, Benjamin EJ, et al. Congestive heart failure in subjects with normal versus reduced left ventricular ejection fraction:

prevalence and mortality in a population-based cohort. J Am Coll Cardiol 1999;33(7):1948–55.

62. Bhatia RS, Tu JV, Lee DS, et al. Outcome of heart failure with preserved ejection fraction in a population-based study. N Engl J Med. 2006;355(3): 260–9.

63. George TL, Hiok CT, Leonard K. Type of liver dysfunction in heart failure and its relation to the severity of tricuspid regurgitation. Am J Cardiol 2002; 90(12):1405.

64. Hunt SA, Abraham WT, Chin MH, et al. ACC/AHA 2005 guideline update for the diagnosis and management of chronic heart failure in the adult: a report of the American college of cardiology/ American heart association task force on practice guidelines (writing committee to update the 2001 guidelines for the evaluation and management of heart failure): developed in collaboration with the American college of chest physicians and the international society for heart and lung transplantation: endorsed by the heart rhythm society. Circulation 2005;112(12):e154–235.

65. Demir M, Kanadasi M, Akpinar O, et al. Cardiac troponin t as a prognostic marker in patients with heart failure: a 3-year outcome study. Angiology 2007;58(5):603–9.

66. Parenti N, Bartolacci S, Carle F, et al. Cardiac troponin I as prognostic marker in heart failure patients discharged from emergency department. Intern Emerg Med 2008;3:44–7.

67. Peacock WF, Emerman CE, Doleh M, et al. Retrospective review: the incidence of non-ST segment elevation MI in emergency department patients presenting with decompensated heart failure. Congest Heart Fail 2003;9(6):303–8.

68. Missov E, Calzolari C, Pau B. Circulating cardiac troponin I in severe congestive heart failure. Circulation 1997;96(9):2953–8.

69. Glauser J, Erickson J, Bhatt D, et al. Elevated serum cardiac markers predict coronary artery disease in patients with a history of heart failure who present with chest pain: insights from the i*tracs registry. Congest Heart Fail 2007;13(3):142–8.

70. Dormans TP, van Meyel JJ, Gerlag PG, et al. Diuretic efficacy of high dose furosemide in severe heart failure: bolus injection versus continuous infusion. J Am Coll Cardiol 1996;28(2):376–82.

71. Pivac N, Rumboldt Z, Sardelic S, et al. Diuretic effects of furosemide infusion versus bolus injection in congestive heart failure. Int J Clin Pharmacol Res 1998;18(3):121–8.

72. Lahav M, Regev A, Ra'anani P, et al. Intermittent administration of furosemide vs continuous infusion preceded by a loading dose for congestive heart failure. Chest 1992;102(3):725–31.

73. Salvador DR, Rey NR, Ramos GC, et al. Continuous infusion versus bolus injection of loop diuretics in

congestive heart failure. Cochrane Database Syst Rev 2005;(3):CD003178.

74. Packer M, Coats AJS, Fowler MB, et al. Effect of carvedilol on survival in severe chronic heart failure. N Engl J Med 2001;344(22):1651–8.

75. Effect of metoprolol CR/XL in chronic heart failure: metoprolol CR/XL randomised intervention trial in congestive heart failure (MERIT-HF). Lancet 1999; 353(9169):2001–7.

76. Hjalmarson A, Goldstein S, Fagerberg B, et al. Effects of controlled-release metoprolol on total mortality, hospitalizations, and well-being in patients with heart failure: the metoprolol CR/XL randomized intervention trial in congestive heart failure (MERIT-HF). JAMA 2000;283(10):1295–302.

77. The cardiac insufficiency bisoprolol study II (CIBIS-II): a randomised trial. Lancet 1999;353(9146):9–13.

78. Kao W, Surjancev BP. Management of acute heart failure exacerbation. Crit Care Clin 2001;17(2):321–35.

79. Cleland JGF, Bristow MR, Erdmann E, et al. Beta-blocking agents in heart failure: should they be used and how? Eur Heart J 1996;17(11):1629–39.

80. Gattis WA, O'Connor CM, Gallup DS, et al. Predischarge initiation of carvedilol in patients hospitalized for decompensated heart failure: results of the initiation management predischarge: process for assessment of carvedilol therapy in heart failure (IMPACT-HF) trial. J Am Coll Cardiol 2004;43(9):1534–41.

81. Chadda K, Goldstein S, Byington R, et al. Effect of propranolol after acute myocardial infarction in patients with congestive heart failure. Circulation 1986;73(3):503–10.

82. Metra M, Torp-Pedersen C, Cleland JG, et al. Should beta-blocker therapy be reduced or withdrawn after an episode of decompensated heart failure? Results from COMET. Eur J Heart Fail 2007;9(9):901–9.

83. Shamimi-Noori S WD, Dasgupta A, Adams S, et al. [abstract]. Beta blocker dose adjustment upon hospitalization for acute decompensated heart failure. J Am Coll Cardiol 2007;40(11 Suppl A):1028–66.

84. Garg R, Yusuf S. Overview of randomized trials of angiotensin-converting enzyme inhibitors on mortality and morbidity in patients with heart failure. Collaborative Group on ACE Inhibitor trials. JAMA 1995;273(18):1450–6.

85. Nony P, Boissel JP, Girard P, et al. Relative efficacy of angiotensin converting enzyme inhibitors on mortality of patients with congestive heart failure: implications of randomized trials and role of the aetiology (ischaemic or non-ischaemic) of heart failure. Eur Heart J 1992;13(8):1101–8.

86. Lee VC, Rhew DC, Dylan M, et al. Meta-analysis: angiotensin-receptor blockers in chronic heart failure and high-risk acute myocardial infarction. Ann Intern Med 2004;141(9):693–704.

87. Yusuf S, Pfeffer MA, Swedberg K, et al. Effects of candesartan in patients with chronic heart failure and preserved left-ventricular ejection fraction: the CHARM-preserved trial. Lancet 2003; 362(9386):777–81.

88. Morris SA, Hatcher HF, Reddy DK. Digoxin therapy for heart failure: an update. Am Fam Physician 2006;74(4):613–8.

89. Ahmed A, Rich MW, Fleg JL, et al. Effects of digoxin on morbidity and mortality in diastolic heart failure: the ancillary digitalis investigation group trial. Circulation 2006;114(5):397–403.

90. Rathore SS, Curtis JP, Wang Y, et al. Association of serum digoxin concentration and outcomes in patients with heart failure. JAMA 2003;289(7):871–8.

91. Adams KF Jr, Patterson JH, Gattis WA, et al. Relationship of serum digoxin concentration to mortality and morbidity in women in the digitalis investigation group trial: a retrospective analysis. J Am Coll Cardiol 2005;46(3):497–504.

92. Loeb HS, Johnson G, Henrick A, et al. Effect of enalapril, hydralazine plus isosorbide dinitrate, and prazosin on hospitalization in patients with chronic congestive heart failure. The V-HeFT VA cooperative studies group. Circulation 1993;87(Suppl.6):VI78–87.

93. Cohn JN, Johnson G, Ziesche S, et al. A comparison of enalapril with hydralazine-isosorbide dinitrate in the treatment of chronic congestive heart failure. N Engl J Med 1991;325(5):303–10.

94. Taylor AL, Ziesche S, Yancy C, et al. Combination of isosorbide dinitrate and hydralazine in blacks with heart failure. N Engl J Med 2004;351(20):2049–57.

95. Patrick K, Noonan LZB. The bioavailability of oral nitroglycerin. J Pharm Sci 1986;75(3):241–3.

96. Colucci WS, Elkayam U, Horton DP, et al. Intravenous nesiritide, a natriuretic peptide, in the treatment of decompensated congestive heart failure. Nesiritide study group. N Engl J Med 2000; 343(4):246–53.

97. Silver MA, Horton DP, Ghali JK, et al. Effect of nesiritide versus dobutamine on short-term outcomes in the treatment of patients with acutely decompensated heart failure. J Am Coll Cardiol 2002;39(5):798–803.

98. Sackner-Bernstein JD, Skopicki HA, Aaronson KD. Risk of worsening renal function with nesiritide in patients with acutely decompensated heart failure. Circulation 2005;111(12):1487–91.

99. Sackner-Bernstein JD, Kowalski M, Fox M, et al. Short-term risk of death after treatment with nesiritide for decompensated heart failure: a pooled analysis of randomized controlled trials. JAMA 2005;293(15):1900–5.

100. Hauptman PJ, Schnitzler MA, Swindle J, et al. Use of nesiritide before and after publications suggesting drug-related risks in patients with acute decompensated heart failure. JAMA 2006;296(15):1877–84.

101. Topol EJ. Nesiritide—not verified. N Engl J Med 2005;353(2):113–6.

102. Teerlink JR, Massie BM. Nesiritide and worsening of renal function: the emperor's new clothes? Circulation 2005;111(12):1459–61.

103. Shlipak MG, Massie BM. The clinical challenge of cardiorenal syndrome. Circulation 2004;110(12):1514–7.

104. Witteles RM, Kao D, Christopherson D, et al. Impact of nesiritide on renal function in patients with acute decompensated heart failure and pre-existing renal dysfunction: a randomized, double-blind, placebo-controlled clinical trial. J Am Coll Cardiol 2007;50(19):1835–40.

105. Riter HG, Redfield MM, Burnett JC, et al. Nonhypotensive low-dose nesiritide has differential renal effects compared with standard-dose nesiritide in patients with acute decompensated heart failure and renal dysfunction. J Am Coll Cardiol 2006;47(11):2334–5.

106. Fonarow GC, Heywood JT, Heidenreich PA, et al. Temporal trends in clinical characteristics, treatments, and outcomes for heart failure hospitalizations, 2002 to 2004: findings from Acute Decompensated Heart Failure National Registry (ADHERE). Am Heart J 2007;153(6):1021.

107. Costanzo MR, Saltzberg M, O'Sullivan J, et al. Early ultrafiltration in patients with decompensated heart failure and diuretic resistance. J Am Coll Cardiol 2005;46(11):2047–51.

108. Costanzo MR, Guglin ME, Saltzberg MT, et al. Ultrafiltration versus intravenous diuretics for patients hospitalized for acute decompensated heart failure. J Am Coll Cardiol 2007;49(6):675–83.

109. Kannel WB, Plehn JF, Cupples LA. Cardiac failure and sudden death in the Framingham study. Am Heart J 1988;115(4):869–75.

110. Packer M. Lack of relation between ventricular arrhythmias and sudden death in patients with chronic heart failure. Circulation 1992;85(Suppl. I):I50–6.

111. Moss AJ, Zareba W, Hall WJ, et al. Prophylactic implantation of a defibrillator in patients with myocardial infarction and reduced ejection fraction. N Engl J Med 2002;346(12):877–83.

112. Bardy GH, Lee KL, Mark DB, et al. Amiodarone or an implantable cardioverter-defibrillator for congestive heart failure. N Engl J Med 2005;352(3):225–37.

113. AVID Investigators. The antiarrhythmics versus implantable defibrillators I. A comparison of antiarrhythmic-drug therapy with implantable defibrillators in patients resuscitated from near-fatal ventricular arrhythmias. N Engl J Med 1997;337(22):1576–84.

114. Buxton AE, Lee KL, Fisher JD, et al. A randomized study of the prevention of sudden death in patients with coronary artery disease. N Engl J Med 1999;341(25):1882–90.

115. Peacock WF. Using the emergency department clinical decision unit for acute decompensated heart failure. Cardiol Clin 2005;23(4):569–88, viii.

116. Deborah Diercks P, Frank W. Short stay management of heart failure. Philadelphia: Lippincott Williams & Wilkins; 2006.

117. Meldon S, Ma OJ, Woolard R, American college of emergency medicine. Geriatric emergency medicine. 1st edition. New York: McGraw-Hill, Health Professions Division; 2004.

118. Peacock W, Frank AJH, Craig Mary T, et al. Predictors of unsuccessful treatment for congestive heart failure in the emergency department observation unit. Acad Emerg Med 1997;4(5):493–4.

119. Johnson D, Jin Y, Quan H, et al. Beta-blockers and angiotensin-converting enzyme inhibitors/receptor blockers prescriptions after hospital discharge for heart failure are associated with decreased mortality in Alberta, Canada. J Am Coll Cardiol 2003;42(8):1438–45.

120. Koelling TM, Johnson ML, Cody RJ, et al. Discharge education improves clinical outcomes in patients with chronic heart failure. Circulation 2005;111(2):179–85.

121. Rich MW, Beckham V, Wittenberg C, et al. A multidisciplinary intervention to prevent the readmission of elderly patients with congestive heart failure. N Engl J Med 1995;333(18):1190–5.

122. Krumholz HM, Amatruda J, Smith GL, et al. Randomized trial of an education and support intervention to prevent readmission of patients with heart failure. J Am Coll Cardiol 2002;39(1):83–9.

123. Phillips CO, Wright SM, Kern DE, et al. Comprehensive discharge planning with postdischarge support for older patients with congestive heart failure: a meta-analysis. JAMA 2004;291(11):1358–67.

124. Lightwood J, Fleischmann KE, Glantz SA. Smoking cessation in heart failure: it is never too late. J Am Coll Cardiol 2001;37(6):1683–4.

125. Suskin N, Sheth T, Negassa A, et al. Relationship of current and past smoking to mortality and morbidity in patients with left ventricular dysfunction. J Am Coll Cardiol 2001;37(6):1677–82.

126. Lancaster T, Stead L, Silagy C, et al. Effectiveness of interventions to help people stop smoking: findings from the cochrane library. BMJ 2000;321(7257):355–8.

127. Simpson E, Beck C, Richard H, et al. Drug prescriptions after acute myocardial infarction: dosage, compliance, and persistence. Am Heart J 2003;145(3):438–44.

Observation Unit Economics

Sandra G. Sieck, RN, MBA[a],*, Mark G. Moseley, MD, MHA[b,c]

KEYWORDS

- Observation medicine • Economics
- Heart failure • Emergency Department

With an aging population (projected 16.5% of the population over the age of 65 in 2020), the United States health care delivery system is struggling to handle an onslaught of chronic disease burden.[1–3] Heart failure (HF) is one such chronic disease process whose incidence is increasing as patients with chronic cardiac disease are living longer because of improved technologic and therapeutic advances. While longevity with chronic disease is desirable to an individual patient, it increasingly places a burden on providers, payers, and the health care infrastructure that must continue to render care for those with decompensated disease states in economically uncertain times. As a result, the delivery of care for acute exacerbations of chronic disease on an ongoing basis continues to strain an already fragile and increasingly fragmented delivery system ill equipped to handle this burden.

Nowhere is this realized more painfully from an economic perspective, than for acute care facilities treating patients with acute heart failure (AHF). Such facilities face the tenuous balancing act between offering improved inpatient therapeutic modalities (mechanical and pharmacologic), while attempting to maintain economic viability under the microscope of use review and prospective payment systems.[4] As payment from all payer sources is increasingly linked to outcome metrics (pay-for-performance), defining and implementing optimal care that is cost-effective and results in the best clinical outcomes has become critical. With this said, improved therapy for AHF has come at the price of increased costs for delivery of care

without the promise of increased reimbursement for the same. Thus, there is a dichotomy for acute care facilities to insure the provision of cost-efficient care while concomitantly maintaining a high quality of care.[4] As a result, the health care delivery and reimbursement system is at a crossroads, where the care for patients with chronic disease states demands innovations that better match patient care needs with economically feasible care models.

BURDEN OF DISEASE

In light of the above, it is not surprising that the clinical and financial burden to the United States health care system and acute care facilities is staggering. Relevant examples of this burden include the following:

- In 2005, the American Heart Association estimated that there were almost 5 million people with HF in the United States.[5]
- In 2001, there were almost 1 million hospitalizations in the United States with a first listed discharge diagnosis of HF (**Fig. 1**).
- Nearly 20% of hospital admissions among persons older than 65 are because of HF, making it responsible for more elderly patient hospitalizations than any other disease.[6]
- Readmission rates were as high as 20% at 30 days.[7]
- HF is the most commonly used Medicare diagnosis-related group (DRG).[3]
- HF accounts for 12 to 15 million physician office visits annually.[8]

[a] Sieck HealthCare Consulting, Mobile, AL, USA
[b] The Ohio State University, OH, USA
[c] The Ohio State University Medical Center, Columbus, OH, USA
* Corresponding author. Sieck HealthCare Consulting, 9431 Jeff Hamilton Road, Mobile, AL 36695, USA.
E-mail address: ssieck@sieckhealthcare.com (S.G. Sieck).

Heart Failure Clin 5 (2009) 101–111
doi:10.1016/j.hfc.2008.08.008
1551-7136/08/$ – see front matter © 2008 Published by Elsevier Inc.

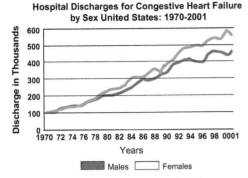

Hospital Discharges for Congestive Heart Failure by Sex United States: 1970-2001

Fig. 1. Trends in United States hospital discharge rates. (*Data from* American Heart Association. Heart Disease and Stroke Statistics—2004 update. Dallas (TX): American Heart Association; 2003.)

- HF was estimated to have contributed $25.8 billion in 2004 in direct and indirect costs in the United States.[9]
- HF accounts for over 10% of total costs for all cardiovascular conditions (**Table 1**). The majority of the expenditures are related to acute hospitalizations (**Fig. 2**).

While this data represents an overview of the impact to the health care system as a whole, it is easy to extrapolate the burden to the level of an individual acute care facility.

REIMBURSEMENT CONSIDERATIONS

Until recently, the majority of AHF patients were admitted to the hospital with first point of contact being the Emergency Department (ED). In fact, the ED served as the initial interface for three out of every four AHF patients admitted to the hospital, and once there, average length of stay (LOS) was 7 days.[10,11] As a result of prospective payment systems initiated by governmental payers in the late 1990s, facilities are reimbursed for AHF patients based on a fixed payment system using the DRG system.[4] This system financially rewards facilities that have a shorter overall LOS, discharging patients more quickly and leading to less cost for the same fixed payment. Under the Inpatient Prospective Payment System (IPPS), the average Medicare payment for DRG 127 (AHF) is $5,456. With the break-even point for most hospitals at about 5 days, and an average LOS of 7 days as noted above, hospitals are not reimbursed sufficiently in most cases to cover their costs: by one estimate, losing $1,288 per AHF patient.[12,13] Today, DRG 127 has been transitioned to three Medical Severity DRGs (MS-DRG):[14] While under the old Centers for Medicare and Medicaid Services (CMS)-DRG system, all patients with a principle diagnosis of congestive heart failure (CHF) were grouped to DRG 127 and the hospital was paid based on the diagnosis, regardless of illness severity. Under the new system, the same patients will be split into three MS-DRGs, stratified by the presence of major complications and comorbidities (MCC), or simply complications and comorbidities (CC). The resulting level of severity illness category is then multiplied by a weighting code to determine the final

Table 1
Cardiovascular disease costs (in $billion) in the United States

	Coronary Heart Disease	Hypertension	Congestive Heart Failure	Total Cardiovascular Disease[a,b]
Direct Costs				
Hospital	$37.0	$5.5	$13.6	$101.7
Nursing home	9.7	3.8	3.5	38.1
Physicians/other professionals	9.6	9.6	1.8	33.4
Drugs/other medical durables	8.5	21.0	2.7	43.3
Home health care	1.4	1.5	2.1	10.3
Total expenditures[b]	$66.3	$41.5	$23.7	$226.7
Indirect costs				
Lost productivity/morbidity	9.1	7.2	–	33.6
Lost productivity/mortality[c]	57.8	6.8	2.1	108.1
Grand totals[b]	$133.2	$55.5	$25.8	$368.4

[a] Original table included stroke and heart disease, which are included in the total cardiovascular disease figures.
[b] Totals may not add up because of rounding and overlap.
[c] Lost future earnings of persons who will die in 2004, discounted at 3%.
Data from American Heart Association. Heart Disease and Stroke Statistics—2004 update. Dallas (TX): American Heart Association; 2003.

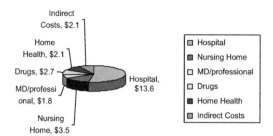

Fig. 2. Costs for heart failure in the United States (in $ billions). (*Data from* American Heart Association. Heart Disease and Stroke Statistics—2004 update. Dallas (TX): American Heart Association; 2003.)

reimbursement. Note that the highest severity is reimbursed at more than twice the rate of the lowest.

> MS-DRG 291, CHF with at least one MCC present Weight: 1.4850 ($7,923)
> MS-DRG 292, CHF with at least one CC present Weight: 1.0216 ($5,450)
> MS-DRG 293, CHF with no MCC or CC present Weight: 0.7317 ($3,903)

Hospitals today are struggling to balance clinical outcomes and financial sustainability. This has forced hospital administrators to place greater pressure on the financial side of the equation, attempting to cut to a profit in a system that historically has rewarded facilities for shorter LOS. CMS has developed new target areas focused on the IPPS 1-day stays, including DRG 127 (heart failure and shock) and DRG 143 (chest pain) listed in the top four. One-day stays excluding transfers and medical 1-day stays and 1-day stays that have prior observation (revenue code 760 or 762) of greater than 24 hours (as reported on the claim) will be excluded from the count of audited 1-day stays, as these admissions do not represent true "1-day stays." Additionally, analysis of payment errors for 1-day stays has identified that 1-day stays with prior observation of 24 hours or greater have a lower incidence of unnecessary admissions than other 1-day stays.[15]

Further compounding a hospital's misery is the fact that Medicare is focusing on inappropriate payments for unnecessary 1-day LOS, readmissions on the same day, and at 7 or 30 days to the same or different facility.[15] This leaves hospitals at jeopardy to potentially treat such patients at their own expense, noting again that nearly 20% of HF patients discharged after an acute hospitalization are readmitted within 30 days, and 50% are readmitted within 6 months.[7,16] An estimated 5.2 million Americans, and more than

550,000 new cases, are diagnosed annually.[7,17] Each year heart failure is responsible for approximately 1 million hospitalizations. The economic burden of heart failure is substantial. In 2007, the projected direct and indirect costs of heart failure are $33.2 billion.[17] Hospitalization accounts for the largest portion of these costs (54%).[18] These overwhelming numbers have prompted hospitals to re-evaluate the current treatment paradigm for AHF, with an emphasis on front-end diagnosis and management in the ambulatory setting.

THE OBSERVATION UNIT

Because of the reimbursement difficulties posed by the inpatient environment, there has been a considerable effort to push more and more services to the outpatient or ambulatory setting. For instance, chest pain centers began to emerge in the late 1990s as an alternative to inpatient admission for patients presenting to the ED with chest pain, as a more efficient way of ruling out acute coronary syndrome in low-risk patient subsets.[4] Not only was this method more efficient and cost effective when compared with a longer admission for patients of the same risk group, but quality of care was not compromised, allowing the same level of care in the ambulatory setting as offered in a traditional inpatient environment.

As a result of the above, the CMS has targeted disease processes, such as HF, chest pain, and asthma for ambulatory diagnosis and therapeutic intervention. Using the positive experience of chest pain centers and the ED based observation unit (OU), observation has been defined as a service provided "on-hospital premises, including use of a bed and periodic monitoring by nursing or other staff, which are reasonable and necessary to evaluate an outpatient's condition or determine the need for possible admission as an inpatient."[19] As such, OUs serve two distinct patient populations:

> Those with diagnostic uncertainty as to the nature of the disease process, who need an intensive period of diagnostic testing to either rule in or exclude the disease process. Example: chest pain for a rule out of acute coronary syndromes.
> Those with a confirmed disease process that requires intensive therapeutic interventions to improve the disease process, sufficient to enable continued outpatient management. Example: HF or asthma.

Approximately 80% of patients placed under an observation level of care can be discharged from the ED, thus preventing inpatient admission

(Robbin Dick, MD, personal communication, 2008). As a result, use of the OU has dramatically increased over the last few years (**Table 2**). Between 2002 and 2003 there was an 85% increase in OU use. Chest pain represented the most common condition seen in an OU, followed by gastrointestinal disorders and asthma, whereas AHF accounted for 5% of OU conditions in 2002 to 2003.[20] In 2007, the CMS also reported an upward trend in the number of observation claims being processed (**Table 3**). Furthermore, in a recent report on the state of the emergency care system in the United States, the Institute of Medicine listed ED-based observation units as a specific intervention hospitals should use to increase operational efficiency, appropriate resource use, and patient care.[21]

The Ambulatory Patient Classification (APC) code 0339 was originally created by the CMS in 2002, designed to relieve some of the pressures of treating HF patients aggressively on the front end of the process (ie, the OU) versus admitting the patients into an acute care setting. In 2008, the CMS deleted APC 0339 and created two new composite APC codes (8002 and 8003). APC 8002 Level I: Extended Assessment and Management (observation following a direct admission or clinic visit) is reimbursed at $351. APC 8003 Level II: Extended Assessment and Management (observation following an emergency level 4 or 5 visit) is reimbursed at $639. APC 8003 includes both ED visits and observation visits (**Table 4**).[22] Noted within these data, the number of claims filed will shift from APC 0600/0604 (low level codes; 30% Medicare claims) to APC 8002/8003 (extended assessment and management; 70% Medicare claims) making available a substantial positive financial shift of allocated reimbursement dollars. The new composite APCs encompass any medical diagnosis that meets medical necessity for observation services targeting high risk areas, such as HF and chest pain where noninvasive cardiac testing, such as stress testing, nuclear imaging, and echocardiography, remain standards of clinical practice. The existing minimal requirements

Table 3
Use of observation claims

Year	Total Number of Observation Claims
2003	56,000
2004	77,000
2005	124,300
2006	271,200

Data from Federal Register/Vol. 72, No. 227/Tuesday, November 27, 2007/Rules and Regulations 66,647 CMS-1392-FC. Available at: http://www.cms.hhs.gov/quarterlyproviderupdates/downloads/cms1392fc.pdf. Accessed November 27, 2007.

for receiving observation payments remain unchanged. In general, these requirements include a stay less than 48 hours but greater than 8 hours. In addition, most diagnostic tests that are performed during the OU stay are billable and reimbursable separately from the OU stay (**Table 5**).[4] The key to optimizing these new composite APCs is to "redesign the care process" with front-loaded activities.

APC 8002/8003 also benefits the hospital in that readmissions, meeting medical necessity and occurring within 30 days after an OU visit, are reimbursable.[4] There is no limit to the number of claims that can be submitted for a patient if billed under the APC outpatient system. In addition, no penalty exists if a patient is admitted to an OU and then requires an inpatient hospital admission at that same point of contact. A strong front-loaded case management model could ensure appropriate observation status. Thereafter, if the patient requires an inpatient admission the hospital does not get the APC reimbursement, but instead receives the DRG reimbursement. Additionally, the OU allows the hospital to save vital inpatient capacity, affording the opportunity to liberate inpatient beds for appropriate ED admissions, direct admissions, and transfer patients. In a study by Ross and colleagues,[23] making the LOS assumptions noted below, the investigators noted that an OU bed was the numerical patient equivalent of about three inpatient (IP) beds:

Observation LOS equals 15 hours, discharge 24 hours per day
IP LOS equals 2.2 days, discharge only during daytime hours
With this LOS, a 14-bed unit made 30 to 50 IP beds available: 8 to 13 monitored beds or 22 to 37 medical/surgical beds
Results: 1 observation bed equals 2.2 to 3.5 IP beds

Table 2
Use of observation units

Year	Total Number of Observation Services	Total Patients for HF Observation Services
2002	30,094	1,603
2003	66,276	3,749

Data from Medicare Outpatient Prospective Payment System Data: Observation Services Claims Data (G244, G263).

Table 4
Observation FY 2005

Comparison of Medicare Reimbursements for AHF FY 2005

APC 0339 – CHF Inpatient			DRG 127 – CHF Outpatient		
Level V< 8 hours		$239	Avg. Reimbursement		$4 617
APC 0339> 8 hours		$408	Mean Cost		$5905
			Medicare Benchmark LOS		5.3 days
UB92	**Billable**	**Reimbursable**	**UB92**	**Billable**	**Reimbursable**
EKG	Yes	Yes	EKG	Yes	No
Labs	Yes	Yes	Labs	Yes	No
ECHO	Yes	Yes	ECHO	Yes	No
CXR	Yes	Yes	CXR	Yes	No
IV Infusion	Yes	Yes	IV infusion	Yes	No
Drug therapy	Yes	Yes	Drug therapy	Yes	No
			***No = bundled under the service provided		
Total		$1300/1400			
Fixed Cost (FC)		($570)	Fixed Cost (FC)	($1498)	
FC varies per institution			FC varies per institution	usually 3 x outpatient	
Mean Variable Cost (V C)		($252)	Mean Variable Cost (VC)	($1168)	
			All diagnostics are bundled under corresponding DRG		
	$478 profit per case			**($1288) loss per case**	

From Hospital Outpatient Prospective Payment System and CY 2008 payment rates, etc., 66,580–67,225 [07–5507]. Available at: http://www.access.gpo.gov/su_docs/fedreg/a071127c.html. Accessed August 16, 2007.

The ED and inpatient physician providers also benefit from observation level of care. The OU allows for more efficient ED operations, and has been demonstrated to decrease hours of ambulance diversion, decrease ED LOS, and improve patient satisfaction with their care (Robbin Dick, MD, personal communication, 2008).[24,25] Observation current procedural terminology codes exist for additional reimbursement (thus increase in relative value unit compensation) for services provided, and the increased ED efficiency allows for more rapid bed turnover, leading to additional volume and reimbursement (Michael Granovsky, MD, personal communication, 2008). In addition, longer periods of monitoring for OU patients allows for a reasonable reduction in medical-legal risk through improved diagnostic accuracy, allowing specialty consultation (ie, cardiologist) for disease processes like HF. Finally, inpatient physicians benefit by taking care of fewer admissions directly from the ED that do not meet inpatient criteria, saving time and resources.

COST-EFFECTIVENESS OF THE OBSERVATION UNIT

The OU allows for the provision of intense therapy and observation services with close monitoring for response to treatment. In the Acute Decompensated Heart Failure Registry (ADHERE) data

registry, the time to initiation of administration of certain intravenous medicines specifically directed at acute HF was 1 hour if the patient's treatment was initiated in the ED, compared with 22 hours if therapy was begun in an inpatient unit (**Table 6**).[26] The OU has definitive protocols for both treatment and timely adjustments in treatment plans based on the clinical parameters being observed. Such a methodology leads to more intense and timely initiation of therapy. This drastic variation in timing can have remarkable differences in clinical outcomes, as well as a dramatic impact on financial implications.

Treatment of AHF in an OU has resulted in reduced 30-day readmissions and hospitalizations, and decreased LOS if a subsequent hospitalization is required.[27] The ADHERE data show that early initiation of intravenous vasoactive therapy can reduce the hospital LOS from an average of 7 days to 4.5 days.[28] Because LOS is the major contributor to facility costs for AHF patients, and because between 70% and 75% of patients admitted to an OU with HF can be dispositioned to home, the potential impact on hospital bed use can be significant.[13,29] The OU experience with AHF at the Cleveland Clinic showed the following positive outcomes:[30] revisits were reduced by 44%; ED observation discharges increased by 9%; HF rehospitalizations were reduced by 36%; and observation rehospitalizations were reduced by 39%.

Table 5
Comparison of medicare reimbursements for acute heart failure FY 2005

APC 0339–CHF Inpatient			DRG 127–CHF Outpatient		
Level V < 8 hours		$239	Average reimbursement		$4,617
APC 0339 > 8 hours		$408	Mean cost		$5,905
			Medicare benchmark		LOS 5.3 days

UB92	Billable	Reimbursable	UB92	Billable	Reimbursable
EKG	Yes	Yes	EKG	Yes	No
Labs	Yes	Yes	Labs	Yes	No
ECHO	Yes	Yes	ECHO	Yes	No
CXR	Yes	Yes	CXR	Yes	No
IV Infusion	Yes	Yes	IV Infusion	Yes	No
Drug therapy	Yes	Yes	Drug therapy	Yes	No

Total	$1,300/1,400	Fixed Cost (FC)	($1,498)
FC	($570)	FC varies per institution	Usually 3 × outpatient
FC varies per institution		Mean Variable Cost	($1,168)
Mean Variable Cost	($252)	All diagnostics are bundled under corresponding DRG	
$478 profit per case		($1,288) loss per case	

Abbreviation: No, bundled under the service provided.
Data from Sieck SG. The process and economics of heart failure. In: Peacock WF, editor. Short stay management of heart failure. Philadelphia: Lippincott Williams and Wilkins; 2006.

The authors believed this impact on outcomes was because of application of testing upon presentation to the OU and early and aggressive treatment with pharmacologic therapies. Using this strategy, APC reimbursement can result in better profitability (see **Table 4**). Although reimbursement for APC 8002/8003 is smaller compared with the DRG reimbursement for a hospitalization, the operational expense for an OU stay are also smaller and overhead costs are generally less (see **Table 4**).[4] Therefore, intensive therapy for AHF started in the OU results in a shorter, more profitable stay for the facility. However, the ability to profit from this patient cohort still requires attention to prospective use review and protocol-driven care for an appropriately selected patient.[4]

Because observation status is not geographically fixed, patients may be coded as observation anywhere in the hospital. However, to this end, there is a distinction between ED based OUs and the delivery of observation level of service provided in traditional inpatient beds. The ED observation unit is protocol driven and focused on efficient and timely bed turnover. This is contrasted to traditional inpatient care, where "standard management" rules often apply. Fiscally, even if a patient is ultimately admitted from an inpatient unit within 24 hours while assigned to observation level of care (thus initially saving the hospital the penalty for inpatient denial of service), this ties up an inpatient bed, whereas more than 75% of patients are reported to be discharged from the ED-based OU (Robbin Dick, MD, personal communication, January 2008). In the setting of limited inpatient capacity and ED overcrowding, such liberation of capacity is both compelling and fundamental to profitability. In addition, there are certain soft dollars that often fail to be calculated into the economic equation of OU development. These include: improvement in the case mix index (the average reimbursement for each case, unique to each hospital and based on that specific hospital's average severity of illness) increases; more inpatient beds allocated for high-acuity patients; bad debt decreases, including less overhead costs for self pays, patient co-pays, and out-of-network verifications; and a decrease in overall DRG 1-day stays.

CLINICAL OUTCOMES

Governmental agencies are increasingly pressuring providers and facilities to reduce patient morbidity and mortality and to improve quality-of-care outcomes (pay-for-performance).

Table 6
Use and cost differences based on Medicare reimbursement type

DRG 127 Inpatient	APC 0339 Outpatient
Average LOS 7.0 days	Average LOS 4.5 days
Average drug therapy initiation = 22 hrs	Average drug therapy initiation = 1.1 hrs
Average contribution margin per case = ($1,288)	Average contribution margin per case = $871
Mortality = 10.9%	Mortality = 4.3%
	Bonus reimbursement for APC 0339 = $408

Average LOS and mortality data based on the ADHERE registry.
Data from Sieck SG. The process and economics of heart failure. In: Peacock WF, editor. Short stay management of heart failure. Philadelphia: Lippincott Williams and Wilkins; 2006.

With the incidence of new cases of HF on the rise, these patients often present to acute care hospital EDs for diagnosis and treatment. Improved disease management and an emphasis on process are critical toward attaining improved clinical outcomes in this set of patients. Some argue that attempts to increase quality of care are inherently more costly because of the use of more therapeutic and diagnostic interventions. One study estimates up to 30% of health care spending pays for ineffective, inappropriate, or redundant care.[31] Additional studies are needed for support of comparative research and quality versus cost, and are essential to improving health care quality while improving the affordability of care. This suggests the overall impact of high quality care can potentially reduce total costs by diminishing unnecessary health care use that results from inappropriate or inadequate care.

The Joint Commission on Accreditation of Healthcare Organizations has created a set of quality performance indicators for HF. These indicators include objective measurement of ejection fraction, angiotensin converting enzyme inhibitor treatment if tolerated, provision of complete discharge instructions, and smoking-cessation counseling.[32] In an analysis of the ADHERE registry data, only 30% of AHF patients meet these quality requirements.[26] Although OU management has been shown to reduce morbidity and provide a trend toward reduced mortality, the impact on quality metrics for observation level of care needs additional study.[13,33] While regulatory bodies and research have focused on improved clinical outcomes, payers (insurance companies and employers) increasingly seek to link quality of care with cost reductions. Payers continue to aggressively explore pay-for-performance programs that financially reward providers and facilities for providing higher quality care in the hopes that such practices will reduce costs.[4]

Y-MODEL

As the health care system transforms from "paying for services" to "paying for care," acute-care facilities must align quality and reimbursement to create a viable operational plan and sustainable competitive advantage. While this is a common concept in the business world, it is not yet common practice in the health care marketplace. The Y-model is an approach that allows facilities to closely examine different aspects of operations within their systems, while encompassing the concept of care delivered across a continuum from point-of-entry to discharge from the system.[34] This model can be applied to the overall operations of these systems or to one specific disease, such as HF. By applying variations of the model, which focus on two end-points (quality and cost), facilities can recognize ways to turn HF from a negative contribution margin to one that breaks-even or contributes favorably.[4]

A comparison of health care to the industrial setting can be made using the Y-model. Industrial facilities precisely detail the exact route from raw material to finished product, with the end product priced to the market based on the operating costs within the process.[4] If the manufacturing process varies greatly over time, production costs rise and are passed on to the consumer. To maintain price control, variance must be eliminated from the system. If this doesn't occur, profitability is jeopardized. Thus, the aim is to maximize the contribution margin by reducing operational costs without compromising quality.

This model can be similarly applied to an AHF patient presenting for care within a health care delivery system. The patient interfaces with different care units within the acute hospital setting, which are analogous to the industrial setting's business units. Each unit's operational strategies potentially affect each subsequent care unit from point-of-entry to discharge. Thus, a seamless transfer of patient care in both outpatient and inpatient settings is needed to optimize quality improvement and positive economic value. Without each care unit providing vital information to others in this holistic approach, moving patients efficiently through the system is challenged.[4]

The current processes in the health care delivery to the AHF patient are more characteristic of a "zig-zag model" (**Fig. 3**). An AHF patient enters through the ED and receives treatment and evaluation through multiple disconnected care units, represented by nursing, the EKG department, radiology, pharmacy, laboratory, and so forth. Each unit is viewed and acts as a single independent business entity from the standpoint of the hospital. The outputs of these units' activities are collated by the provider, once the patient has been admitted to an inpatient bed where treatment plans are initiated. The zig-zag model is a fragmented and disorganized delivery model.

The Y-Model represents a different strategy, and allows for a template by which to optimize

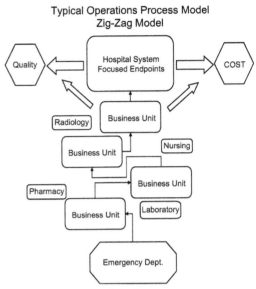

Fig. 3. The zig-zag model of care.

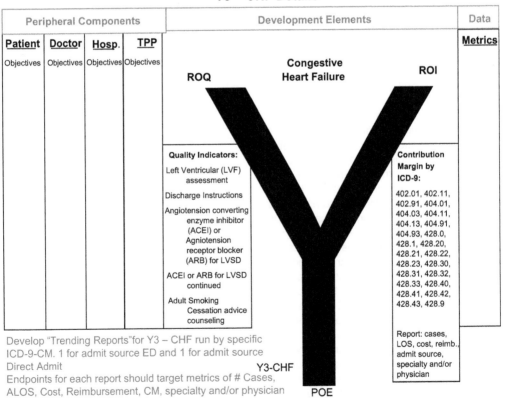

Fig. 4. Y- Model (Inpatient Disease Management Process Improvement Tool).

care costs by placing resources at the front end of the delivery process (at point-of-entry). The model integrates a financial strategy that meets quality metrics and produces positive net value by point-of-entry clinical case management. Beginning in the ED, this concept emphasizes an efficient, rapid assessment and action centered on a seamless integration of ancillary services, such as the laboratory, diagnostic imaging, and skilled nursing, while understanding the economic impacts on decisions made as the patient is directed through the system.[4] Prospective case management at the initial point-of-care determines "what happens next" for the ED patient: discharge, observation level of service, or inpatient admission (and to what level of care).

The Y-Model can positively impact quality, costs, efficiency, and clinical outcomes by providing drill downs on the exact volume by ICD-9 codes instead of the inpatient DRG. This facilitates a more accurate picture of the number of patients processed in the ambulatory setting within the system. Patients who require inpatient admission are admitted to an appropriate level of care, while those who can be effectively treated in the ambulatory setting are treated and released. As inappropriate admissions are weeded out of the system, the inpatient setting experiences a positive increase in the case-mix-index (because the average inpatient is sicker and this results in greater per case reimbursement) (Robbin Dick, MD, personal communication, January 2008).

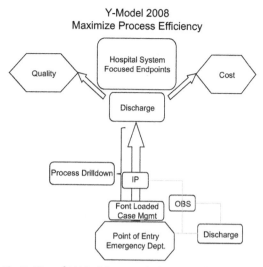

Fig. 5. Use of Y-Model to maximize cost-efficiency.

Patients with AHF can be appropriately risk stratified and identified for an ideal level of care using the Y-model in a manner that positively impacts the contribution margins (**Fig. 4**). This model emphasizes a multidisciplinary team approach to align the "care units" that affect an AHF patient's progress through the current system. The emphasis is on front-end case management to support the physician in establishing the pathway the patient will follow (**Fig. 5**). A patient is not arbitrarily admitted to an inpatient bed, treated, and then discharged. Rather, risk-stratified

Fig. 6. Quality and cost focus of the Y-Model. *POE = point of entry.

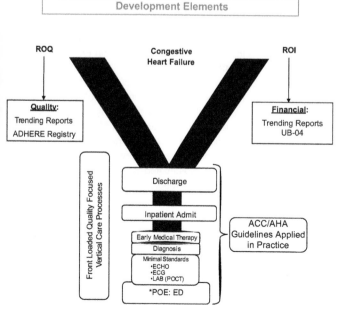

patients are determined to need additional resources, and case management establishes the most ideal venue to undergo specific therapies.[4] By integrating the clinical and financial pathways, facilities can realize the financial implications of making decisions based on standard management versus protocol driven care. The Y-model places an emphasis on process improvement while targeting the end-points of quality and contribution margin (**Fig. 6**).

One medical center has reported its experience in successfully implementing part of the model for an Acute Coronary Syndrome (ACS) Process Improvement Project.[35] Before the initiative the hospital had a "zig-zag" model of care. Patients entered through the ED and were admitted to the acute care bed, diagnostics were completed, and treatment was then initiated. With initiation of the Y-model, stratification was performed and appropriate therapy initiated in the ED with point-of-care testing in a patient-centric improvement effort. The new design resulted in improvements in turnaround time for therapy, reduced LOS, enhanced patient placement in the most appropriate bed venue (eg, critical care unit, telemetry, or clinical decision unit), and improved patient satisfaction.[35] Improvements demonstrated by the ACS redesign can be translated to the AHF setting. Similar to the ACS patient, not every HF patient requires inpatient admission. And similarly, not all HF patients are candidates for the OU. Point-of-entry triaging to the most appropriate care unit where an individualized treatment plan is rendered allows a facility to better merge quality care with positive financial outcomes.[4,35]

SUMMARY

The current process of regulatory oversight and pay-for-performance reimbursement is a reality in today's health care delivery system. To maintain profitability, facilities must be willing to implement new strategies that marry operational redesign, quality care, and cost-effective treatment. Nowhere is this truer than with patients with AHF. Clinical care that is in the wrong setting, using the wrong treatment algorithms, is doomed for clinical and financial failure. As payers increasingly favor outpatient strategies for patient management, inpatient facilities must develop effective strategies to shift inpatient care into ambulatory settings. The Y-model offers a solution that is fixed on process improvement techniques that levy positive economic impact. The model is based on aligning quality and finance targets with attention to clinical outcomes and is suggested as an innovation of a redesigned care process for the AHF patient population.

REFERENCES

1. U.S. Census Bureau. Avaliable at: http://www.census.gov/. Accessed November 20, 2007.
2. Peacock WF, Albert NM. Observation unit management of heart failure. Emerg Med Clin North Am 2001;19:209–32.
3. Massie BM, Shah NB. Evolving trends in epidemiologic factors of heart failure: rationale for preventative strategies and comprehensive disease management. Am Heart J 1997;133:703–12.
4. Sieck SG. The process and economics of heart failure. Short Stay Management of Heart Failure, vol. 5. Philadelphia: Lippincott Williams & Wilkins; 2006.
5. American Heart Association. Heart disease and stroke statistics—2005 update. Dallas (TX): American Heart Association; 2005.
6. Jessup M, Brozena S. Epidemiology and causes of heart failure. N Engl J Med 2003;348(20):2007–18.
7. Aghababian RV. Acutely decompensated heart failure: opportunities to improve care and outcomes in the emergency department. Rev Cardiovasc Med 2002;3(Suppl 4):S3–9.
8. O'Connell JB, Bristow M. Economic impact of heart failure in the United States: time for a different approach. J Heart Lung Transplant 1993;13:S107–12.
9. Heart disease and stroke statistics: 2004 update. Available at: http://www.americanheart.org. Accessed August 24, 2007.
10. ADHERE Registry data on file; January 2004.
11. Graff L, Orledge J, Radford MJ, et al. Correlation of the Agency for Health care Policy and Research congestive heart failure admission guideline with mortality: peer review organization voluntary hospital association initiative to decrease events (PROVIDE) for congestive heart failure. Ann Emerg Med 1999;34:429–37.
12. Emerman CL. Treatment of the acute decompensation of heart failure: efficacy and pharmacoeconomics of early initiation of therapy in the emergency department. Rev Cardiovasc Med 2003;4:S13–20.
13. Peacock WF. Heart failure management in the emergency department observation unit. Prog Cardiovasc Dis 2004;46:465–85.
14. Centers for Medicare and Medicaid services. Available at: http://www.cms.hhs.gov/MLNGenInfo. Accessed September 22, 2007.
15. Short-term acute care program for evaluating payment patterns electronic report (ST PEPPER) user's guide. October 2007. Available at: http://www.hpmpresources.org/LinkClick.aspx?fileticket=H5IICGIqbvM%3d&;tabid=1059&mid=1052. Accessed November 10, 2007.

16. Jong P, Vowinckel E, Liv PP, et al. Prognosis and determinants of survival in patients newly hospitalized for heart failure: a population-based study. Arch Intern Med 2002;162:1689–94.

17. American Heart Association. Heart disease and stroke statistics: 2007 update at-a-glance. Available at: http://www.americanheart.org/downloadable/heart/1166711577754HS_StatsInsideText.pdf. Accessed January 14, 2007.

18. Vinson JM, Rich MW, Sperry JC, et al. Early readmission of elderly patients with congestive heart failure. J Am Geriatr Soc 1990;38:1290–5.

19. Medicare observation status reference volume. Issue IV; Jan 3, 2003.

20. Mace S, Graff L, Mikhail M, et al. A national survey of observation units. Am J Emerg Med 2003;21(7):529–33.

21. Institute of Medicine. The future of emergency care: hospital based emergency care at the breaking point; June 2006. Washington DC: National Academies Press; 2006.

22. Hospital outpatient prospective payment system and CY 2008 payment rates, etc. 66580–67225 [07–5507]. Available at: http://www.access.gpo.gov/su_docs/fedreg/a071127c.html. Accessed August 16, 2007.

23. Ross M, Wilson AG, McPherson M, et al. The impact of an ED observation bed on inpateint bed availability. Acad Emerg Med 2001;8:576.

24. Roberts R, Graff L. Economic issues in observation unit medicine. Emerg Med Clin North Am 2001;19(1):19–33.

25. Tackling the capacity crisis: successful bed management strategies. HFMA sponsored by McKesson Corporation. March 2006. Available at: www.hfma.org/NR/rdonlyres/E581803B-4E58-4E41-8E5A-DE4F4E262322/0/hfma_bedmgmt.pdf. Accessed August 7, 2007.

26. Fonarow GC, for the ADHERE Scientific Advisory Committee. The Acute Decompensated Heart Failure Registry (ADHERE): opportunities to improve care of patients hospitalized with acute decompensated heart failure. Rev Cardiovasc Med 2003;4:S21–30.

27. Peacock WF, Remer EE, Aponte J, et al. Effective observation unit treatment of decompensated heart failure. Congest Heart Fail 2002;8:68–73.

28. Peacock WF, Emerman CL, Costanzo MR, et al. Early initiation of intravenous therapy improves heart failure outcomes; an analysis from the ADHERE registry database. Ann Emerg Med 2003;42(4):S26 [abstract 92].

29. Peacock WF, Albert NM. Patient outcome and costs following an acute heart failure (HF) management program in an emergency department (ED) observation unit [abstract 240]. J Heart Lung Transplant 1999;18:92.

30. Peacock F. Management of acute decompensated heart failure in the emergency department. J Am Coll Cardiol 2003;4:336A.

31. Fisher E, Wennberg D, Stukel T, et al. The implications of regional variations in medicare spending: part 2, health outcomes and satisfaction with care. Ann Intern Med 2003;138:288–98.

32. The Joint Commission. Available at: www.jcaho.org. Accessed August 16, 2007.

33. Peacock WF. Acute emergency department management of heart failure. Heart Fail Rev 2003;8:335–8.

34. Sieck Healthcare Consulting. Available at: www.sieckhealthcare.com. Accessed August 15, 2007.

35. Holland J, Holt T, Nord G, et al. Enhancing outcomes of acute coronary syndrome. Abstracts from the Eighth Annual Society of Chest Pain Centers Scientific Sessions. Clinical Pathways in Cardiology 2005;4(4):193–4.

Special Cases in Acute Heart Failure Syndromes: Atrial Fibrillation and Wide Complex Tachycardia

Peter S. Pang, MD*, Mihai Gheorghiade, MD

KEYWORDS

- Acute heart failure syndromes • Atrial fibrillation
- Wide complex tachycardia

Hospitalization for acute heart failure syndromes (AHFS) portends a significant in-hospital and post-discharge morbidity and mortality.[1–5] Management of these patients presents significant challenges, given the heterogeneity of the patient population and the differing and complex etiologies why patients present with acute decompensation.[4] Approximately 50% of the AHFS population has preserved systolic function; a significant number have underlying coronary artery disease, are female, have diabetes, renal insufficiency, and present with hypertension; with only a very small percentage who present with cardiogenic shock.[2,3,6]

Approximately 30% of patients with AHFS present with atrial fibrillation (**Tables 1** and **2**).[6–9] This arrhythmia may be the precipitating cause of AHFS or may merely reflect the underlying substrate of a patient with chronic HF who now presents with acute decompensation.[10] In either case, management of the arrhythmia occurs within the overall context of HF management.

In contrast, although wide complex tachycardias, if defined broadly by premature ventricular contractions, nonsustained ventricular tachycardia, ventricular tachycardia (VT), polymorphic ventricular tachycardia, accelerated idioventricular rhythms, supraventricular tachycardia with aberrancy, or ventricular fibrillation, are relatively common in the chronic HF population at large,[11–13] it has rarely been addressed in the setting of AHFS outside of textbooks (see **Table 1**).[11]

The pathophysiology of both AF and HF has been extensively discussed elsewhere.[5,14–16] This article focuses on both AF and WCT with specific principles of emergency department (ED) management reviewed in the setting of AHFS.

AF is defined as a "supraventricular tachyarrhythmia characterized by uncoordinated atrial activation with consequent deterioration of mechanical function."[14] How the ventricle responds to this atrial activation depends on (1) properties of the atrioventricular node, (2) presence of accessory pathways if any, (3) vagal and sympathetic tone, and (4) effects of medications.[1] The authors will focus on the management of AF with rapid ventricular response (RVR) in the setting of ED AHFS.

For patients with either AF or HF, developing the other condition predicts a worse prognosis, although in advanced HF some debate exists as to whether development of AF at this late juncture imputes a worse prognosis.[14,17–22] In general, rate versus rhythm control does not confer a mortality benefit.[23–25] However, some controversy still exists within the setting of HF, given the worse prognosis of those with HF who develop

Northwestern Memorial Hospital, Chicago, IL, USA
* Corresponding author. Department of Emergency Medicine, Northwestern Memorial Hospital, 259 East Erie Street, Suite 100, Chicago, IL 60611.
E-mail address: ppang@northwestern.edu (P.S. Pang).

Heart Failure Clin 5 (2009) 113–123
doi:10.1016/j.hfc.2008.08.009

Table 1
Arrhythmia in the history or at presentation

Registry	Author and Year of Publication	Number of Patients	AF/Flutter (%)	Presentation NSVT (%)	VT (%)	VF (%)	Other
EPICAL[37]	Zannad et al, 1999	499	25.6 in nonsinus rhythm				
EuroHeart[32]	Cleland et al, 2003	11,327	42 (9% of patients presented with rapid AF)		VT + 8	VF =	→ Syncope 15%
Swiss Registry[38] (two centers)	Rudiger 2005	312	29.2 (in 15% of cases AF was new and triggered the AHF)				→ 7% cases triggered by symptomatic bradycardia
OPTIMIZE-HF[39]	Fonarow et al (initial pub 2004)	48,000	31				
IMPACT-HF[40]	O'Conner et al, 2005	567	35.4 (in 8% of cases AF caused the AFH)		VT + 11.5	VF =	→ 50% on β-blocker, 36% on ACEI on admission → 12.5% arrhythmic deaths by 60 d
ADHERE[7]	Adams et al, 2005	110,000	31		8	1	

Abbreviations: ACEI, angiotensin-converting enzyme inhibitor; AF, atrial fibrillation; AHF, acute heart failure; NSVT, nonsustained ventricular tachycardia; VF, ventricular fibrillation; VT, ventricular tachycardia.
From Chicos AB, Kadish AH. Arrhythmia in acute heart failure. In: Mebazaa A, Gheorghiade M, Zannad FM, editors. Acute heart failure. London: Springer-Wilson; 2008. With kind permission of Springer Science + Business Media.

Table 2 on page 115

Table 2
Epidemiology of arrhythmia in acute heart failure: data from selected acute heart failure trials

Trial	Intervention	No. Patients	Arrhythmia in the History or at Presentation				New Arrhythmias During Hospitalization				
			Afib/ Flutter (%)	NSVT (%)	Sust. VT (%)	VF (%)	Afib/ Flutter (%)	NSVT (%)	Sust. VT (%)	VF (%)	Other
OPTIME-CHF[41]	Milrinone versus placebo	949	32		10	3	M 0.5 P 4.6		2.1	1.2	
VMAC[42]	Nesiritide versus NTG versus placebo	489	35		13	6					34% had frequent PVSs
LIDO[43]	Levosimendan versus dobutamine	203	13		7	1	L 4 D 2	L 1 D 2	L 1 D 2		
RITZ-2[44]	Tezosen versus placebo	285	24.6								
RITZ-4[45]	Tezosen versus placebo	192					T 5.2 P 2.1		T 5.2 P 6.3		Patients excluded if heart rate >130/min
RITZ-5[46]	Tezosen versus placebo	84	21.4								
PRECEDENT[47]	N1 versus N2 versus dobutamine	255	27	26	7.5			N1 6 N2 5 D 13			
IMPACT-HF[48]	Start carvedilol	363	22		VT + VF = 9						

Abbreviations: D, dobutamine; L, levosimendan; M, milrinone; N1, nesiritide, 0.015 µg/kg/min; N2, nesiritide, 0.03 µg/kg/min; NGT, nitroglycerin; NSVT, nonsustained ventricular tachycardia; P, placebo; Sust. VT, sustained ventricular tachycardia; T, tezosentan; VF, ventricular fibrillation.
From Chicos AB, Kadish AH. Arrhythmia in acute heart failure. In: Mebazaa A, Gheorghiade M, Zannad FM, editors. Acute heart failure. London: Springer-Wilson; 2008. With kind permission of Springer Science + Business Media.

AF.[18,26,27] Whether or not maintaining or restoring sinus rhythm confers a mortality benefit has not been prospectively investigated in a large randomized controlled trial, however, although the Atrial Fibrillation and Congestive Heart Failure trial is currently underway and was designed to answer this question.[26,28,29]

Three general considerations determine management: (1) rate control, (2) rhythm control, and (3) prevention of thromboembolism. Prioritization of rate versus rhythm control strategy depends on the clinical presentation.[14]

DEMOGRAPHICS OF ATRIAL FIBRILLATION IN ACUTE HEART FAILURE SYNDROMES

Significant overlap exists in terms of risk factors for developing either AF or HF.[14,21,30] Not surprisingly, epidemiologic evidence of an association between the two has been demonstrated.[20,21,30] Data from the Framingham Heart Study suggest that HF is the strongest independent risk factor for the development of AF.[20,30,31]

HF registry data provide further insight into the characteristics of patients with AF and AHFS. In the EuroHeart Failure Survey-I, 42% of patients had a history of AF with 9% of patients observed to have AF with RVR during their hospitalization.[32] EuroHeart Failure Survey-I was not a survey of admissions, however, but of deaths and discharges.

Approximately 31% of patients in both the Acute Decompensated Heart Failure National Registry and the Organized Program to Initiate Life-Saving Treatment in Hospitalized Patients with Heart Failure had a history of AF.[6–9] From Acute Decompensated Heart Failure National Registry, 20% of patients had an initial EKG of AF, with 29% having some other abnormal rhythm.[8]

In a large nationwide Italian registry (N = 2807) of AHFS patients admitted to a hospital with an intensive cardiac care unit, 44% of patients had de novo HF with the remainder as acute-on-chronic HF.[3] At time of admission, 798 patients had AF with 21% of the total study population having a history of paroxysmal AF. Of the patients presenting with AF, 59.5% had a RVR greater than 100 beats per minute.[33]

The Finnish Acute Heart Failure study was a national prospective observational study of 620 patients hospitalized for AHFS. Of these patients, 27% had a history of chronic AF. A significant number (29.4%) had AF as the precipitating factor for AHFS in 24.8% of those with chronic HF and a cause of de novo HF in 34.3%. One third of all patients with de novo AF were determined to have AF as the precipitating cause.[34]

In a retrospective cohort study of 216 patients who presented to an emergency department with acute pulmonary edema (mean age, 75.3 years), 24.3% had AF (14.6% as paroxysmal AF and 9.7% as chronic).[3] AF at the time of admission did not affect survival.[35]

THE EFFECT OF ATRIAL FIBRILLATION WITH RAPID VENTRICULAR RESPONSE

Four main adverse effects from AF with RVR were outlined in the 2005 American College of Cardiology and American Heart Association guidelines for chronic HF management:[16] (1) loss of atrial kick to ventricular filling with subsequent decrease in cardiac output, (2) rapid HR might increase demand and decrease coronary perfusion, (3) RVR may diminish both cardiac contraction and cardiac relaxation, and (4) stasis of blood may predispose to embolic phenomenon. These adverse effects outline potential targets and provide a rationale for therapy.

ATRIAL FIBRILLATION AND ACUTE HEART FAILURE SYNDROMES

Evidence for the management of AF and AHFS in the ED is limited.[10,18] Given the lack of prospective data in chronic HF and AF, it is not surprising that evidence-based management in AHFS is lacking. Management is guided largely by principles as opposed to best evidence (**Tables 3** and **4**).

Management Principles

Rate control, consideration of rhythm control, and prevention of thromboembolism are the main considerations during acute management, with rate or rhythm control being dependent on the acute clinical picture.[11,14,18] Acutely, rate versus rhythm control is often the primary decision, with keen attention to the risk and prevention of thromboembolism.[14] Correction of any electrolyte abnormalities or other causes of AF (ie, thyrotoxicosis) should be performed.

In some cases, elucidating whether AF is the cause of AHFS versus a manifestation of sympathetic overdrive in patients who present with AHFS may be difficult to determine. In general, in patients with chronic HF and chronic persistent AF, mitigation of their acute HF symptoms (ie, dyspnea) by therapies to relieve congestion may decrease the RVR, assuming they are compliant with their medications at baseline. In patients with de novo HF and AF, it is much more likely that AF is the cause of AHFS. Regardless, optimal arrhythmia management requires excellent HF management.[10]

Table 3

Studies assessing cardioversion of acute atrial fibrillation in patients with chronic heart failure

Study Author	Type of Study	N	% Ventricular Function	Duration of AF	Initial Heart Rate (Beats. Min^{-1}) Mean ± SD	Drug administered/ Dose	Conversion to Sinus Rhythm/ Time to Conversion	Adverse Event
DAAF trial Group, 1997[49]	Double-blind, randomized, placebo controlled[a]	28 Dig:15 Placebo:13	Not given	21.7 ± 30.4 h[b]	122 ± 23 bmp[c]	Dig IV 0.88 ± 0.35 mg (mean ± SD)	6/15—Dig group, 5/13—placebo group time to conversion not given	None
Hou et al, 1996[50]	Single blind, randomized, placebo controlled[a]	50 Dig:24 Am:26	Mean FS: Dig:27 Am:26	Dig: 4 h Am: 14 h (median)	Dig: 163 ± 26 Am: 157 ± 20	Dig: 0.013 mg/kg × 3 at 2 h intervals Am: IV 300 mg in 1 h, 960 mg over next 23 h	Dig: 17/24 (71%) 6.5 h (median) Am: 24/26 (92%) 2.5 h (median)	Dig:-none Am:-2 patients
Clemo et al, 1998[51]	Retrospective	38	EF: 40 ± 16	23/38 patients (61%) had an AF/SVT of <24 h	149 ± 13	Am, IV: 242 ± 137 mg at 1 h (range, 60–1000) At 24 h 1137 ± 280 mg (range, 99–2500)	11/38 (30%) in 24 h/time not given	1 (non-CVS side effect)
Kumar, 1996[52]	Retrospective	8	<15 (EF)	>30 min	159 ± 9	Am. IV: 300 mg in 1 h	7/8 (87.5%) reversion 27 ± 13 min (mean)	None
Andrivet et al, 1994[53]	Prospective, randomized[d]	16	Not given	Not given[e]	140 for both groups (mean)	Oralgroup—2026 ± 79 mg in 24 h, IVgroup—1038 ± 62 mg in 24 h	7/16 (44%) using either oral or IV route/ time not given	None

Abbreviations: AF, atrial fibrillation; AFL, atrial flutter; Am, amiodarone; BMD, betamethyldigoxin; bmp, beats per minute; CHF, chronic heart failure; CVS, cardiovascular; D, dofetilide; DAAF, Digoxin in Acute Atrial Fibrillation Trial Group; Dig, digoxin; Dilt, diltiazem; EF, ejection fraction; FS, fraction shortening; I, ibutilide; IV, intravenous; NYHA, New York Heart Association Class; SD, standard deviation; SVT, supraventricular tachycardia.

a Subgroup of atrial fibrillation patients with coronary heart failure in a trial of 239 patients.

b Mean ± standard deviation for all patients.

c Mean ± standard deviation for all patients.

d Open label trial comparing oral with intravenous amiodarone, subgroup of chronic heart failure patients (16 of 72 patients in trial).

e 56% of all patients in trial had atrial fibrillation duration of <48 h.

From Khand AU, Rankin AC, Kaye GC, et al. Systematic review of the management of atrial fibrillation in patients with heart failure. Eur Heart J 2000;21:614; with permission.

Table 4
Studies assessing ventricular rate control of acute atrial fibrillation in patients with chronic heart failure

Study author, Year, Reference	Type of Study	N	% Ventricular Function	Duration of AF	Initial Heart Rate (bmp)	Drug Administered/ Dose	Heart Rate Slowing Effect of Drug	Adverse Event
Hou et al, 1995[50]	Single-blind, randomized, digoxin-controlled	50 Dig: 24 Am: 26	Means FS: Dig: 27 Am: 26	Median: Dig: 4 h Am: 14 h	Dig: 163 ± 26 Am: 157 ± 20	Dig: 0.013 mg/ kg × 3 at 2-h intervals Am: IV 300 mg in 1 h, 960 mg over next 23 h	Dig: 150 bpm Am: 122 bmp (at 1 h)	Dig: 0 Am: 2 (1 worsening heart failure and 1 death)
Goldenberg et al, 1994[54]	Randomized, double-blind, placebo-controlled	37 Dilt: 22 Placebo:15	36 (EF)	—	>120	Dilt IU (first dose 0.25 mg/ kg over 2 min, if not effective then 0.35 mg/kg)	Dilt: 36/37 response rate[a] Placebo: 0/15 Median response time: 5 min	3 (8%) symptomatic hypotension No worsening of chronic heart failure
Clemo et al, 1998[51]	Retrospective	38	40 ± 16 (EF)	23/38 patients (61%) had an AF for <24 h	149 ± 13 (mean ± SD)	Am, IV: 1 h, 242 ± 137 mg (range, 60–1000)At 24 h 1137 ± 280 mg (range, 99–2500)	15 min 134 ± 14 1-h: 109 ±18 24 h: 99 ± 15 (bmp, mean ± SD)	1
Heywood et al, 1998[55]	Uncontrolled study	9	34 ± 18 (mean EF ± SD)	—	142 (mean)	Dilt IV/ initial dose 0.25 mg/ kg (0.30 mg/ kg) given if heart rate reduction <10%)	114 bmp Median response time 5 min	None

Abbreviations: AF, atrial fibrillation; Am, amiodarone; bmp, beats per minute; Dig, digoxin; Dilt, diltiazem; EF, ejection fraction; FS, fraction shortening; SD, standard deviation.

[a] Response rate defined as 20% reduction in baseline heart rate or heart rate less than 100 achieved. Figures for diltiazem incorporate all placebo nonresponders who are given diltiazem.

From Khand AU, Rankin AC, Kaye GC, et al. Systematic review of the management of atrial fibrillation in patients with heart failure. Eur Heart J 2000;21:614; with permission.

GUIDELINE RECOMMENDATIONS

Various guideline recommendations help inform the acute management of AF and AHFS and are presented as consensus recommendations given the paucity of data in AF and ED AHFS.[5]

European Society of Cardiology

Rate versus rhythm control depends on the clinical picture and duration of the AF. The European Society of Cardiology guidelines on AHF recommend cardioversion if possible, after weighing the risks and benefits.[5] Pharmacologically, digoxin, β-blockers, and amiodarone are recommended along with anticoagulation.[5] Both verapamil and diltiazem are to be avoided because of the risk of inducing heart block or worsening of HF,[5] although β-blockers may have similar effects. If underlying systolic function is known, rate control was further emphasized in those patients with diastolic dysfunction.[5] If AF is secondary to AHF, digoxin is recommended as a Class IIb, level of evidence B recommendation.[5]

American College of Cardiology and American Heart Association: Chronic Heart Failure Guidelines

Specific guidelines addressing acute HF management have not yet been published by the American College of Cardiology and American Heart Association.[16] In chronic HF, digoxin and β-blockers are recommended, although caution is advised regarding β-blockers in those with clinical decompensation.[16] Both verapamil and diltiazem are not recommended;[16] however, it should be emphasized that these are recommendations for the chronic setting.

American College of Cardiology, American Heart Association, European Society of Cardiology, European Heart Rhythm Association, and Heart Rhythm Society Guidelines

AF guidelines endorsed by the aforementioned societies had the following Class I recommendations in regards to AF in HF in those without an accessory pathway: (1) intravenous β-blockers or nondihydropyridine calcium channel antagonists (verapamil, diltiazem) are recommended for rate control acutely, but caution is needed in those with hypotension or HF (level of evidence: B); (2) intravenous digoxin or amiodarone are recommended for rate control in those patients with AF and HF (level of evidence: B); and (3) oral digoxin is recommended to control the heart rate at rest in patients with AF and is indicated for patients with HF and left ventricular dysfunction (level of evidence: C).[14]

Of note, avoiding intravenous nondihydropyridine calcium channel blockers (verapamil and diltiazem) in those patients with decompensated HF and AF for risk of exacerbating hemodynamic compromise is a class III recommendation (risk outweighs benefit).[14]

Absent hemodynamic instability, direct-current cardioversion was given a Class I, level of evidence C recommendation for those patients with RVR refractory to pharmacologic therapy with ongoing myocardial ischemia, systemic hypotension, angina, or HF.[14]

Despite warnings against nondihydropyridine therapy, a systematic review of AF in chronic heart failure conducted in 2000 by Khand and colleagues[10] suggests the efficacy of diltiazem without safety concerns in the setting of AF and HF, although the data are limited. Acute AF was defined as AF of less than 48 hours in duration from time of onset.[10] They systematically reviewed both pharmacologic and electrical therapy on AF in HF (see **Tables 3** and **4**).

SCENARIOS OF ATRIAL FIBRILLATION AND ACUTE HEART FAILURE SYNDROMES
Cardiogenic Shock

For the patient with hemodynamically unstable AF and AHFS, immediate cardioversion is recommended, consistent with Advanced Cardiac Life Support (ACLS) guidelines. Pharmacologic therapies may worsen hypotension and although risk of thromboembolism merits careful consideration, treatment of the life-threat is paramount. Concomitant use of pharmacologic therapies or immediately after cardioversion may be required to maintain sinus rhythm or rate control. In addition, thromboembolic prophylaxis is required, even if sinus rhythm is restored. It should be remembered that end stage or advanced HF patients may present with alarming hemodynamic numbers, but may in fact be maintaining adequate perfusion.

Rhythm Control Strategy

Rhythm control should be considered in the following AF and AHFS patients with careful consideration of the risks of thromboembolism with pretreatment or concomitant thromboembolic prophylaxis that must be continued after restoration of sinus rhythm: cardiogenic shock, hemodynamic instability with failure to respond promptly to pharmacologic therapy,[14] and de novo AHFS secondary to AF with definitive knowledge of AF duration less than 48 hours. Alternatively, a rate control strategy might also be used with delayed cardioversion if indicated at a later date.

Rate Control Strategy

In general, rate control should be the predominant strategy in management of AHFS and AF. Available data to guide pharmacologic management in the ED are limited.[10,18] Based on the work by Khand and colleagues,[10] intravenous diltiazem is more effective than intravenous digoxin without any negative safety signals, although diltiazem has strong cautions per established society recommendations. Less data exist for intravenous β-blockers; however, after weighing the risk-benefit profile and still considered, use of short-acting agents (ie, esmolol) is recommended.

Atrial Fibrillation in Chronic Heart Failure Patients with Acute Decompensation

This category represents most patients who present with AHFS. Many have a history of underlying AF; acute decompensation opens the door for AF with RVR as a result of sympathetic overdrive. In general, treatment of the HF by relief of congestion often results in rate control.

For patients with new-onset AF and chronic HF, restoration of sinus rhythm should be considered assuming both thromboembolic risks and duration of AF less than 48 hours is clearly established. Rate control often is sufficient, however, and improved diastolic filling may improve hemodynamics and symptoms.

In addition, certain management strategies for HF may predispose to arrhythmias, especially with inotropic agents. Other AHFS therapies, may adversely affect electrolytes (eg, IV loop diuretics), which may facilitate the development of arrhythmias. These disturbances require correction.

For those AHFS patients who present with AF and preserved systolic function, rate control improves diastolic filling time, decreases filling pressure, and subsequently improves forward flow. Agents, such as β-blockers and nondihydropyridine calcium channel blockers, might all be considered, although the use of verapamil or diltiazem should be cautiously considered, given guideline recommendations.

De Novo Heart Failure and Atrial Fibrillation

A rhythm control strategy might also be considered. If another etiology of either the HF or AF is present, however, patients may relapse back into AF (ie, severe hypokalemia; hypomagnesemia; thyrotoxicosis; toxicities, such as cocaine). Assuming hemodynamic stability and absent of worsening HF, a rate control strategy might also be pursued.

Summary

Deciding between rate or rhythm control and thromboembolic risk management are among the initial decisions in AF and AHFS management. In general, guideline recommended pharmacologic management for AF and AHFS is limited to digoxin and amiodarone, with a specific warning against use of nondihyrdopyridine calcium channel blockers.[14]

WIDE COMPLEX TACHYCARDIA

WCT is defined as a rate greater than 100 beats per minute with a QRS complex greater than or equal to 120 milliseconds.[36] Despite diagnostic criteria or algorithms, none are perfect, and diagnostic uncertainty in regards to the WCT is the norm. All WCT should be assumed to be of ventricular origin until proven otherwise. Immediate next actions depend on hemodynamic stability and the clinical picture.

Apart from ACLS recommendations for WCT and cardiac arrest or hemodynamic instability, evidence-based management for the treatment of WCT and ED AHFS is limited. Epidemiologically, WCT, defined by nonsustained ventricular tachycardia, VT, ventricular fibrillation, premature ventricular contractions, and accelerated idioventricular rhythm in the chronic HF patient is common.[12,13] Similar to AF, some general management principles are presented.

Differentiation Between Supraventricular Tachycardia and Wide Complex Tachycardia

Although this is a topic unto itself, it is worth reviewing briefly given the potential for differences in management. Concordance throughout the limb leads, namely monophasic R or monophasic QS complexes with the same polarity, suggests VT.[36] AV dissociation, with no association between P and QRS complexes or where the atrial rate is slower than the ventricular rate, suggests VT.[36] Dressler beats seen during the WCT also suggest VT.[36] Other algorithms and diagnostic rules and aids are available.[36] Essentially, treatment of VT with supraventricular tachycardia therapies has potentially catastrophic results, whereas the converse is not true. In patients with HF, it is more likely to be a genuine ventricular arrhythmia as opposed to a supraventricular tachycardia with aberrant features.

General Management

WCT in AHFS presents significant challenges. Treatment of hypotension in AHFS might involve therapies that are proarrhythmic, such as milrinone, dopamine, or dobutamine.[11] Use of procainamide or amiodarone to treat VT may worsen hypotension, an undesirable side effect in the AHFS patient.[11]

An important first question to answer is whether the WCT is the cause of AHFS or merely a marker of known underlying HF. In the chronic setting, asymptomatic nonsustained ventricular tachycardia has not been identified as a marker for increased risk of sudden death.[13] In the emergency department or other acute setting, in general, it is safer to assume the WCT is malignant before an otherwise benign assumption.

Similar to AF, electrolyte disturbances, such as hypokalemia and hypomagnesemia, should be actively sought and treated with due consideration of other precipitants (ie, ischemia) of the ventricular arrhythmia.

Treatment

Patients who are hemodynamically unstable require immediate cardioversion. In stable patients with ventricular cause of their WCT, procainamide or amiodarone is recommended, with amiodarone preferred because of lesser likelihood of subsequent hypotension. β-blockers and nondihydropyridine calcium channel blockers in the setting of ventricular arrhythmias and AHFS should be avoided.

SUMMARY

There is a paucity of evidence to guide management in patients who present with arrhythmias and ED AHFS, making definitive recommendations difficult. Hemodynamically unstable patients require immediate cardioversion per ACLS guidelines. Management of both AF and WCT occurs within the overall context of AHFS management. In AF, a rate versus rhythm control strategy with consideration of thromboembolic risks is the first decision branch point. Management of HF will reduce the sympathetic drive in some cases and thus lead to a decrease in the ventricular rate. In WCT and AHFS, clinicians should assume ventricular origin of the arrhythmia until proved otherwise. Further research is needed to provide better evidence for the management of these common arrhythmias in AHFS.

REFERENCES

1. Fonarow GC, Adams KF Jr, Abraham WT, et al. Risk stratification for in-hospital mortality in acutely decompensated heart failure: classification and regression tree analysis. JAMA 2005;293:572.
2. Fonarow GC, Heywood JT, Heidenreich PA, et al. Temporal trends in clinical characteristics, treatments, and outcomes for heart failure hospitalizations, 2002 to 2004: findings from acute decompensated heart failure national registry (ADHERE). Am Heart J 2007; 153:1021.
3. Fonarow GC, Stough WG, Abraham WT, et al. Characteristics, treatments, and outcomes of patients with preserved systolic function hospitalized for heart failure: a report from the OPTIMIZE-HF Registry. J Am Coll Cardiol 2007;50:768.
4. Gheorghiade M, Zannad F, Sopko G, et al. Acute heart failure syndromes: current state and framework for future research. Circulation 2005;112:3958.
5. Nieminen MS, Bohm M, Cowie MR, et al. Executive summary of the guidelines on the diagnosis and treatment of acute heart failure: the Task Force on Acute Heart Failure of the European Society of Cardiology. Eur Heart J 2005;26:384.
6. Gheorghiade M, Filippatos G, De Luca L, et al. Congestion in acute heart failure syndromes: an essential target of evaluation and treatment. Am J Med 2006;119:S3.
7. Adams KF Jr, Fonarow GC, Emerman CL, et al. Characteristics and outcomes of patients hospitalized for heart failure in the United States: rationale, design, and preliminary observations from the first 100,000 cases in the Acute Decompensated Heart Failure National Registry (ADHERE). Am Heart J 2005;149:209.
8. ADHERE Scientific Advisory Committee. Acute Decompensated Heart Failure National Registry (ADHERE) Core Module Q1 2006 final cumulative national benchmark report. In: Scios, Inc, 2006.
9. Fonarow GC. The Acute Decompensated Heart Failure National Registry (ADHERE): opportunities to improve care of patients hospitalized with acute decompensated heart failure. Rev Cardiovasc Med 2003;4(Suppl 7):S21.
10. Khand AU, Rankin AC, Kaye GC, et al. Systematic review of the management of atrial fibrillation in patients with heart failure. Eur Heart J 2000;21: 614.
11. Chicos AB, Kadish AH. Arrhythmia in acute heart failure. In: Mebazaa A, Gheorghiade M, Zannad FM, editors. Acute heart failure. London: Springer-Wilson; 2008.
12. Doval HC, Nul DR, Grancelli HO, et al. Nonsustained ventricular tachycardia in severe heart failure: independent marker of increased mortality due to sudden death. GESICA-GEMA Investigators. Circulation 1996;94:3198.
13. Teerlink JR, Jalaluddin M, Anderson S, et al. Ambulatory ventricular arrhythmias in patients with heart failure do not specifically predict an increased risk

of sudden death. PROMISE (Prospective Randomized Milrinone Survival Evaluation) Investigators. Circulation 2000;101:40.

14. Fuster V, Ryden LE, Cannom DS, et al. ACC/AHA/ ESC 2006 guidelines for the management of patients with atrial fibrillation–executive summary: a report of the American College of Cardiology/ American Heart Association Task Force on Practice Guidelines and the European Society of Cardiology Committee for Practice Guidelines (writing committee to revise the 2001 guidelines for the management of patients with atrial fibrillation). J Am Coll Cardiol 2006;48:854.

15. Heart Failure Society of America. Executive summary: HFSA 2006 comprehensive heart failure practice guideline. J Card Fail 2006;12:10.

16. Hunt SA, Abraham WT, Chin MH, et al. ACC/AHA 2005 guideline update for the diagnosis and management of chronic heart failure in the adult: a report of the American College of Cardiology/American Heart Association Task Force on Practice Guidelines (writing committee to update the 2001 guidelines for the evaluation and management of heart failure): developed in collaboration with the American College of Chest Physicians and the International Society for Heart and Lung Transplantation: endorsed by the Heart Rhythm Society. Circulation 2005;112:e154.

17. Crijns HJ, Tjeerdsma G, de Kam PJ, et al. Prognostic value of the presence and development of atrial fibrillation in patients with advanced chronic heart failure. Eur Heart J 2000;21:1238.

18. Efremidis M, Pappas L, Sideris A, et al. Management of atrial fibrillation in patients with heart failure. J Card Fail 2008;14:232.

19. Folkeringa JR, Crijns HJ, Van Veldhuisen DJ. Prognosis of atrial fibrillation in congestive heart failure. Circulation 2004;109:e11.

20. Heist EK, Ruskin JN. Atrial fibrillation and congestive heart failure: risk factors, mechanisms, and treatment. Prog Cardiovasc Dis 2006;48:256.

21. Wang TJ, Larson MG, Levy D, et al. Temporal relations of atrial fibrillation and congestive heart failure and their joint influence on mortality: the Framingham Heart Study. Circulation 2003;107: 2920.

22. Wasywich CA, Whalley GA, Gamble GD, et al. Does rhythm matter? The prognostic importance of atrial fibrillation in heart failure. Heart Lung Circ 2006;15:353.

23. Cain ME. Atrial fibrillation: rhythm or rate control. N Engl J Med 2002;347:1822.

24. Van Gelder IC, Hagens VE, Bosker HA, et al. A comparison of rate control and rhythm control in patients with recurrent persistent atrial fibrillation. N Engl J Med 2002;347:1834.

25. Wyse DG, Waldo AL, DiMarco JP, et al. A comparison of rate control and rhythm control in patients with atrial fibrillation. N Engl J Med 2002;347:1825.

26. Al-Khatib SM, Shaw LK, Lee KL, et al. Is rhythm control superior to rate control in patients with atrial fibrillation and congestive heart failure? Am J Cardiol 2004;94:797.

27. Kareti KR, Chiong JR, Hsu SS, et al. Congestive heart failure and atrial fibrillation: rhythm versus rate control. J Card Fail 2005;11:164.

28. AF-CHF Investigators. Rationale and design of a study assessing treatment strategies of atrial fibrillation in patients with heart failure: the Atrial Fibrillation and Congestive Heart Failure (AF-CHF) trial. Am Heart J 2002;144:597.

29. Hagens VE, Crijns HJ, Van Veldhuisen DJ, et al. Rate control versus rhythm control for patients with persistent atrial fibrillation with mild to moderate heart failure: results from the RAte Control Versus Electrical Cardioversion (RACE) study. Am Heart J 2005;149:1106.

30. Van den Berg MP, Tuinenburg AE, Crijns HJ, et al. Heart failure and atrial fibrillation: current concepts and controversies. Heart 1997;77:309.

31. Benjamin EJ, Levy D, Vaziri SM, et al. Independent risk factors for atrial fibrillation in a population-based cohort. The Framingham Heart Study. JAMA 1994;271:840.

32. Cleland JG, Swedberg K, Follath F, et al. The EuroHeart failure survey programme–a survey on the quality of care among patients with heart failure in Europe. Part 1: patient characteristics and diagnosis. Eur Heart J 2003;24:442.

33. Tavazzi L, Maggioni AP, Lucci D, et al. Nationwide survey on acute heart failure in cardiology ward services in Italy. Eur Heart J 2006;27:1207.

34. Siirila-Waris K, Lassus J, Melin J, et al. Characteristics, outcomes, and predictors of 1-year mortality in patients hospitalized for acute heart failure. Eur Heart J 2006;27:3011.

35. Bentancur AG, Rieck J, Koldanov R, et al. Acute pulmonary edema in the emergency department: clinical and echocardiographic survey in an aged population. Am J Med Sci 2002;323:238.

36. Podrid P, Ganz L. Approach to the diagnosis and treatment of wide QRS complex tachycardia. Available at: www.UpToDate.com, Vol Online 15.3. Accessed October 1, 2008.

37. Zannad F, Briancon S, Juilliere Y, et al. Incidence, clinical and etiologic features, and outcomes of advanced chronic heart failure: the EPICAL Study. Epidemiologie de l'Insuffisance Cardiaque Avancee en Lorraine. J Am Coll Cardiol 1999;33:734.

38. Rudiger A, Harjola VP, Muller A, et al. Acute heart failure: clinical presentation, one-year mortality and prognostic factors. Eur J Heart Fail 2005;7:662.

39. Fonarow GC, Abraham WT, Albert NM, et al. Organized program to initiate lifesaving treatment in hospitalized patients with heart failure (OPTIMIZE-HF): rationale and design. Am Heart J 2004;148:43.

40. O'Connor CM, Stough WG, Gallup DS, et al. Demographics, clinical characteristics, and outcomes of

patients hospitalized for decompensated heart failure: observations from the IMPACT-HF registry. J Card Fail 2005;11:200.

41. Cuffe MS, Califf RM, Adams KF Jr, et al. Short-term intravenous milrinone for acute exacerbation of chronic heart failure: a randomized controlled trial. JAMA 2002;287:1541.

42. VMAC Investigators. Intravenous nesiritide vs nitroglycerin for treatment of decompensated congestive heart failure: a randomized controlled trial. JAMA 2002;287:1531.

43. Follath F, Cleland JG, Just H, et al. Efficacy and safety of intravenous levosimendan compared with dobutamine in severe low-output heart failure (the LIDO study): a randomised double-blind trial. Lancet 2002;360:196.

44. Torre-Amione G, Young JB, Colucci WS, et al. Hemodynamic and clinical effects of tezosentan, an intravenous dual endothelin receptor antagonist, in patients hospitalized for acute decompensated heart failure. J Am Coll Cardiol 2003;42:140.

45. O'Connor CM, Gattis WA, Adams KF Jr, et al. Tezosentan in patients with acute heart failure and acute coronary syndromes: results of the randomized intravenous TeZosentan study (RITZ-4). J Am Coll Cardiol 2003;41:1452.

46. Kaluski E, Kobrin I, Zimlichman R, et al. RITZ-5: randomized intravenous TeZosentan (an endothelin-A/B antagonist) for the treatment of pulmonary edema: a prospective, multicenter, double-blind, placebo-controlled study. J Am Coll Cardiol 2003;41:204.

47. Burger AJ, Horton DP, LeJemtel T, et al. Effect of nesiritide (B-type natriuretic peptide) and dobutamine on ventricular arrhythmias in the treatment of patients with acutely decompensated congestive heart failure: the PRECEDENT study. Am Heart J 2002;144:1102.

48. Gattis WA, O'Connor CM, Gallup DS, et al. Predischarge initiation of carvedilol in patients hospitalized for decompensated heart failure: results of the initiation management predischarge: process for assessment of carvedilol therapy in heart failure (IMPACT-HF) trial. J Am Coll Cardiol 2004;43:1534.

49. The Digitalis in Acute Atrial Fibrillation (DAAF) Trial Group. Intravenous digoxin in acute atrial fibrillation. Results of a randomized, placebo-controlled multicentre trial in 239 patients. Eur Heart J 1997; 18:649.

50. Hou ZY, Chang MS, Chen CY, et al. Acute treatment of recent-onset atrial fibrillation and flutter with a tailored dosing regimen of intravenous amiodarone: a randomized, digoxin-controlled study. Eur Heart J 1995;16:521.

51. Clemo HF, Wood MA, Gilligan DM, et al. Intravenous amiodarone for acute heart rate control in the critically ill patient with atrial tachyarrhythmias. Am J Cardiol 1998;81:594.

52. Kumar A. Intravenous amiodarone for therapy of atrial fibrillation and flutter in critically ill patients with severely depressed left ventricular function. South Med J 1996;89:779.

53. Andrivet P, Boubakri E, Dove PJ, et al. A clinical study of amiodarone as a single oral dose in patients with recent-onset atrial tachyarrhythmia. Eur Heart J 1994;15:1396.

54. Goldenberg IF, Lewis WR, Dias VC, et al. Intravenous diltiazem for the treatment of patients with atrial fibrillation or flutter and moderate to severe congestive heart failure. Am J Cardiol 1994;74:884.

55. Heywood JT, Graham B, Marais GE, et al. Effects of intravenous diltiazem on rapid atrial fibrillation accompanied by congestive heart failure. Am J Cardiol 1991;67:1150.

Nursing Considerations for the Management of Heart Failure in the Emergency Department

Elsie M. Selby, MSN, ARNP, CCRN, CCNS[a],
Robin J. Trupp, PhD(c), MSN, ARNP, CCRN[b],*

KEYWORDS

- Heart failure • Emergency department nursing
- Patient education

RAPID TRIAGE AND EARLY TREATMENT

The morbidity and mortality benefits resulting from rapid triage and intervention for acute myocardial infarction have been well documented. A similar approach to acute decompensated heart failure (AHF) has demonstrated benefits as well. Analysis of the Acute Decompensated Heart Failure Registry database revealed that patients receiving vasoactive therapy had a mean door-to-treatment time of 2 hours if treatment was initiated in the emergency department (ED) versus a dismal 23 hours for treatment initiated in inpatient units.[1,2] It is postulated that initiating vasoactive therapy in the ED can decrease acute care length of stay by as much as 3 days.[3,4] More importantly to patients, early treatment means faster symptom improvement. To accomplish this, ED nurses play important roles in triaging and facilitating the prompt delivery of evidence-based therapies in this population.

NURSING CONSIDERATIONS
Nurses as Detectives—Making the Connection and Leading the Way

Heart failure (HF) represents a complex syndrome that is a challenge for both clinicians and patients to manage. Patients face an extensive list of medications for treating HF and its symptoms, such as angiotensin converting enzyme inhibitors, diuretics, beta-blockers, and electrolyte supplements. When the common comorbidities seen in this population are factored in, such as hypertension, diabetes, or dyslipidemias, adherence to prescribed pharmacologic and non-pharmacologic therapies becomes even more difficult. Patients typically receive verbal or written instructions on medications and dietary restrictions, as well as other important information on topics such as exercise, when to seek care, and smoking cessation. Because of the breadth of information required to optimally manage their disease and symptoms is great, it is critical that this data be reviewed with patients at every opportunity, whether in conjunction with routine care or while in the ED or observation unit (OU) during a HF exacerbation.[5] Within the ED and OU, education must be tailored for the patient and their family, taking into consideration the severity and symptoms of the acute illness, any associated stress or anxiety, and the brevity of the interaction. For these reasons, the nurse must focus and concentrate on key concerns.

Unfortunately, there are no trials of ED- or OU-based education programs for patients with HF. However, some research has suggested that these patient-care locations may serve as a suitable environment to initiate education on lifestyle

[a] Ephraim McDowell Regional Medical Center, Danville, KY, USA
[b] Comprehensive CV Consulting LLC, Columbus, OH, USA
* Corresponding author. 8640 Craigston Court, Dublin, OH 43017-9780.
E-mail address: rjtrupp@gmail.com (R.J. Trupp).

Heart Failure Clin 5 (2009) 125–128
doi:10.1016/j.hfc.2008.08.007

changes because patients may "make the connection" between decisions made about diet or medications and the consequences of their choices.[6,7] Given that medication and dietary nonadherence have been documented as significant causes of decompensation and hospitalization, the role of education on adherence cannot be over-emphasized.[8] On many occasions, AHF can be directly linked to a choice made about the recommended treatment plan. For example, a patient may decide to skip a dose of diuretic because they are going on an outing and do not want to make frequent bathroom stops, may eat a food that is high in sodium, or may take a nonsteroidal anti-inflammatory drug (NSAID) for arthritic pain. All of these choices could ultimately lead to excess extracellular volume, worsening symptoms, and an ED visit.

ED and OU nurses should always maintain a high index of suspicion for dietary or medication indiscretions in patients diagnosed with AHF. In order to make the connection, targeted questions about diet and medications must be asked. For example, rather than asking "Have you been eating a low-sodium diet?", "What did you eat for lunch and dinner yesterday?" provides more detailed information on sodium consumption. "Tell me what medications you have taken today" is more informative than "Have you taken your medications today?" Asking the family similar questions can yield valuable information as well. Inquiring about prescribed and over-the-counter medications or herbal supplements may also reveal hidden sources of sodium or contraindicated therapies.

It is estimated that only about 10% of patients actually take their medications as prescribed.[9] Barriers to adherence can be multifaceted and include such things as costs, forgetfulness, and real or perceived side effects.[10] Additional medication issues include the use of contraindicated medications, such as NSAIDs, calcium channel blockers, or specific antibiotics. Adherence to a low sodium diet is perhaps the most significant nonpharmacologic treatment used in the management of HF symptoms. Yet, despite its importance, compliance is meager at best. Reported barriers include a lack of understanding of any diet restrictions, poor taste of food, and lack of self-control as reasons for not adhering to a low-sodium diet.[5] Irrespective of the short-stay interaction during an ED visit, the ED nurse can impact a patient's future disease management skills by embracing the opportunity to deliver education directed at specific issues identified in the patient/family interview.

Learning from past experience is superior to reading information in a pamphlet or receiving oral instructions. Therefore, linking behavioral decisions with the ensuing adverse consequences assists the patient in making the connection that ideally will lead to better choices in the future. Education can then be targeted around the identified area of concern. Unfortunately, there is limited evidence on patient education and adherence issues specific to the acute-care setting. In the majority of studies, patient education is one of a number of outpatient interventions targeting adherence, reduced health care expenditures, or both. Therefore, nurses must extrapolate and implement results demonstrating efficacy in other health care settings. Fortunately, the current body of literature suggests that patient education, usually in the setting of multidisciplinary HF management programs, can enhance medication compliance, which in turn is associated with decreased hospital utilization and improved quality-of-life. In the ED, the short-term interaction of the visit may preclude the nurse from addressing each of these issues individually, although the OU nurse would be expected to have greater opportunity for intervention irrespective of the geographic location. Connecting the patient to resources, such as a social worker, disease management clinic, telemedicine program, home health agency or alerting the inpatient nurse to these problems may be beneficial.

Self-Monitoring of Symptoms

Patients with heart failure often report difficulty in identifying worsening signs and symptoms of HF, which may lead to a delay in seeking medical treatment.[11,12] This delay results in worsening symptoms that eventually send the patient to the ED. Patient-reported barriers to recognizing signs and symptoms of decompensation and to reporting them include failure to recognize the symptoms as being related to HF, lack of knowledge about worsening symptoms, and the desire not to "bother" their health care provider or to "worry" family.[13,14]

Teaching patients to recognize early signs and symptoms of worsening HF and to report them to their health care provider should prevent unnecessary ED visits and hospitalizations. This early communication alerts the health care provider of a potential event so that treatment can be initiated to prevent further decompensation and ultimately avoid an ED visit or hospitalization. Unfortunately, the common signs and symptoms of HF are neither specific nor sensitive enough for complete accuracy, making a definitive diagnosis and treatment plan challenging for providers.[15]

While the ED is not the ideal location for in-depth instruction on self-monitoring, a targeted review of symptoms leading up to the current ED visit can present another teachable moment for the patient in the OU. Early signs and symptoms include decreased appetite, increased fatigue, abdominal bloating, early satiety, and sleeping difficulties.[12] Later signs and symptoms consist of increased dyspnea, increased peripheral edema, increased abdominal girth, orthopnea, and cough.[12] The OU nurse can assist the patient in identifying those signs and symptoms that have just been experienced. By helping the patient to acknowledge the recent signs and symptoms of worsening HF and relating it to the current hospital visit, the OU nurse can assist the patient in making the connection and potentially impact future decompensation events.

Social Considerations

Support systems that include family, friends, and health care agencies play a vital role in the overall management of HF patients.[13] Stable support systems help patients with the complex adherence issues related to medications, diet, and self-monitoring.[13] Although the ED stay does not allow for a thorough review of a patient's available support system, the OU can provide this opportunity, and the nurse may make an initial assessment and alert the social worker for further follow-up. Furthermore, a social worker or a case manager in the OU may provide additional support for these patients in collaboration with the ED nurse.

Additional Barriers to Self-Care

Because of the complexity of the management of HF, many patients face numerous barriers to self-care. Although some issues are likely too great for the ED nurse to undertake, there are some simple and fixable barriers that could easily be addressed in the OU. In addition to the issues discussed previously, other considerations include the availability of home scales for daily weights and challenges associated with the complex medication regimen. Maintaining a supply of scales and medication organizers in the OU, for patients who do not have the resources to obtain these things on their own, would be simple and beneficial.

SUMMARY

Despite a lack of trials examining the impact of educational interventions in the ED and OU, there is ample evidence in other health care settings supporting its use in the management of patients with HF. Given the large volume of these patients

that present to the hospital, implementation of strategies to increase the understanding and management of HF, thereby reducing morbidity and improving quality-of-life, are warranted. Therefore, the challenge for the ED and OU nurse is to adapt these interventions to fit realistically within their fast-paced environment. Future research is necessary to provide evidence supporting the influence of education within the ED and OU setting.

REFERENCES

1. American Heart Association. Heart Disease and Stroke Statistics—2005 Updated. Dallas (TX): American Heart Association 2005.
2. Fonarow GC, For the ADHERE Scientific Advisory Committee. The Acute Decompensated Heart Failure National Registry (ADHERE): opportunities to improve care of patients hospitalized with acute decompensated heart failure. Rev Cardiovasc Med 2003;4(Suppl 7):S21–9.
3. Aghababian R. Acutely decompensated heart failure: opportunities to improve care and outcomes in the Emergency Department. Rev Cardiovasc Med 2002;3(Suppl 4):S3–9.
4. Emerman CL, Peacock F, Fonarow GC. Effect of emergency department initiation of vasoactive infusion therapy on heart failure length of stay. Ann Emerg Med 2002;40:S46.
5. Adams KF, Lindenfeld J, Arnold JMO, et al. Executive Summary: HFSA 2006 comprehensive heart failure practice guideline. J Card Fail 2006; 12:10–38.
6. Williams S, Brown A, Patton R, et al. The half-life of the "teachable moment" for alcohol misusing patients in the emergency department. Drug Alcohol Depend 2005;77(2):205–8.
7. Dominique J, de Quervain DJF, Roozendaal B, et al. Acute cortisol administration impairs retrieval of long term declarative memory in humans. Nat Neurosci 2000;3:313–4.
8. Dunbar S, Clark P, Deaton C, et al. Family education and support interventions in heart failure. Nurs Res 2005;54(3):158–66.
9. Levanthal MJE, Riegel B, Carlson B, et al Negotiating compliance in heart failure: remaining issues and questions. Eur J Cardiovasc Nurs 2005;4: 298–307.
10. Evangelissta L, Doering LV, Dracup K, et al. Compliance behaviors of elderly patients with advanced heart failure. J Cardiovasc Nurs 2003;18(3): 197–206.
11. Carlson B, Reigel B, Moser DK. Self-care abilities of patients with heart failure. Heart Lung 2001;30(5): 351–9.

12. Frantz AK. Breaking down the barriers to heart failure patient self-care. Home Healthc Nurse 2004; 22(2):109–15.

13. Reigel B, Carlson B. Facilitators and barriers to heart failure self-care. Patient Educ Couns 2002;46: 287–95.

14. Jaarsma T, Huda HA, Dracup K. Self-care behavior of patients with heart failure. Scand J Caring Sci 2000;14:112–9.

15. Dao Q, Krishnaswamy P, Kazanegra R, et al. Sensitivity, specificity and accuracy of signs and symptoms in heart failure. J Am Coll Cardiol 2001;37(2):379–85.

Emergency Department Presentation of Heart Transplant Recipients with Acute Heart Failure

Paul Chacko, MD[a],*, Shibu Philip, MD[b]

KEYWORDS

- Heart transplantation • Acute heart failure
- Emergency department • Cardiac allograft dysfunction
- Cardiac allograft vasculopathy • Arrythmia

Heart failure is a rapidly growing public health problem in the United States. It is estimated that approximately 5.2 million people (2.5% of the United States population) have a diagnosis of heart failure. In addition, 550,000 new cases are diagnosed each year.[1] Advances in medical management (β-blockers, angiotensin-converting enzyme inhibitors, and spironolactone) and the widespread use of defibrillators have improved the quality of life and long-term outcome for patients who have heart failure.[2–5] Despite this, the outlook for patients who have symptomatic class IV heart failure is dismal, with mortality rates as high as 50% at 6 months.[6] Heart transplantation is one of the most effective treatments for patients who have end-stage heart failure and who remain symptomatic despite optimal medical management. Based on the recent report from the Registry of the International Society for Heart and Lung Transplantation (ISHLT), more than 76,000 cardiac transplantations have been performed at 300 transplant centers since 1982.[7] Because heart transplant recipients require immunosuppressive treatment, they are more susceptible to problems related to "under" immunosuppression (allograft rejection and allograft vasculopathy) and "over" immunosuppression (infections and malignancies). Consequently, morbidity and mortality rates are high. Such problems related to immunosuppressive treatment can lead to cardiac allograft dysfunction, which can present as acute heart failure in the emergency department (ED).

HEART TRANSPLANTATION: AN OVERVIEW

In 1967, Christiaan Barnard performed the first human heart transplant using the heterotopic technique, in which the donor heart was "piggy-backed" beside the native heart.[8] Heterotopic transplantation is indicated in recipients who have fixed, high-grade pulmonary hypertension and when a smaller donor heart is transplanted into a larger recipient. The orthotopic technique, which involves the implantation of the donor heart in place of the native heart, has been accepted as the standard procedure in most centers. Depending on the technique of anastomosis between the donor and recipient heart, orthotopic heart transplantation can be classified further as biatrial (donor left and right atria anastomosed to that of the recipient), bicaval (anastomosis of superior and inferior vena cava instead of right atrium), or total (in addition, anastomosis of pulmonary veins instead of left atrium). The bicaval technique is performed at 75% of world heart transplant centers.[9] Indications and contraindications for heart transplant procedure are listed in **Box 1**.[10] Mortality rates

[a] The Ohio State University College of Medicine, Columbus, OH, USA
[b] Jeanes Hospital, Philadelphia, PA, USA
* Corresponding author. Division of Hospital Medicine, Department of Internal Medicine, The Ohio State University College of Medicine, 4510 Cramblett Hall, 456 W. 10th Avenue, Columbus, OH 43210.
E-mail address: paul.chacko@osumc.edu (P. Chacko).

Heart Failure Clin 5 (2009) 129–143
doi:10.1016/j.hfc.2008.08.011
1551-7136/08/$ – see front matter © 2008 Elsevier Inc. All rights reserved.

> **Box 1**
> **Indications and contraindications for heart transplantation**
>
> *Indications for heart transplantation*
>
> Cardiogenic shock with reversible end organ dysfunction.
>
> Low cardiac output state requiring inotropic support.
>
> Symptomatic patients who fit NYHA III/IV category not responding to optimal medical treatment with a LVEF < 20% and a VO2 max < 15mL/kg/min.
>
> Ventricular arrhythmias not responding to medical treatment or implantation of ICD.
>
> Primary cardiac tumor confined to the heart.
>
> *Contraindications for heart transplantation*
>
> Irreversible pulmonary hypertension with PVR > 6 Woods units.
>
> Active infection.
>
> Malignancy.
>
> Recent substance abuse.
>
> Psychological/Social factors that can lead to non compliance.
>
> Irreversible hepatic/ renal failure.
>
> *Abbreviations*: NYHA, New York Heart Association; LVEF, left ventricular ejection fraction; VO2 max, maximal oxygen consumption; ICD, implantable cardioverter-defibrillator; PVR, pulmonary vascular resistance.

are highest in the initial 6 months after the transplantation, followed by a steady mortality of 3.4% per year extending beyond 15 years. The transplant half-life (the time at which 50% of persons receiving a transplant remain alive) has improved from 5.3 years in the early 1980s to 10.3 years from 1992 to 2001. In the first year of heart transplantation, non-cytomegalovirus infection was responsible for 33% of deaths, followed by graft failure (18%) and rejection (12%). Five years after transplantation, 30% of deaths are caused by cardiac allograft vasculopathy, and malignancy contributes to 22%.[7]

Immunosuppression in Heart Transplantation

Allograft rejection is the expected response of the recipient's immune system to allogenic donor heart tissue. This response is prevented by immunosuppression initiated in the immediate perioperative period with high doses of intravenous immunosuppressants that later are converted to oral form. Immunosuppressive therapy can be divided into induction and maintenance regimens. Induction therapy usually is indicated in patients who are at a high risk of acute rejection, which consists of female patients and those who have high titers of panel reactive antibodies (PRA). It is also beneficial in patients who have renal dysfunction by delaying the use of a nephrotoxic immunosuppressant, such as calcineurin inhibitor (CNI). About 40% of heart transplant centers use induction regimens in the form of intraoperative and postoperative intravenous steroids and anti-lymphocyte antibodies. Antilymphocyte antibodies could either be antithymocyte globulin derived from horses (ATGAM) and rabbits (rATG, Thymoglobulin) or monoclonal antibodies directed towards T cells, such as OKT3.[11] These antibodies, given for 10 to 14 days after transplantation, are associated with a high risk of infection, malignancy, or both. Newer induction agents such as interleukin-2 antagonists (daclizumab and basiliximab) are associated with a reduced risk of rejection while avoiding the risk of infection. Maintenance therapy consists of the simultaneous use of three categories of drugs: a CNI, such as cyclosporine or tacrolimus, an anti-metabolite, such as azathioprine or mycophenolate mofetil, and steroids. Combination therapy targets multiple pathways in T-cell activation and allows the administration of drugs at lower doses, resulting in reduced side effects.[12] Mycophenolate mofetil, given at a dose of 500–1500 mg twice daily, has replaced azathioprine in most centers because of the latter's higher risk of malignancy. Because of the long-term adverse effects of steroid use, attempts are made to attain steroid-free immunosuppression by early (within 1 month) or late (6 months after transplantation) steroid withdrawal. Late withdrawal is preferred, because most rejection happens in the first 6 months.[9] Target-of-rapamycin inhibitors (sirolimus and everolimus) are associated with a lower rate of allograft rejection than are azathioprine or cyclosporine. Their use enables a "CNI reduced" or "CNI free" drug regimen with reduction in nephrotoxicity. In addition, cardiac allograft vasculopathy and posttransplantation malignancy are noted to be low.[13]

Prophylaxis for Infection in Heart Transplantation

Increasingly potent immunosuppressive agents exacerbate the heart transplant recipient's susceptibility to infections. The use of these agents leads to the reactivation of herpes simplex virus (HSV) and infection by opportunistic pathogens such as pneumocystis jiroveci (PCP), cytomegalovirus (CMV), aspergillus, and nocardia. In the immediate postoperative period, most infections are nosocomial and are caused by bacteria or fungus. Opportunistic infections by CMV, HSV, epstein barr virus (EBV), PCP, cryptococcus, and mycobacterium are seen predominantly 1 to 6 months after transplantation. Community-acquired infections tend to become more common 6 months after transplantation. Because the risk of infection is highest during the initial year after the transplantation, mandatory prophylaxis is advised. Trimethoprim-sulphamethoxazole, used for prophylaxis against PCP, also is effective in preventing nocardiosis and toxoplasmosis. Antifungal prophylaxis with nystatin or clotrimazole prevents oral candidiasis. Depending on the geographic location or the predilection of the transplantee to invasive fungal infections, prophylaxis is indicated in certain high-risk groups. This category comprises patients who have any of the following conditions: those who undergo retransplantation, hepatic and renal dysfunction, use of greater degree of immunosuppression, surgical complications and bacterial or CMV infections in the posttransplant period.[14,15] Antiviral prophylaxis against CMV with intravenous ganciclovir or oral valgancyclovir is offered in two scenarios: a CMV-seronegative recipient receiving a heart from seropositive donor, and a CMV-seropositive recipient requiring lympholytic therapy. Acyclovir, famciclovir, or valgancyclovir prevents reactivation of herpes in seropositive recipients.[16]

HEART TRANSPLANT RECIPIENTS IN THE EMERGENCY DEPARTMENT

There is limited literature on the ED presentation of heart transplant recipients. Sternbach and colleagues conducted a retrospective review of ED presentation of heart transplant recipients at Stanford University Medical Center from 1988 through 1990. Fever (37%) was the most common presenting symptom, followed by shortness of breath (13%), gastrointestinal symptoms of nausea, vomiting, and diarrhea (10%), and chest pain (9%).[17] Syndromes that need to be considered in the differential diagnosis of patients who present with dyspnea are listed in **Box 2**.

A high index of suspicion for allograft rejection and infections is required, even when transplant recipients present with vague complaints. Unlike a kidney transplant rejection, which can be managed with supportive measures such as hemodialysis, allograft dysfunction in a cardiac transplantee can be fatal. Therefore heart transplant recipients must be given emergency-category status, irrespective of their stable vital signs, and they should

---

Box 2
Differential diagnosis of shortness of breath in heart transplant recipients

Cardiac
    Allograft dysfunction
    Pericardial effusion and tamponade
    Constrictive pericarditis

Pulmonary
    Infections
        Pneumocystis jiroveci
        Cytomegalovirus
        Herpes simplex virus
        Aspergillus
        Nocardia
        Mycobacterial infections
        Community-acquired pneumonia

    Tumors
        Bronchogenic carcinoma
        Kaposi sarcoma

    Drug toxicity
        Sirolimus-associated interstitial pneumonitis

Renal
    Calcineurin inhibitor–induced nephrotoxicity
    Nephropathy secondary to steroid induced diabetes
    Hypertensive renal disease

Hematology
    Anemia of chronic disease

---

be considered for hospital admission. ED care of heart transplant recipients must include a multidisciplinary approach to streamline management. This approach involves early recognition of signs and symptoms of rejection by the triage nurse, checking baseline investigations prior to a detailed history and physical evaluation, early consultation with the heart transplantation team, and pharmacy consultation to avoid adverse drug interactions. Although isolation is not required, frequent hand washing and avoiding all exposure to active infection is advised. Endocarditis prophylaxis also is recommended before any invasive procedure except endotracheal intubation.[18] Recipients taking maintenance steroids are at an increased risk of chronic adrenal insufficiency and must receive corticosteroid replacement in adequate doses.[19]

CARDIAC ALLOGRAFT DYSFUNCTION

Dysfunction of the allograft may occur because of left ventricular (LV) and/or right ventricular (RV) dysfunction. RV dysfunction usually is seen immediately after heart transplantation and is related to high pulmonary artery pressure and resistance in the recipient caused by long-standing heart failure. The right ventricle, however, adapts to pulmonary pressure and resistance, leading to normalization of RV function.[20] LV dysfunction, which can be diastolic or systolic, is of major concern. The majority of the work that has been done has focused on the systolic function of the transplanted heart. Diastolic dysfunction is addressed in a later section of this article. Data on the evolution of LV systolic function after heart transplantation are scarce and conflicting. Some studies showed a decline in LVEF, whereas others have demonstrated the EF to be maintained as long as 4 years after transplantation.[21,22] In one of the largest studies by Hershberger and colleagues, the mean EF using radionuclide ventriculography decreased from 63.8% to 55.6% in the first year after transplantation and remained stable thereafter.[23] LV dysfunction can be divided further by the time from transplantation into early (observed intraoperatively and in the immediate postoperative period) and late (after the first few postoperative weeks to years after surgery). In the first year after transplantation, cardiac allograft rejection, infections, and malignancies involving the myocardium are responsible for late LV dysfunction, whereas allograft coronary artery disease primarily is responsible for LV dysfunction that occurs later on. Other causes of LV dysfunction include atrioventricular valve regurgitation, arrhythmias, recurrence of the original disease such as in infiltrative disorders (amyloidosis, sarcoidosis, and hemochromatosis), and myocarditis (giant cell or lymphocytic).[24] The causes of cardiac dysfunction in heart transplant recipients are shown in **Fig. 1**.

Cardiac Allograft Rejection

Rejection is an important cause of morbidity and mortality in the first year after transplantation, with the incidence declining thereafter over time. Based on the time after transplantation, rejection is classified as hyperacute (within minutes to hours after transplantation), acute (weeks to months after transplantation), or chronic (months to years after transplantation). Acute rejection is divided further into acute cellular rejection and acute humoral rejection. Acute cellular rejection, mostly seen within the first 3 to 6 months, is a T-cell–mediated response.[25] Most of these events are diagnosed by surveillance endomyocardial biopsy in asymptomatic recipients who have normal LV function. Occasionally, severe hemodynamic compromise is noted in 5% of recipients who have either LV or RV dysfunction.[26] Diagnosis and treatment are based on the ISHLT grading of endomyocardial biopsy, which was introduced in 1990 and was revised in 2004.[27] Hemodynamically stable grade 1R rejection is not treated. Grade 2R rejection is managed with a transient increase in the steroid dose. Severe rejections (hemodynamic

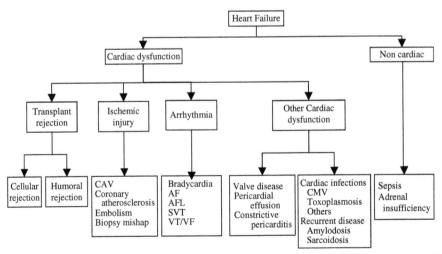

Fig. 1. Differential diagnosis of heart failure in heart transplant recipients. AF, atrial fibrillation; AFL, atrial flutter; CAV, cardiac allograft vasculopathy; CMV, cytomegalovirus; SVT, supraventricular tachycardia; VF, ventricular fibrillation; VT, ventricular tachycardia. (*Data from* Semigram MJ, Stevenson LW. Case 37–2007: a 47 year old man with left ventricular dysfunction after heart transplant. N Engl J Med 2007;357:2286–97.)

compromise or grade 3R) are treated with lympholytic therapy with antithymocyte globulin (Thymoglobulin or ATGAM) or OKT3.[28] Acute humoral or antibody-mediated rejection, caused by antibodies against donor HLA or endothelial cell antigen, constitutes only 7% of all rejections. Antibody-mediated rejection often occurs in the first 4 months after transplantation and is associated with a high rate of hemodynamic compromise (29%–47%), graft loss (15%), and death (64%). Diagnosis is made by demonstrating immunoglobulins and complement in blood vessels by immunofluorescence or immunoperoxidase staining. The presence of endothelial cell swelling with intravascular macrophage accumulation on hematoxylin and eosin stain also is suggestive of the diagnosis. Assessment of circulatory antibodies is restricted to patients who have hemodynamic compromise. Treatment involves removal of antibodies with plasmapheresis and suppression of B-lymphocyte activity with high doses of steroids, lympholytic therapy, and intravenous immunoglobulin.[29]

Allograft Coronary Artery Disease

LV dysfunction after heart transplantation can result from coronary artery disease caused by cardiac allograft vasculopathy or coronary atherosclerosis. Cardiac allograft vasculopathy or chronic rejection is a rapidly progressive atherosclerosis reported in 7% of survivors at 1 year, in 32.3% at 5 years, and in 45.7% of survivors at 8 years after transplantation.[7] It differs from atherosclerosis by being concentric and diffuse, involving the entire length of epicardial vessels. LV dysfunction is produced by myocardial infarction (which can be silent) or as a result of myocardial hibernation, often noticed because of the reduction of myocardial blood supply. Coronary angiograms usually are needed to diagnose cardiac allograft vasculopathy, but the concentric involvement of the coronary vessels results in under diagnosis. Intravascular ultrasound is the most sensitive test, but widespread use is limited by its cost and invasive nature and the need for expertise. The most sensitive noninvasive test is dobutamine stress echocardiography. Exercise nuclear imaging is specific and can be used to confirm positive dobutamine echocardiograms. The roles of cardiac CT and MRI in this setting are emerging.[30] Treatment with angioplasty, stenting, and coronary artery bypass has a limited role in diffuse disease; retransplantation is the definitive option. Prevention is the best strategy and includes avoiding injury to the donor heart before transplantation and aggressive treatment of cardiac risk factors

such as diabetes, hypertension, and hyperlipidemia. Prevention and treatment of CMV infection and of allograft rejection also are important.[31] Coronary atherosclerosis, seen in nontransplanted hearts, also can occur in transplanted hearts. Compared to cardiac allograft vasculopathy, coronary atherosclerosis is more localized, proximal, and eccentric, so it is more amendable to coronary intervention. Other rare causes leading to ischemic heart failure are myocardial infarction following endomyocardial biopsy, left anterior descending myocardial bridge, coronary vasospasm, and thrombosis.[32–35]

Arrhythmias

Arrhythmias can be a manifestation of cardiac dysfunction as well as a precipitating factor inducing LV dysfunction. The common dysrhythmias encountered in cardiac transplant patients are summarized in the following sections. Although tachyarrhythmias commonly are related to LV dysfunction, failure to maintain adequate cardiac output in bradycardia is known to present as congestive heart failure. Dysrhythmias encountered in heart transplant patients are categorized as early and late, depending on whether they occur within or after 2 weeks of transplantation. Because most early arrhythmias are observed in the immediate postoperative period, this discussion focuses on late-onset arrhythmias that often pose a challenge to ED physicians.

Bradyarrhythmias

The incidence of bradyarrhythmias varies from 14% to 44% in United States and European studies but is as low as 11% in a study reported from Taiwan.[36] Most clinicians consider sinus bradycardia in the setting of heart transplantation to be a heart rate less than 80 beats/min, instead of the usual threshold of 60 beats/min, given that the resting heart rate in transplant recipients often is very high. Sinus node dysfunction is the most common type encountered, while junctional bradycardia and atrioventricular blocks (AVB) are responsible for the rest. Bradycardia that occurs in the early period often resolves on its own and is related mainly to ischemia during surgery. Late-onset bradyarrhythmias tend to be associated with AVB because of underlying cardiac allograft vasculopathy or rejection.[37] Long-term follow-up of a cohort of heart transplant recipients who experienced symptomatic bradycardia as a result of late-onset AVB revealed the absence of sinoatrial nodal artery.[38] Hence late-onset bradyarrhythmias must be evaluated in detail with coronary angiography and biopsy to rule out possible rejection.

Hemodynamically unstable situations warrant use of isoproterenol while arrangements are made for the implantation of a permanent pacemaker. It is important to bear in mind that vagolytics (eg, atropine) have no effect on the atrioventricular node because of denervation. A trial with methylxanthines can be attempted in stable conditions, but insertion of a permanent pacemaker often is needed in addition to addressing the underlying ischemia caused by cardiac allograft vasculopathy or rejection. Current guidelines restrict the use of a permanent pacemaker to (1) symptomatic bradycardia not resolving with drugs, or (2) awake, asymptomatic third-degree AVB with associated periods of asystole lasting 3 seconds or longer or escape rhythms of less than 40 beats/min.[39] The optimal mode of pacing is still debated, but the general consensus is to encourage atrioventricular synchronization and to provide rate-responsive pacing. Further discussion of mode settings is beyond the scope of this article.

Supraventricular Tachyarrhythmias

Studies evaluating the incidence of supraventricular tachyarrhythmia have been inclusive of both early and late-onset arrhythmias. In a recent evaluation of 167 heart transplant recipients, Ahmari and colleagues noted the incidence of late-onset atrial fibrillation and atrial flutter to be 9.5% and 15%, respectively.[40] Postoperative inflammation and altered hemodynamics may explain the higher incidence noted in initial studies, considering their frequent observation in the early period. Late-onset atrial fibrillation and atrial flutter, however, have a strong correlation with rejection and cardiac allograft vasculopathy.[40,41] Macroentry circuits as a mechanism for atrial flutter have been demonstrated by Krishnan and colleagues.[42]

Because late-onset atrial fibrillation is related to an increased all-cause mortality, the identification and treatment of the trigger factors is pivotal to prevent cardiac dysfunction.[43] To date, no clear guidelines have been established for treating these dysrhythmias. As in non–heart transplant patients, the choice between rate control and rhythm control is an important consideration, because the persistence of atrial fibrillation can lead to LV dysfunction, even in the absence of cellular rejection, humoral rejection, or cardiac allograft vasculopathy.[44] If there is evidence of hemodynamic instability, cardioversion (via direct-current cardioversion [DCCV] or drugs) or overdrive pacing can be considered. Electric cardioversion is preferred because of its efficacy and quick results. Chemical cardioversion with amiodarone and ibutilide also has been effective, the latter being very beneficial when prior DCCV has been unsuccessful.[45,46] For

chronic arrhythmias, class Ic drugs are used in the absence of an ischemic myocardium. Flecainaide, a class Ia drug, is used where there is coexisting LV dysfunction or cardiac allograft vasculopathy. Rate control can be attained with β-blockers, calcium-channel blockers, or amiodarone. β-Blockers are considered first-choice therapy because of the increased sensitivity of the myocardium to adrenergic chemicals after heart transplantation. Non-hydropyridines such as diltiazem need to be used cautiously because their interaction with cyclosporine poses a difficulty in maintaining immunosuppression. Because of the risk of torsades, drugs that cause Q-T prolongation need to be administered carefully whenever there is concurrent use of tacrolimus. The benefits of anticoagulation should be weighed against the risk of bleeding, because heart transplant recipients are at a high risk for embolic events. Aspirin is the choice for lower-risk recipients, but all others need to be treated with warfarin. In patients who experience atrial flutter, electro-anatomic mapping offers an advantage in identifying the re-entry circuit, and radiofrequency ablation offers a good response. In resistant scenarios, the option of atrioventricular nodal ablation and the placement of a permanent pacemaker is always reserved.

The incidence of other supraventricular tachyarrhythmias such as atrioventricular nodal re-entry tachycardia (AVNRT) and atrioventricular re-entry tachycardia have been described in heart transplant recipients in either case reports or case series.[47,48] Collins and colleagues noted a 1% incidence of AVNRT and a 2% incidence of ectopic atrial tachycardia among pediatric heart transplant recipients.[49] The higher incidence of dual atrioventricular pathways in heart transplant recipients puts them at elevated risk for AVNRT. The presence of excitable myocardial tissue across suture lines in the atria can facilitate genesis of ectopic atrial tachycardia.[50] Myocardial damage resulting from rejection or ischemia also can act as the site of focal atrial tachycardia. All these types of supraventricular tachycardia need to be evaluated promptly with further invasive tests.

Treatment options are similar to those in patients who have not had heart transplants. Synchronized DCCV is the first choice in unstable patients; drugs are offered in stable patients. Adenosine is the drug of first choice, but the dose needs to be half the usual dose or less because of the increased adenosine sensitivity in heart transplant recipients. Vagal maneuvers and digoxin tend to be ineffective because of the parasympathetic denervation following heart transplantation. β-Blockers and calcium-channel blockers are useful, but their ability to exaggerate LV dysfunction needs to be considered. If tachycardia persists despite initial measures, electrophysiologic evaluation can identify pathways amenable to radiofrequency ablation, which often is curative.

Ventricular Tachyarrhythmias

Premature ventricular complexes (PVC) in the form of isolated beats, ventricular couplets, and multifocal PVC have been observed to decrease in frequency with time after heart transplantation. The same decrease is noted for accelerated idioventricular rhythm and nonsustained ventricular tachycardia.[51] It has been suggested that episodes occurring early after transplantation are caused by increased catecholamine presence or by rejection. Later episodes, however, have been correlated with cardiac allograft vasculopathy. A recent report of frequent PVCs resulting in cardiomyopathy and its reversal with radiofrequency ablation has demonstrated the importance of treating these events. As shown in these reports, focal radiofrequency ablation can be used to rectify the rhythm disturbance, but underlying rejection and cardiac allograft vasculopathy must be ruled out.

With the advent of better immunosuppression, ventricular tachycardia and ventricular fibrillation have decreased from an initial incidence of 25%.[52] Treatment modalities are those used for non–heart transplant patients and include direct current cardioversion and antiarrhythmics such as amiodarone, procainamide, and, rarely, lidocaine. Sudden cardiac death as a result of fatal arrhythmias is believed to occur in 10% to 27% of transplant survivors because of underlying rejection or cardiac allograft vasculopathy.[53,54] Data regarding the use of an internal cardiac defibrillator to prevent this outcome are limited by small sample size and the availability of only retrospective analyses. Montpetit and colleagues suggested that the threshold for internal cardiac defibrillator insertion be lowered to include patients who have an EF less than 40%, considering the higher incidence of sudden cardiac death in that subgroup.[55] Until prospective trials provide clear data, clinicians must rely on existing recommendations for defibrillator implantation in heart transplant recipients.

In summary, all patients who have a history of heart transplantation and who present to the ED with cardiac dysfunction need to be evaluated in detail with ECG and telemetry monitoring. Early consultation with an electrophysiologist and a transplant cardiologist is advised to identify arrhythmias that can appear benign but reflect significant underlying cardiac pathology such as rejection or cardiac allograft vasculopathy. In many cases, treatment of these dysrhythmias has reversed the cardiomyopathy and thereby offered a better prognosis and quality of life.

Pericardial Diseases

A moderate to large pericardial effusion is seen in 20% to 35% of recipients after heart transplant surgery and usually resolves within 3 months postoperatively. Rarely it can lead to pericardial tamponade in the postoperative period, thus requiring drainage.[56] Cardiac tamponade presents with dyspnea, orthopnea, jugular venous engorgement, reduced heart sounds, and hypotension. Because of the increased risk of infections and malignancies in heart transplant recipients, diagnostic pericardiocentesis must be considered in late pericardial effusion even in the absence of tamponade. Constrictive pericarditis usually occurs 3 months to 2 years after transplantation and may be related to pericardial effusion or hematoma, postpericardiotomy syndrome, mediastinitis, or intrathoracic infections.[57] Immunosuppression leads to an increased risk for infectious constrictive pericarditis such as purulent, tuberculous, or fungal pericarditis.[58,59] Restrictive pericarditis physiology leads to a clinical presentation with symptoms of fluid overload and decreased cardiac output. Use of echocardiography as a diagnostic modality can identify this pathology at the bedside; however, CT and MRI of the heart, as well as invasive hemodynamic measurement, can be helpful in difficult scenarios. Transient constriction as a sequel to postpericardiotomy syndrome, infections, or malignancy may improve with a variety of agents including nonsteroidal anti-inflammatory drugs, steroids, antibiotics, chemotherapy, angiotensin-converting enzyme inhibitors, and diuretics. Symptoms that persist after 2 to 3 months of conservative treatment or that occur in patients who have hemodynamic compromise may require pericardiectomy.[60]

Myocarditis and Infections

Immunosuppression leads to increased susceptibility to latent as well as new infections that can rarely involve the cardiac allograft. In addition to the usual organisms (echovirus and coxsackie virus), CMV, EBV, toxoplasmosis, and Chagas disease can lead to clinical and subclinical myocarditis in heart transplant recipients.[61] Aspergillus and parvovirus B19 also have been reported to cause myocarditis.[62,63] CMV infections can be acquired from reactivation of endogenous viruses or via donated allograft and blood products from seropositive donors. In addition, CMV is implicated in LV dysfunction by direct myocardial infection besides being associated with the pathogenesis of acute rejection and cardiac allograft vasculopathy.[64,65] Sepsis also can cause LV dysfunction.[66] Serologic tests are of limited use in an immunocompromised host. Nucleic acid–based molecular assay (PCR) and antigen assay (pp65 in CMV) are of limited value in the ED. Because symptoms are few and atypical, tissue histology is needed for the diagnosis of infections. The reference standard test for the diagnosis of myocarditis is endomyocardial biopsy. Effective treatments can be achieved with the use of ganciclovir or valgancyclovir for CMV, trimethoprim-sulphamethoxazole for toxoplasmosis, and broad-spectrum antibiotics when sepsis is a consideration.[67]

Malignancy

The incidence of malignancy in transplant recipients is noted to be about 5% to 6%. Because of immunosuppression, the risk of malignancy is about 100 times greater in heart transplant recipients than in the general population.[68] Posttransplantation lymphoproliferative disorder, seen in 2% to 5% of heart transplant recipients, is associated with EBV exposure and the use of immunosuppressants such as CNIs, azathioprine, and OKT3. Extranodal involvement is common; allograft involvement may be in the form of a cardiac mass or myocardial infiltration resulting in LV dysfunction. Diagnosis is made on tissue biopsy from the endomyocardium, lymph node, or bone marrow. Treatment modalities include reducing the extent of immunosuppression, surgical excision, chemotherapy, and rituximab.[69]

Valvular Disease

Tricuspid valve regurgitation (TR) is the most frequent valvular abnormality seen after orthotopic heart transplantation, with a prevalence of 67% to 85% as detected by echocardiogram. Risk factors for the development of TR are size mismatch between the donor heart and pericardial cavity, biatrial technique, high-grade rejection, repeated endomyocardial biopsy, pulmonary hypertension, and ischemic injury to the right ventricle.[70] Most cases of TR are mild and asymptomatic. Moderate to severe TR, seen in 25% to 34% of transplant recipients, presents with symptoms of RV volume overload. Surgical repair or replacement is required in 4% of transplant recipients for refractory right-sided heart failure.[71] Left-sided valvular regurgitations are less common. Roig and colleagues observed mitral regurgitation in 8 (6%) of 141 heart transplant recipients and noted associations with cardiac allograft vasculopathy and mortality.[72]

Diastolic Heart Failure

Diastolic dysfunction, measured by Doppler echocardiogram or pulmonary artery catheter, occurs frequently after transplant surgery but resolves within the first 4 to 8 weeks after transplantation.[73,74] It may persist or even reappear later because of allograft rejection, constrictive or effusive-constrictive pericarditis, recurrence of infiltrative disorders, and increased incidence of hypertension following the use of CNIs.[75] Aziz and colleagues found a restrictive filling pattern defined by mitral deceleration time in 41 of the 152 recipients at 24 months after transplantation.[76] Using a pulmonary artery catheter, Tallaj and colleagues found diastolic dysfunction in 11% of recipients at 1 year after transplantation.[77] Siostrzonek and colleagues described a case in which cyclosporine withdrawal led to relief of diastolic dysfunction.[78] Lobato and colleagues reported a case of postoperative pulmonary edema caused by diastolic dysfunction.[79]

EVALUATION OF ALLOGRAFT DYSFUNCTION

LV dysfunction is suspected in heart transplant recipients presenting with shortness of breath, orthopnea, fatigue, palpitations, and signs of left- or right-sided heart failure on physical examination. Asymptomatic LV dysfunction can be found on routine diagnostic tests such as echocardiograms, radionuclide ventriculography, or right heart catheterization. Natriuretic peptide, cardiac markers, ECG, and chest radiographs are helpful in identifying this pathology, but endomyocardial biopsy has the advantage of identifying the cause.

History and Physical Examination

Allograft rejection and cardiac allograft vasculopathy, the two main causes of LV dysfunction, present with nonspecific symptoms. Most allograft rejection is diagnosed at surveillance endomyocardial biopsy. A few cases present with LV dysfunction, arrhytmias, or gastrointestinal symptoms caused by hepatic congestion. Because of the denervation of the transplanted heart, the classical symptoms of ischemia are absent. Even though 10% to 30% of heart transplant recipients have partial reinnervation and may present with angina, cardiac allograft vasculopathy rarely presents as chest pain. Most patients present late with silent myocardial infarction, congestive heart failure, arrhythmias, or sudden death.[80] A detailed medication history, including compliance, dosing, and timing of immunosuppressive drugs, must be taken for proper adjustment of immunosuppressive drugs. Blood draws for drug-level monitoring are necessary also.

Natriuretic Peptides

Serum natriuretic peptide (BNP) and N-terminal proBNP (NT-proBNP) are established in the diagnosis of heart failure in patients who present to the ED with shortness of breath.[81,82] Their role in heart transplant recipients is not clear, however. High levels of BNP are seen within the first month after heart transplantation, followed by a gradual decline, but rarely do the levels return to normal. In one of the largest studies to date, Park and colleagues observed that the BNP level was elevated three- to fourfold, with a median level of 153 pg/mL, in stable heart transplant recipients.[83] Similarly the mean NT-proBNP level was 4032 pg/mL within 6 months after heart transplantation, compared with 480 pg/mL beyond 6 months after transplantation. This elevation, observed despite a normal systolic function, could be attributed to high pulmonary capillary wedge pressure, high transpulmonary gradient, diastolic dysfunction, RV enlargement or dilatation, or significant TR.[84]

BNP has been extensively studied as a noninvasive marker of allograft performance to detect allograft rejection. Masters and colleagues showed a correlation between a BNP level higher than 400 pg/mL and grade 2 or higher rejection in 10 patients. Similarly, Herva and colleagues demonstrated a correlation between elevated natriuretic peptide levels with a rejection of grade 2 and higher among transplantees in the initial 90 days following their heart transplantation. This correlation was supported by the observation of Hammerer-Lercher and her colleagues as well as Wu and her team, who noticed the association between elevated BNP levels and high-grade rejection. (grade ≥ 3). In a review of six other studies, no significant increase in natriuretic peptide was seen during acute allograft rejection.[85] Thus the association between BNP and rejection is seen only in severe rejection (grade ≥ 3), especially during the first 6 months after transplantation. Therefore BNP cannot be used as a marker of rejection in stable heart transplant recipients and is unlikely to replace or reduce the use of endomyocardial biopsy in detecting rejection.

Cardiac Markers

Creatinine kinase (CK), its myocardial band isoform (CK-MB), myoglobin, lactate dehydrogenase, and aspartate dehydrogenase have no role in the noninvasive detection of rejection or cardiac allograft vasculopathy because of lack of specificity. Cardiac troponin I and cardiac troponin T are cardiac myofibrillar proteins that can be detected in blood with very small amounts of myocardial necrosis (<1 g). The role of troponin in cardiac rejection has been investigated extensively, with conflicting results, and its use in evaluation of allograft rejection cannot be recommended.[86] Elevated troponin levels, however, can identify a subset of recipients who are at increased risk for the development of cardiac allograft vasculopathy.[87] The role of troponin in acute settings has not been well studied, but increasing levels, compared with baseline, may suggest myocardial injury resulting from rejection or coronary artery disease.

Electrocardiogram

Denervation and the loss of autonomic nervous system control in transplanted hearts leads to higher resting heart rates at around 100 beats/min, with tachycardia occurring in more than half of recipients. A resting heart rate of less than 130 beats/min usually has no significant adverse effects. In recipients who have a biatrial transplant, two P waves may be seen because of the retained recipient's right atrium.[88] Right bundle branch block, the most common ECG abnormality, is seen in approximately 50% of recipients and carries a benign prognosis.[89] New-onset bradyarrhythmias (sinus bradycardia, advanced atrioventricular block) or tachyarrhythmias (atrial flutter and fibrillation) warrant evaluation for rejection or underlying cardiac allograft vasculopathy.[88]

Radiology

Chest radiographs may show cardiomegaly and pulmonary edema suggestive of LV dysfunction. Conventional CT and MRI have limited roles in the diagnosis of allograft rejection and cardiac allograft vasculopathy. MRI coronary angiograms can be used to visualize coronary arteries and their branches and can be used as a screening tool to reduce the number of coronary angiograms. CT coronary artery calcium scoring has a high negative predictive value (up to 97%) and may be useful in ruling out cardiac allograft vasculopathy. The main role of imaging in heart transplant recipients admitted with shortness of breath is to rule out infections and malignancies involving the lung and heart.[90]

Drug-Level Monitoring

Nonadherence to immunosuppressive regimens is a risk factor for rejection and cardiac allograft vasculopathy.[91] Optimal immunosuppression is ensured by frequent drug-level monitoring. Trough levels are drawn for tacrolimus, mycophenolate mofetil, and sirolimus, whereas a 2-hour postdose level was found to be best for cyclosporine. Adequate immunosuppression is achieved when the target level is within the range shown in **Table 1**. At present no monitoring tool is available for steroids. Azathioprine is initiated at the dose of 1–2mg/kg/d, and the dose is decreased if the white blood cell count is less than 3000–4000 mm³.[12]

Endomyocardial Biopsy

The endomyocardial biopsy remains the reference-standard investigation for diagnosing acute cellular rejection following heart transplantation and is an important element of rejection surveillance. Tissue fragments are procured from the RV septum using a bioptome via a percutaneous transvenous route. The surveillance biopsies are performed routinely once a week for the first month, every 2 weeks for the next 6 weeks, monthly for the next 3 months. Thereafter, it is repeated every 3 months until the end of first year, three or four times per year in the second year, and then one or two times per year in the subsequent years. Once an episode of rejection is identified and treated, follow-up biopsies are obtained after 1 to 2 weeks to assess the adequacy of therapy.[92,93] Endomyocardial biopsy also is useful in diagnosing other conditions leading to ventricular dysfunction such as myocarditis, infiltrative lesions (amyloidosis and sarcoidosis), ischemia, and infarction.[94] Complication occurs in 1% to 1.7% of biopsies with TR being the most common.

Molecular Testing

Endomyocardial biopsy, although definitive in diagnosing rejection, has inherent limitations: it is invasive, is not reproducible, can produce false-negative results, and is associated with a low but finite risk of TR or myocardial infarction. These disadvantages have generated searches for noninvasive markers of rejection including gene-expression profiling (GEP) using DNA microarray technology and real-time PCR measurement.

Allomap (XDx, Inc.), a commercially available GEP test, utilizes peripheral blood mononuclear cells as the DNA source to analyze 20 gene expressions (11 informative, 9 control). The test uses a score ranging from 0 to 40 with a lower score suggesting a low risk of moderate/severe acute cellular rejection (grade ≥ 3A/2R, according to the original/revised ISHLT classification). The Cardiac Allograft Rejection Gene Expression Observational study compared GEP scores with endomyocardial biopsy during the posttransplantation period at eight heart transplant centers. Scores below 34 had a negative predictive value of more than 99% in identifying grade 3A/2R or higher acute cellular rejection in clinically stable cardiac transplant recipients 6 months or longer after transplantation. Potentially, GEP can avoid the need for surveillance biopsy.[95] At present, however, there is no recommendation for its use in heart transplant recipients presenting with signs and symptoms of rejection. Therefore its use in the ED to diagnose allograft rejection cannot be recommended. Further studies are needed, and bedside molecular tests must be developed before GEP can be used for the rapid diagnosis of rejection in the ED.

Echocardiogram

Common echocardiogram findings in stable heart transplant recipients include an increase in left atrial size, abnormal interventricular septal motion, increased LV mass, valvular regurgitation, and abnormal diastolic filling. Doppler echocardiogram and tissue Doppler have shown diastolic dysfunction in acute rejection, but its role as a noninvasive test is not clear. In the detection of cardiac allograft vasculopathy, resting wall abnormality was found to be specific (65%–100%), whereas dobutamine stress echocardiogram was found to be sensitive (50%–100%). Dobutamine stress echocardiogram has advantages over angiogram or intravascular ultrasound for the detection of cardiac allograft vasculopathy involving microvasculature and may have a role

Table 1
Target levels for immunosuppressive drugs after heart transplantation

Drug	Early (<2 Years)	Late (>2 Years)
Tacrolimus	10–15 ng/mL	5–10 ng/mL
Cyclosporine	300–350 ng/mL	200 ng/mL
Sirolimus	5–15 ng/mL during both periods	
Mycophenolate	2.5–5 μg/mL during both periods	

in screening recipients before these invasive procedures.[96]

MANAGEMENT OF ALLOGRAFT DYSFUNCTION

Despite literature highlighting RV failure in the immediate and early postoperative period, there is a paucity of data pertaining to acute decompensated heart failure in stable recipients. Consequently, an approach similar to that used in the nontransplant patient is considered. This approach includes the use of supplemental oxygen, diuretics, vasodilators, inotropic support, and short-term positive pressure ventilation. The altered neurohormonal environment in heart transplant patients causes the inotropic effect of norepinephrine to be more pronounced, the effect of dopamine to be lesser, and that of dobutamine to be unchanged when compared with nontransplant hearts.

Invasive measures such as intra-aortic balloon pulsation, an intraventricular assist device, or extracorporeal membrane oxygenation may be used to maintain tissue oxygenation when the response to conservative measures is poor.[97] Every attempt should be made to diagnose the cause of LV dysfunction and to direct treatment to the specific cause. Because rejection is an important cause of LV dysfunction in the first year after transplantation, most centers start presumptive treatment with high-dose steroids (methyl prednisone in doses of 500 to 1000 mg intravenously) until the result of endomyocardial biopsy is available. **Fig. 2** shows the management algorithm in a transplant recipient presenting with symptoms of heart failure. Specific treatment of allograft rejection, cardiac allograft vasculopathy, myocarditis, and malignancy involving the heart have been described in detail in previous sections.

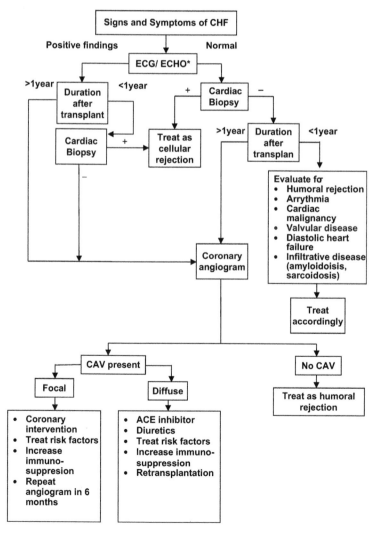

Fig. 2. Algorithmic approach to evaluate cardiac allograft dysfunction. ACE, angiotensin converting enzyme; CAV, cardiac allograft vasculopathy; ECG/ECHO*: electrocardiogram and echocardiogram to evaluate for ischemia; ECHO, echocardiogram.

SUMMARY

With an increasing number of heart transplantations being performed around the world and the
improvement in the survival rates, more transplant
recipients may present to the ED with comorbidities unique to the transplanted heart and related
immunosuppression, including heart failure. This
article is aimed at enabling the ED physician identify and better manage this unique group of patients for whom time is life. In this endeavor,
physicians must strive to uphold Alexander Pope's
words:

*"A wise physician, skill'd our wounds to heal,
Is more than armies to the public weal."*

REFERENCES

1. Rosamond W, Flegal K, Friday G, et al. Heart disease and stroke statistics—2007 update: a report from the American Heart Association Statistics Committee and Stroke Statistics Subcommittee. [erratum appears in Circulation. 2007;115(5):e172]. Circulation 2007;115(5):e69–171.
2. Shibata MC, Flather MD, Wang D. Systematic review of the impact of beta blockers on mortality and hospital admissions in heart failure [see comment]. Eur J Heart Fail 2001;3(3):351–7.
3. Garg R, Yusuf S. Overview of randomized trials of angiotensin-converting enzyme inhibitors on mortality and morbidity in patients with heart failure. Collaborative group on ACE inhibitor trials [erratum appears in JAMA 1995 Aug 9;274(6):462]. JAMA 1995;273(18):1450–6.
4. Pitt B, Zannad F, Remme WJ, et al. The effect of spironolactone on morbidity and mortality in patients with severe heart failure. Randomized Aldactone evaluation study investigators [see comment]. N Engl J Med 1999;341(10):709–17.
5. Rivero-Ayerza M, Theuns DAMJ, Garcia-Garcia HM, et al. Effects of cardiac resynchronization therapy on overall mortality and mode of death: a meta-analysis of randomized controlled trials [see comment]. Eur Heart J 2006;27(22):2682–8.
6. Aaronson KD, Mancini DM. Mortality remains high for outpatient transplant candidates with prolonged (>6 months) waiting list time. J Am Coll Cardiol 1999;33(5):1189–95.
7. Taylor DO, Edwards LB, Boucek MM, et al. Registry of the International Society for Heart and Lung Transplantation: twenty-fourth official adult heart transplant report—2007. J Heart Lung Transplant 2007;26(8):769–81.
8. Barnard CN. The operation. A human cardiac transplant: an interim report of a successful operation performed at Groote Schuur hospital, Cape Town. S Afr Med J 1967;41:1271–4.
9. Al-khaldi A, Robbins RC. New directions in cardiac transplantation. Annu Rev Med 2006;57:455–71.
10. Zakliczynski M, et al. New guidelines in the selection of patients with heart insufficiency for heart transplantation—discussion of standards of the International Society of Heart and Lung Transplantation (ISHLT) in 2006. Kardiol Pol 2006;64(12):1462–4.
11. Woodley SL, Renlund DG, O'Connell JB, et al. Immunosuppression following cardiac transplantation. Cardiol Clin 1990;8(1):83–96.
12. Lindenfeld J, Miller GG, Shakar SF, et al. Drug therapy in the heart transplant recipient: part II: immunosuppressive drugs. Circulation 2004;110(25):3858–65.
13. Gustafsson F, Ross HJ. Proliferation signal inhibitors in cardiac transplantation. Curr Opin Cardiol 2007;22(2):111–6.
14. Playford EG, Webster AC, Sorell TC, et al. Antifungal agents for preventing fungal infections in solid organ transplant recipients. Cochrane Database Syst Rev 2004;(3):CD004291.
15. Villacian JS, Paya CV. Prevention of infections in solid organ transplant recipients [see comment]. Transpl Infect Dis 1999;1(1):50–64.
16. Lindenfeld J, Page RL 2nd, Zolty R, et al. Drug therapy in the heart transplant recipient: part III: common medical problems. Circulation 2005;111(1):113–7.
17. Sternbach GL, Varon J, Hunt SA. Emergency department presentation and care of heart and heart/lung transplant recipients. Ann Emerg Med 1992;21(9):1140–4.
18. Zavotsky KE, Sapienza J, Wood D. Nursing implications for ED care of patients who have received heart transplants (CE). J Emerg Nurs 2001;27(1):33–9.
19. Coursin DB, Wood KE. Corticosteroid supplementation for adrenal insufficiency. JAMA 2002;287(2):236–40.
20. Bacal F, Pires PV, Moreira LF, et al. Normalization of right ventricular performance and remodeling evaluated by magnetic resonance imaging at late follow-up of heart transplantation: relationship between function, exercise capacity and pulmonary vascular resistance. J Heart Lung Transplant 2005;24(12):2031–6.
21. Hartmann A, Maul FD, Huth A, et al. Serial evaluation of left ventricular function by radionuclide ventriculography at rest and during exercise after orthotopic heart transplantation. Eur J Nucl Med 1993;20(2):146–50.
22. Tischler MD, Lee RT, Plappert T, et al. Serial assessment of left ventricular function and mass after orthotopic heart transplantation: a 4-year longitudinal study. [erratum appears in J Am Coll Cardiol

1994 Jan;23(1):281]. J Am Coll Cardiol 1992;19(1): 60–6.

23. Hershberger RE, Ni H, Toy W, et al. Distribution and declines in cardiac allograft radionuclide left ventricular ejection fractions in relation to late mortality. J Heart Lung Transplant 2001;20(4):417–24.

24. Jarcho JA, Mark EJ. Case 17-1998. A 53-year-old man with left ventricular dysfunction four years after a heart transplantation. N Engl J Med 1998; 338(22):1608–16.

25. Lindenfeld J, Miller GG, Shakar SF, et al. Drug therapy in the heart transplant recipient: part I: cardiac rejection and immunosuppressive drugs. Circulation 2004;110(24):3734–40.

26. Mills RM, Naftel DC, Kirklin JK, et al. Heart transplant rejection with hemodynamic compromise: a multiinstitutional study of the role of endomyocardial cellular infiltrate. Cardiac Transplant Research Database. J Heart Lung Transplant 1997;16(8): 813–21.

27. Stewart S, Winters GL, Fishbein MC, et al. Revision of the 1990 working formulation for the standardization of nomenclature in the diagnosis of heart rejection [see comment]. J Heart Lung Transplant 2005; 24(11):1710–20.

28. Delgado JF, Sanchez V, de la Calzada CS. Acute rejection after heart transplantation. Expert Opin Pharmacother 2006;7(9):1139–49.

29. Uber WE, Self SE, Van Bakel AB, et al. Acute antibody-mediated rejection following heart transplantation. Am J Transplant 2007;7(9):2064–74.

30. Kass M, Allan R, Haddad H. Diagnosis of graft coronary artery disease. Curr Opin Cardiol 2007;22(2): 139–45.

31. Kass M, Haddad H. Cardiac allograft vasculopathy: pathology, prevention and treatment. Curr Opin Cardiol 2006;21(2):132–7.

32. Drobinski G, et al. Myocardial infarction after endomyocardial biopsy in a heart transplant patient. J Interv Cardiol 2002;15(5):403–5.

33. Pittaluga J, Dorent R, Ghossoub J-J, et al. Left anterior descending coronary artery bridge. A cause of early death after cardiac transplantation. Chest 1997;111(2):511–3.

34. Lipski A, Sahar G, De Bruyne Y, et al. Acute myocardial infarction immediately after heart transplantation. J Heart Lung Transplant 1993;12(6 Pt 1): 1065–6.

35. Semigran MJ, Stevenson LW, Passeri JJ, et al. Case records of the Massachusetts General Hospital. Case 37-2007. A 47-year-old man with left ventricular dysfunction after heart transplantation. N Engl J Med 2007;357(22):2286–97.

36. Lai CL, Chen WJ, Wang SS, et al. Bradyarrhythmias and cardiac pacing after orthotopic heart transplantation in a Chinese population. Transplant Proc 2002;34(8):3232–5.

37. Cui G, Kobashigawa J, Margarian A, et al. Cause of atrioventricular block in patients after heart transplantation. Transplantation 2003;76(1):137–42.

38. Weinfeld MS, Kartashov A, Piana R, et al. Bradycardia: a late complication following cardiac transplantation. Am J Cardiol 1996;78(8):969–71.

39. Gregoratos G, Abrams J, Epstein AE, et al. ACC/AHA/NASPE 2002 guideline update for implantation of cardiac pacemakers and antiarrhythmia devices: summary article: a report of the American College of Cardiology/American Heart Association Task Force on Practice Guidelines (ACC/AHA/NASPE Committee to Update the 1998 Pacemaker Guidelines). Circulation 2002;106(16):2145–61.

40. Ahmari SA, Bunch TJ, Chandra A, et al. Prevalence, pathophysiology, and clinical significance of post-heart transplant atrial fibrillation and atrial flutter. J Heart Lung Transplant 2006;25(1):53–60.

41. Cui G, Tung T, Kobashigawa J, et al. Increased incidence of atrial flutter associated with the rejection of heart transplantation. Am J Cardiol 2001;88(3):280–4.

42. Krishnan SC, Falsone JM, Sanders WE, et al. Catheter ablation of atrial flutter in a heart transplant recipient. Pacing Clin Electrophysiol 2002;25(8): 1262–5.

43. Pavri BB, O'Nunain SS, Newell JB, et al. Prevalence and prognostic significance of atrial arrhythmias after orthotopic cardiac transplantation. J Am Coll Cardiol 1995;25(7):1673–80.

44. Woo GW, Schofield RS, Klodell CT, et al. Atrial fibrillation as a cause of left ventricular dysfunction after cardiac transplantation. J Heart Lung Transplant 2006;25(1):131–3.

45. Oral H, Souza JJ, Michaud GF, et al. Facilitating transthoracic cardioversion of atrial fibrillation with ibutilide pretreatment. N Engl J Med 1999;340(24): 1849–54.

46. Franco V, Tallaj JA, Rayburn BK, et al. 259: ibutilide is safe and efficacious in heart transplant recipients. J Heart Lung Transplant 2007;26(2 Suppl 1):S153.

47. Rothman SA, Hsia HH, Bove AA, et al. Radiofrequency ablation of Wolff-Parkinson-White syndrome in a donor heart after orthotopic heart transplantation. J Heart Lung Transplant 1994;13(5):905–9.

48. Padder FA, Wilbur SL, Kantharia BK, et al. Radiofrequency catheter ablation of atrioventricular nodal reentrant tachycardia after orthotopic heart transplantation. J Interv Card Electrophysiol 1999; 3(3):283–5.

49. Collins KK, Thiagarajan RR, Chin C, et al. Atrial tachyarrhythmias and permanent pacing after pediatric heart transplantation. J Heart Lung Transplant 2003;22(10):1126–33.

50. Lai W, Kao A, Silka MJ, et al. Recipient to donor conduction of atrial tachycardia following orthotopic heart transplantation. Pacing Clin Electrophysiol 1998;21(6):1331–5.

51. Scott CD, Dark JH, McComb JM. Arrhythmias after cardiac transplantation. Am J Cardiol 1992;70(11): 1061–3.

52. Tagusari O, Kormos RL, Kawai A, et al. Native heart complications after heterotopic heart transplantation: insight into the potential risk of left ventricular assist device. J Heart Lung Transplant 1999; 18(11):1111–9.

53. Patel VS, Lim M, Massin EK, et al. Sudden cardiac death in cardiac transplant recipients. Circulation 1996;94(9 Suppl):II273–7.

54. Alexander RT, Steenbergen C. Cause of death and sudden cardiac death after heart transplantation. An autopsy study. Am J Clin Pathol 2003;119(5): 740–8.

55. Montpetit M, Singh M, Muller E, et al. 340: sudden cardiac death in heart transplant patients: is there a role for defibrillators? J Heart Lung Transplant 2007;26(2 Suppl 1):S182.

56. Al-Dadah AS, Guthrie TJ, Pasque MK, et al. Clinical course and predictors of pericardial effusion following cardiac transplantation. Transplant Proc 2007; 39(5):1589–92.

57. Copeland JG, Riley JE, Fuller J. Pericardiectomy for effusive constrictive pericarditis after heart transplantation. J Heart Transplant 1986;5(2):171–2.

58. Canver CC, Patel AK, Kosolcharoen P, et al. Fungal purulent constrictive pericarditis in a heart transplant patient. Ann Thorac Surg 1998;65(6):1792–4.

59. Puius YA, Scully B. Treatment of Candida albicans pericarditis in a heart transplant patient. Transpl Infect Dis 2007;9(3):229–32.

60. Mehta A, Mehta M, Jain AC. Constrictive pericarditis. Clin Cardiol 1999;22(5):334–44.

61. Brady WJ, Ferguson JD, Ullman EA, et al. Myocarditis: emergency department recognition and management. Emerg Med Clin North Am 2004;22(4): 865–85.

62. Rueter F, Hirsch HH, Kunz F, et al. Late Aspergillus fumigatus endomyocarditis with brain abscess as a lethal complication after heart transplantation. J Heart Lung Transplant 2002;21(11):1242–5.

63. Heegaard ED, Eiskjaer H, Baandrup U, et al. Parvovirus B19 infection associated with myocarditis following adult cardiac transplantation. Scand J Infect Dis 1998;30(6):607–10.

64. Gonwa TA, Capehart JE, Pilcher JW, et al. Cytomegalovirus myocarditis as a cause of cardiac dysfunction in a heart transplant recipient. Transplantation 1989;47(1):197–9.

65. Partanen J, Nieminen MS, Krogerus L, et al. Cytomegalovirus myocarditis in transplanted heart verified by endomyocardial biopsy. Clin Cardiol 1991; 14(10):847–9.

66. Kumar A, Haery C, Parrillo JE. Myocardial dysfunction in septic shock. Crit Care Clin 2000;16(2):251–87.

67. Fishman JA. Infection in solid-organ transplant recipients. N Engl J Med 2007;357(25):2601–14.

68. Ippoliti G, Rinaldi M, Pellegrini C, et al. Incidence of cancer after immunosuppressive treatment for heart transplantation. Crit Rev Oncol Hematol 2005;56(1): 101–13.

69. Everly MJ, Bloom RD, Tsai DE, et al. Posttransplant lymphoproliferative disorder. Ann Pharmacother 2007;41(11):1850–8.

70. Aziz TM, Burgess MI, Rahman AN, et al. Risk factors for tricuspid valve regurgitation after orthotopic heart transplantation. Ann Thorac Surg 1999;68(4): 1247–51.

71. Badiwala MV, Rao V. Tricuspid valve replacement after cardiac transplantation. Curr Opin Cardiol 2007; 22(2):123–7.

72. Roig E, Jacobo A, Sitges M, et al. Clinical implications of late mitral valve regurgitation appearance in the follow-up of heart transplantation. Transplant Proc 2007;39(7):2379–81.

73. StGoar FG, Gibbons R, Schnittger I, et al. Left ventricular diastolic function. Doppler echocardiographic changes soon after cardiac transplantation. Circulation 1990;82(3):872–8.

74. Young JB, Leon CA, Short HD 3rd, et al. Evolution of hemodynamics after orthotopic heart and heart–lung transplantation: early restrictive patterns persisting in occult fashion. J Heart Transplant 1987; 6(1):34–43.

75. Mena C, Wencker D, Krumholz HM, et al. Detection of heart transplant rejection in adults by echocardiographic diastolic indices: a systematic review of the literature. J Am Soc Echocardiogr 2006;19(10):1295–300.

76. Aziz TM, Burgess MI, Haselton PS, et al. Transforming growth factor beta and diastolic left ventricular dysfunction after heart transplantation: echocardiographic and histologic evidence. J Heart Lung Transplant 2003;22(6):663–73.

77. Tallaj JA, Kirklin JK, Brown RN, et al. Post-heart transplant diastolic dysfunction is a risk factor for mortality. J Am Coll Cardiol 2007;50(11): 1064–9.

78. Siostrzonek P, Teufelsbauer H, Kreiner G, et al. Relief of diastolic cardiac dysfunction after cyclosporine withdrawal in a cardiac transplant recipient. Eur Heart J 1993;14(6):859–61.

79. Lobato EB, Tang YS, Cole PJ. Postoperative pulmonary edema secondary to diastolic dysfunction in a patient with a previous heart transplant. J Clin Anesth 1998;10(4):331–7.

80. Aranda JM Jr, Hill J. Cardiac transplant vasculopathy. Chest 2000;118(6):1792–800.

81. Maisel AS, McCord J, Nowak RM, et al. Bedside B-type natriuretic peptide in the emergency diagnosis of heart failure with reduced or preserved ejection fraction. Results from the Breathing Not Properly

multinational study [see comment]. J Am Coll Cardiol 2003;41(11):2010–7.

82. Januzzi JL Jr, Camargo CA, Anwaruddin S, et al. The N-terminal Pro-BNP investigation of dyspnea in the emergency department (PRIDE) study. Am J Cardiol 2005;95(8):948–54.

83. Park MH, Scott RL, Uber PA, et al. Usefulness of B-type natriuretic peptide levels in predicting hemo-dynamic perturbations after heart transplantation despite preserved left ventricular systolic function. Am J Cardiol 2002;90(12):1326–9.

84. Park MH, Uber PA, Scott RL, et al. B-type natriuretic peptide in heart transplantation: an important marker of allograft performance. Heart Fail Rev 2003;8(4):359–63.

85. Shaw SM, Williams SG. Is brain natriuretic peptide clinically useful after cardiac transplantation? J Heart Lung Transplant 2006;25(12):1396–401.

86. Dengler TJ, Gleissner CA, Klingenberg R, et al. Bio-markers after heart transplantation: nongenomic. Heart Fail Clin 2007;3(1):69–81.

87. Faulk WP, Labarrere CA, Torry RJ, et al. Serum car-diac troponin-T concentrations predict development of coronary artery disease in heart transplant pa-tients. Transplantation 1998;66(10):1335–9.

88. Stecker EC, Strelich KR, Chugh SS, et al. Arrhyth-mias after orthotopic heart transplantation. J Card Fail 2005;11(6):464–72.

89. Marcus GM, Hoang KL, Hunt SA, et al. Prevalence, patterns of development, and prognosis of right bundle branch block in heart transplant recipients. Am J Cardiol 2006;98(9):1288–90.

90. Chughtai A, Cronin P, Kelly AM. Heart transplanta-tion imaging in the adult. Semin Roentgenol 2006; 41(1):16–25.

91. De Geest S, Dobbels F, Fluri C, et al. Adherence to the therapeutic regimen in heart, lung, and heart–lung transplant recipients. J Cardiovasc Nurs 2005;20(5 Suppl):S88–98.

92. Stehlik J, Starling RC, Movsesian MA, et al. Utility of long-term surveillance endomyocardial biopsy: a multi-institutional analysis. J Heart Lung Transplant 2006;25(12):1402–9.

93. Miniati DN, Robbins RC. Heart transplantation: a thirty-year perspective. Annu Rev Med 2002;53: 189–205.

94. Cunningham KS, Veinot JP, Butany J. An approach to endomyocardial biopsy interpretation. J Clin Pathol 2006;59(2):121–9.

95. Starling RC, Starling RC, Movsesian MA, et al. Molec-ular testing in the management of cardiac transplant recipients: initial clinical experience. [Erratum ap-pears in J Heart Lung Transplant. 2007;26(2):204]. J Heart Lung Transplant 2006;25(12):1389–95.

96. Thorn EM, de Filippi CR. Echocardiography in the cardiac transplant recipient. Heart Fail Clin 2007; 3(1):51–67.

97. Onwuanyi A, Taylor M. Acute decompensated heart failure: pathophysiology and treatment [see com-ment]. Am J Cardiol 2007;99(6B):25D–30D.

Index

Note: Page numbers of article titles are in **boldface** type.

A

ACE inhibitors, use in observation unit, 94
Aldosterone antagonist, in acute heart failure, 51
Allograft dysfunction, after transplantation, 136–139
    cardiac markers in, 137
    drug-level monitoring in, 137–138
    echocardiogram in, 138
    electrocardiogram in, 137
    endomyocardial biopsy in, 138
    history and physical examination in, 136
    management of, 138–139
    molecular testing in, 138
    natriuretic peptides and, 137
    radiology in, 137
Allograft rejection, in heart transplantation, 132–133
Angiotensin-converting enzyme inhibitors, in acute heart failure, 51
    in heart failure, 22
Arginine vasopressin, heart failure and, 13
Arrhythmias, in acute heart failure, 113
    epidemiology of, 115
    in heart transplantation, 133–134
Atrial fibrillation, 113
    acute, in chronic heart failure, cardioversion in, 117
        guidelines for, 119
        ventricular rate control in, 118
        with acute decompensation, 120
    and de novo heart failure, 120
    effect of, with rapid ventricular response, 116
    in acute heart failure syndromes, 116, 119–120

B

ß-Blockers, in acute heart failure, 51
Balloon pumps, intra-aortic, 55–57
    complications due to, 57
Bradyarrhythmias, in heart transplantation, 133–134
Breathing Not Properly Study, 29–31
Bronchodilators, prehospital, in heart failure, 22

C

Cardiac arrest, internal cardioverter defibrillator and, 70
Cardiac dysfunction, neurohormonal activation in, 12–14

Cardiac dysrhythmia, malignant, defibrillation of cardioversion in, 59
Cardiac troponin I, in heart failure, 32
Cardiogenic shock, 119
Cardiorenal syndrome, in acute decompensated heart failure, 14
Cardiovascular disease, and heart failure, 4–5
    costs of, 102
Cardioversion, or defibrillation, in malignant cardiac dysrhythmia, 59
Cardioverter/defibrillator devices, implantable, in heart failure, 32
Central venous catheter, and internal cardioverter defibrillator, 70
Chest radiography, in heart failure, 26
Circulatory assist devices, in acute heart failure, **55–62**
    intra-aortic balloon pumps, 55–57
    ventricular assist devices, 57–60
Congestive heart failure, 1
Coronary artery disease, allograft, in heart transplantation, 133
    and heart failure, 4
Coronary syndrome, acute, 68, 69

D

Defibrillators, internal cardiac, history and background of, 63–65
    industry representatives for, 24-hour contact numbers, 71
    interrogation for, 65–66
    lead complications of, 67
    presentation and evaluation of, 65
    surgical complications of, 66–67
    internal cardioverter, cardiac arrest and, 70
        central venous catheter and, 70
        "electrical storm" and, 69
        electrocautery and, 70
        ethical issues in, 70
        failure of, 70
        shock due to, evaluation of patient presenting with, 69
        succinylcholine and, 71
Diuretics, in acute heart failure, 44
    in heart failure, 40
    prehospital, in heart failure, 22
Dobutamine, in acute heart failure, 49

Heart Failure Clin 5 (2009) 145–148
doi:10.1016/S1551-7136(08)00148-7

heartfailure.theclinics.com

Moving?

Make sure your subscription moves with you!

To notify us of your new address, find your **Clinics Account Number** (located on your mailing label above your name), and contact customer service at:

E-mail: elspcs@elsevier.com

800-654-2452 (subscribers in the U.S. & Canada)
314-453-7041 (subscribers outside of the U.S. & Canada)

Fax number: 314-523-5170

Elsevier Periodicals Customer Service
11830 Westline Industrial Drive
St. Louis, MO 63146

*To ensure uninterrupted delivery of your subscription, please notify us at least 4 weeks in advance of move.

Printed and bound by CPI Group (UK) Ltd, Croydon, CR0 4YY

03/10/2024

01040360-0013